A Birth That Changed a Nation

Thank you for choosing a SAGE product!
If you have any comment, observation or feedback,
I would like to personally hear from you.
Please write to me at **contactceo@sagepub.in**

Vivek Mehra, Managing Director and CEO, SAGE India.

Bulk Sales

SAGE India offers special discounts
for purchase of books in bulk.
We also make available special imprints
and excerpts from our books on demand.

For orders and enquiries, write to us at

Marketing Department
SAGE Publications India Pvt Ltd
B1/I-1, Mohan Cooperative Industrial Area
Mathura Road, Post Bag 7
New Delhi 110044, India

E-mail us at **marketing@sagepub.in**

Get to know more about SAGE

Be invited to SAGE events, get on our mailing list.
Write today to **marketing@sagepub.in**

This book is also available as an e-book.

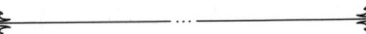

A Birth That Changed a Nation

A New Model of Care and Inclusion

Mithu Alur

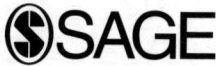

Los Angeles | London | New Delhi
Singapore | Washington DC | Melbourne

First published in 2017 by

 SAGE Publications India Pvt Ltd
B1/I-1 Mohan Cooperative Industrial Area
Mathura Road, New Delhi 110 044, India
www.sagepub.in

SAGE Publications Inc
2455 Teller Road
Thousand Oaks, California 91320, USA

SAGE Publications Ltd
1 Oliver's Yard, 55 City Road
London EC1Y 1SP, United Kingdom

SAGE Publications Asia-Pacific Pte Ltd
3 Church Street
#10-04 Samsung Hub
Singapore 049483

Published by Vivek Mehra for SAGE Publications India Pvt Ltd, typeset in 10/13 pt Palatino Linotype by Diligent Typesetter India Pvt Ltd, Delhi and printed at Saurabh Printers Pvt Ltd, Greater Noida.

Library of Congress Cataloging-in-Publication Data Available

ISBN: 978-93-860-6221-5 (PB)

SAGE Team: Rudra Narayan, Alekha Chandra Jena, Mayukh Lahiri and Ritu Chopra

A Dedication

The growth and development of The Spastics Society of India has been a family movement. Several families came forward when a baby we called Malini was born. Malini was born with cerebral palsy, a disorder that was shrouded in ignorance in those early years. There were many families that contributed; however, it was Malini's family that was particularly involved in beginning a movement around the country. Her mother, fathers, brothers, sisters, aunts, uncles, great-aunts, grandparents, my mother-in-law, all put their shoulders to the wheel to help. In the West, we see that services are initiated by parents; however, in India, because of the strong joint family system a broader group of the extended family came forward.

This book is dedicated to those who loved and served and preferred to remain anonymous, who went beyond themselves, with grit and determination and love and passion for the cause, who sincerely believed that *the right was to work only, not to the fruits.*

To those people then … this book is dedicated: to my late sister, Mita Nundy who left us in August 2014 and left behind a trail of services, a grand institution, but preferred to remain anonymous; to Mrs Shanti Talukdar, her mother-in-law, and to my parents, Sauransu and Bina Bose, born in pre-Independence India, stalwart patriots of Modern India, who taught us to serve the country beyond ourselves; to my brother-in-law, Samiran Nundy, whose support for Malini was invaluable; to my sister-in-law Junie, who wrote about the work, *'it is a far, far, better thing that I do, than I have ever done before.'*

It is also dedicated to all those numerous brave hearts who believed in us, left the fast track of making money and joined the journey to carve out a niche for the neglected and forgotten millions of our country: to our most dedicated and committed Trustees—earlier Nergesh Palkhivala, Radhika Roy, Ranjit Chib and later Shri Kamal Bakshi, Professor Sitanshu Mehta, to name a few; and to the two wonderful people I had the privilege to work with the late Nargis and Sunil Dutt, who gave of themselves generously, loving the cause deeply.

Above all, to my husband Sathi Alur and, my son, Nikhil Chib, both of whom stood stead-fastly behind me through thick and thin, contributing to the cause: to the raison d'être, Malini, who with her cheer and laughter spurred us on; to my brother, my nieces and nephews, who were always there for us, who quietly supported us behind the scenes, and most of all to the children, parents, and people behind this wonderful movement of service within a virgin territory always tough to pioneer. I learnt so much in this journey myself getting much more than I gave.

I end this dedication with a quote from Rabindranath Tagore's poem, *The Little Lamp,*

"Who will do my duties?" said the Setting Sun...
"I shall do what I can, my Master," said the Little Lamp.

Mithu Alur, 2015

Contents

List of Figures

List of Abbreviations

AAC	Augmentative and Alternative Communication
AADI	Action for Ability Development and Inclusion
ADAPT	Able Disabled All People Together
ADHD	Attention Deficit Hyperactive Disorder
ADL	Activity of Daily Living
AHRTAG	Appropriate Health Resources and Technologies Action Group
AIIMS	All India Institute of Medical Sciences
AIRA	All India Regional Alliance
APTP	Advanced Pre-vocational Training Programme
ARG	ADAPT Rights Group
ASER	Annual Status of Education Report
AYJNIHH	Ali Yavar Jung National Institute for the Hearing Handicapped
BCL	British Council Library
BEST	Brihanmumbai Electric Supply and Transport
BIL	Barriers to Inclusion List
BMC	Brihanmumbai Municipal Corporation
BRC	Block Resource Centres
CABE	Central Advisory Board of Education
CAPP	Culturally Appropriate Policy and Practice
CASER	Change Agents for School Education and Research
CAT	Care Attendant Transport
CBM	Christian Blind Mission
CBR	Community-Based Rehabilitation
CDC	Centers for Disease Control and Prevention
CDF	Child Development Fund
CHV	Community Health Volunteer
CIDA	Canadian International Development Agency
CIHD	Centre for International Health and Development
COH	Children's Orthopaedic Hospital
CP	Cerebral Palsy
CPA	Care Programme Approach

CPA	Care Pathway Approach
CSIE	Centre for Studies on Inclusive Education
CSR	Corporate Social Responsibility
CWD	Children with Disabilities
CWSN	Children with Special Needs
DAF	Disability Action Forum
DEE	Disability Equality Education
DFID	Department for International Development
DIET	District Institute of Education and Training
DISE	District Information System for Education
DLU	Disability Legislation Unit
DPEP	District Primary Education Programme
DPO	Disabled Peoples Organisation
DRC	District Resource Centres
DRST	District Resource Support Team
DS	Development Scores
DTP	Desktop Publishing
ECCE	Early Childhood Care and Education
EFA	Education for All
EMG	Electromyogram
EMIS	Educational Management Information System
FIR	First Information Report
FMB	Family Managed Business
GOI	Government of India
HRLN	Human Rights Law Network
HRD	Human Resource and Development
HSC	Higher Secondary Certificate
IAS	Indian Administrative Service
IBM-SPSS	International Business Machine-Statistical Package for the Social Sciences
ICDS	Integrated Child Development Scheme
IDOD	International Day of the Disabled
IECC	Inclusive Education Coordinating Committee
IECYD	Inclusive Education of Children and Youth with Disabilities
IEDC	Integrated Education for the Disabled Children
IEDH	Inclusive Education District Hub
IEDSS	Inclusive Education for Disabled Children at Secondary Stage
IEHNCO	Inclusive Education and Health Needs Coordinator
IEP	Individualized Education Programme
IGNOU	Indira Gandhi National Open University
IICP	Indian Institute of Cerebral Palsy
IOE	Institute of Education
IRB	Institutional Review Board
MAF	Mithu Alur Foundation

MCP	Management in Cerebral Palsy
MHRD	Ministry of Human Resources Development
MICS	Multiple Indicator Cluster Surveys
MOE	Ministry of Education
NAC	National Advisory Council
NCC	National Cadet Corps
NCCP	National Centre for Cerebral Palsy
NCERT	National Council of Educational Research And Training
NCF	National Curriculum Framework
NCTE	National Council For Teacher Education
NDT	Neurodevelopmental Therapy
NEUPA	National University of Educational Planning and Administration
NGO	Non-government Organization
NIOS	National Institute of Open Schooling
NIPCCD	National Institute of Population Control and Community Development
NJDC	National Job Development Centre
NRCI	National Resource Centre for Inclusion
NRHM	National Rural Health Mission
NSD	North South Dialogue
NSS	National Sample Survey
NIDRR	National Institute on Disability and Rehabilitation Research
NSSO	National Sample Survey Organisation
OAI-PMH	Open Archives Protocol for Metadata Harvesting
OBC	Other Backward Classes
ODA	Overseas Development Agency
OECD	Organisation for Economic Co-operation and Development
OOS	Out of School
OPD	Outpatient Department
OT	Occupational Therapy
PCP	Person Centered Planning
PHC	Primary Health Centre
PIED	Project for Integrated Education Development
PIL	Public Interest Litigation
PIP	Project Implementation Plan
PSM	Preventive and Social Medicine
PT	Physical Therapy
PWD	Persons with Disabilities
RAC	Research Action Committee
RBM	Result-based Management
RBSK	Rashtriya Bal Swasthya Karikram
RCI	Rehabilitation Council of India
REACH	Remedial Education Assessment Counselling Handicapped
RMSA	Rashtriya Madhyamik Shikhsha Abhiyan

RTE	Right to Education
SC	Schedule Caste
SCERT	State Council for Education Research and Training
SDC	Skills Development Centre
SI	Sensory Integration
SIDA	Swedish International Development Cooperation Agency
SMART-PT	Statewide Massive and Rigorous Training for Primary Teachers
SRS	School of Rehabilitation Sciences
SSA	Sarva Shiksha Abhiyan
SSC	Secondary School Certificate
SSEI	Spastics Society of Eastern India
SSI	The Spastics Society of India
SSNI	Spastics Society of Northern India
ST	Schedule Tribe
TCS	Tata Consultancy Services
TISS	Tata Institute of Social Sciences
TTC	Teacher Training Course
UGC	University Grants Commission
UNCRPD	United Nations Convention on the Rights of Persons with Disabilities
UNICEF	United Nations Children's Fund
UNESCO	United Nations Educational, Scientific and Cultural Organization
UPE	Universalization of Primary Education
WFP	World Food Programme
WHO	World Health Organization

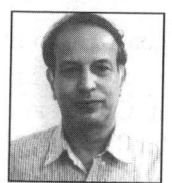
Dr Samiran Nundy

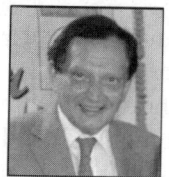
Dr Farokh Udwadia

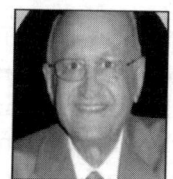
Late Dr Hiralal Desai

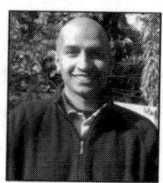
Dr Surajit Nundy

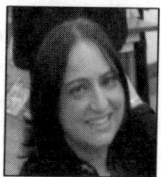
Dr Mithu Alur

Foreword

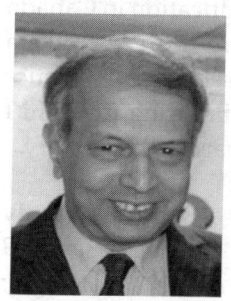
Dr Samiran Nundy

It seems strange to be writing a foreword to a book which is about people and a movement that have been so close to me most of my life. Not only are the main actors my closest relatives, it has been a privilege for me to have been associated with such a cause, the care of the disadvantaged, which, it has been said, is the hallmark of an advanced civilization. I remember when I was in medical school in England many years ago one of my teachers, Professor Ronald MacKeith, a renowned paediatrician, used to say that the members of a family into which a handicapped child was born always became better persons. They changed into more tolerant and sympathetic human beings who, unexpectedly, did not seem to confine their efforts to their own kith and kin but extended their compassion to those outside their immediate environment thus helping to make the world a better place to live. I think this is true of everyone who works with children with cerebral palsy (CP) and is amply exemplified by the story which is recounted in this book.

Malini's birth as such a child spurred Mithu into doing not only what was best for her own daughter but has stimulated her as well as her entire extended family, to which I am proud to belong, to do what they could for other children who were similarly afflicted.

I clearly remember Mithu ringing me up in England in 1967 to fix an appointment with Professor Jack Tizard for her daughter (as well as 'facilitating' my marriage to her sister!) and the subsequent years we spent together in Cambridge and London. It was there in England that Malini received the best care in the world and it was because she witnessed and learnt from this experience that Mithu was determined to bring such standards of care for the differently abled to India, a country which had no such facility at all. It was a place where the association of the word 'spastic' was that it rhymed with 'plastic'; the ignorance was so abysmal that people generally believed that they could do nothing and would be like 'vegetables'. They were excluded from schools, as schools did not admit them. Mithu and her organization have transformed people's attitude to those who are differently abled by changing their segregated 'treatment' from being a medical problem for doctors to becoming a team effort at management whose goals are to fit everyone to live proudly and be integrated into the normal world.

The whole saga of how Mithu met Mrs Indira Gandhi, the small beginnings in Colaba and the subsequent growth into a magnificent institution in Mumbai which has helped set up 28 others in the rest of the country is something which to me, looking back, is absolutely astounding. The birth of a single spastic child to a 23-year-old mother has set off a chain of events which has revolutionized the management of children with CP and, more importantly, has given them an identity, pride and self-confidence.

As Chairman of the Institutional Review Board (IRB), I had the privilege, together with my illustrious colleagues like Dr Farokh Udwadia, to witness at our annual meetings the enthusiasm and single-mindedness of all the workers in the Centre for Inclusive Education for the research projects they were conducting. I had then suggested that the history of The Spastics Society of India (SSI) should be written so that others in similar situations might learn from the challenges the founders faced and how they surmounted the obstacles which they encountered.

I am pleased to say that this wonderful book, which has chronicled this history in great detail, has met all my expectations.

Finally, on behalf of my late mother, Santi Nundy, who studied special education in Canada at the age of 54 and who said that working in the Spastics Society of Eastern India in Kolkata constituted the happiest years of her life, and my late wife, Mita, who set up the Spastics Society of Northern India (AADI) and who helped build its magnificent building in Delhi I can only say thank you to Mithu et al. for giving us the opportunity to be part of this history.

Samiran Nundy
Chairperson, IRB
MA (Cambridge, England); MB, B.Chir (Cambridge); MRCP (Edinburgh);
FRCS (England); M.Chir (Cambridge); FRCP (Edinburgh)

Dr Samiran Nundy, who is chairperson of our IRB, was a medical undergraduate in Cambridge and Guy's Hospital London and then trained, first in Medicine at the Hammersmith Hospital and later in surgery at Guy's, Addenbrooke's Cambridge, the Hammersmith and the Massachusetts General Hospital in Boston. He has taught at the Universities of Cambridge, London and Harvard and returned to Delhi's All India Institute of Medical Sciences (AIIMS) in 1975 where he eventually became Professor and Head of the Department of Gastrointestinal Surgery. He left AIIMS in 1996 to start the Surgical Gastroenterology and Liver Transplantation Department in Sir Ganga Ram Hospital, New Delhi. His clinical and research interests are in the management of complicated diseases of the liver, bowel and pancreas, as well as the quality of Indian medical research and publications and health information available on the web. He has written or edited 37 books and authored or co-authored 248 research papers. He has been the editor of *The National Medical Journal of India, Tropical Gastroenterology, Indian Journal of Medical Ethics* and the website DrRaxa.com and has also served on 24 journal editorial boards including the *British Medical Journal*. He is now dean of the Ganga Ram Institute for Postgraduate Medical Education and Research and editor in chief of Current Medicine Research and Practice and is on the board of trustees of Sir Ganga Ram Hospital.

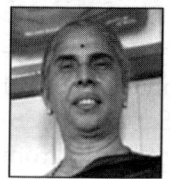
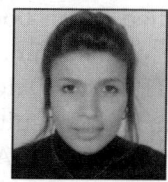
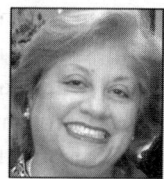
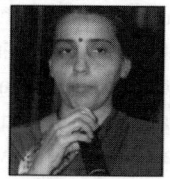
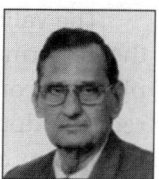

Dr Armida Fernandez   Dr Anaita Hegde   Professor Zenobia Nadirshaw   Dr Anuradha Sovani   Professor J.C. Sharma

Foreword

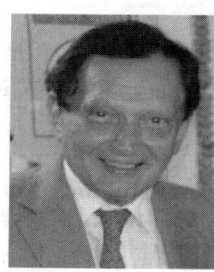

Dr Farokh Udwadia

The problems physically and/or mentally disabled children and their parents who look after them face are immense. These children are sidelined from the mainstream of life, disenfranchized and disempowered because of lack of proper education and care. They remain neglected, segregated and 'the children of a lesser God'.

The origin of this book is in the birth of a child, Malini, with CP to Mithu Alur. Devastating as it was, it threw a challenge to the mother and the challenge evoked a truly splendid and befitting response. The care extended towards this spastic child by the parents as also by the immediate and extended family generated a ripple effect. The fact that there were many children like Malini who needed similar care led to the founding of SSI, now called ADAPT (Able Disabled All People Together) under the aegis of Dr Mithu Alur. This book is a historical retrospective and prospective research study extending over four decades conducted by Dr Mithu Alur and team under the auspices of SSI within the ADAPT school. The study discusses the assessment, overall management and follow-up of physically and/or mentally disabled children by a trained team of very dedicated workers. The historical account detailed in this book shows that a holistic approach to management, which combines education, treatment, training, skills development and psychosocial support in a centre such as ADAPT, can bring such terribly neglected and deprived children into the mainstream of life and living. To be able to desegregate disabled children and succeed in integrating them with other normal children and mainstreaming them as they grow up with the society around them is easier said than done.

Integration of such children brings with it a sense of belonging, security, confidence and an overall enrichment and purpose to their lives. Dr Alur and her colleagues have succeeded in doing this and deserve our plaudits and congratulations for their dedication and work.

The validity and impact of the historical research embodied in this book is best judged by the performance of such children when integrated into the mainstream. Malini is an example—she completed her diploma in desktop publishing (DTP) from Oxford Polytechnic and received double Masters in London. Malini is presently with Tata Consultancy Services (TCS) in London and manages well. Many other disabled students from ADAPT with help from skilled teachers have passed their board examinations with distinction, gone to university and become accountants, librarians and computer experts. A number of them have even set up their own business and are holding jobs successfully.

Dr Alur and her colleagues have blazed a worthy trail which many have followed and many will follow. Her approach to the empowerment of disabled children as detailed in this book may well serve as a model for other workers in this field. This book should be read by doctors, physiotherapists, social workers and all those interested in this field of human endeavour. In fact, it should be read by all who care. Caring for others, in particular for those who are disabled or disenfranchized, enriches the quality of life in this world—enriching both those who are cared for, as also those who care.

I consider it an honour and a privilege to have served on the IRB under the able chairmanship of Dr Samiran Nundy. I feel enriched by this experience.

Dr Farokh Udwadia
Co-Chairperson, IRB
MD, FRCP (Edinburgh), FRCP (London), FAMS, Master FCCP, FACP

Dr Farokh Udwadia is co-chairperson of our IRB. He was awarded a Distinction in medicine at both the MBBS and MD examinations by the University of Bombay. He was elected a Fellow of the Royal College of Physicians, Edinburgh, in 1969 at the age of 38 years—the youngest Indian ever to be so elected. He has been Emeritus Professor of Medicine, Grant Medical College & JJ Group of Hospitals, Mumbai, since 1989. He has several (over 50) publications in international and national journals—chiefly in *Respiratory Medicine, Tropical Eosinophilia, Tetanus* and *Critical Care Medicine*. He has received numerous distinctions and has been awarded the Padma Bhushan for contribution to medicine in 1987.

Preface

Disabled people are not only the most deprived human beings in the developing world, they are also the most neglected.

—Amartya Sen

This book begins with a personal recollection of my own interest in physical disability because of my daughter, Malini, who was born with cerebral palsy (CP), and from whom I have learnt so much. Malini's birth generated a ripple effect, resulting in starting a movement in India. She became the raison d'être for the birth of the organization, which brought about a phenomenal spread of awareness round the country.

The title of this book is *A Birth That Changed a Nation: A New Model of Care and Inclusion*. It is written in a narrative style account of a research study, evidence based, investigating and examining the 40 years of policy and practice developed by a team of professionals for an organization called The Spastics Society of India (SSI). The data for this study was extensive. The methodology used was a combination of quantitative and qualitative research, drawing on multiple sources of information such as desk and field research, tracking documents through historical research from several libraries and archives, involving audiovisual material, observations, questionnaires, interviews and focus group discussions. The sample consisted of 1,445 files. A 'case study' approach was agreed upon by the Institutional Review Board (IRB), examining the organization under 10 domains. Being an action research study, the team of researchers who compiled the data consisted of a group of practitioners and academics, each drawing from their own experience. The data was gathered from available documentation from annual reports, brochures, peer-reviewed publications and books in the archives. The research protocol was approved by the IRB. It was agreed that the usual format of background, methods, results, discussion and conclusion would be followed.

At the core of this book is a new method of *rehabilitation and care* developed in the early 1970s for children with multiple disabilities like CP as well as other physical disabilities: children who were often described as having 'intelligent minds with disobedient bodies'. CP, being a condition which is chronic and lifelong, needed a model of management that was longitudinal and holistic in its engagement with parents and the community. In the 1960s, very little was known about the condition. There were some medical facilities and services which were widely scattered over long distances but no educational service within a school setting. To address this gap, a group consisting essentially of family members and close friends came together and created an innovative model for India, combining education and treatment in a special school setting, which brought the care from hospitals in its folds. That single school became an institution and evolved to become a movement.

This model emerged, unfortunately, from a personal trauma but it led to the creation of a service, bringing in the passion of parents together with professional skills combined with a level of care that transcended the usual service model. Each child was an individual who received individual evaluation, individual treatment and individual care, which was unique in this country. What is particularly interesting is how the birth of one child shook the nation, resulting in an entire extended family responding and coming forward to play a part in virgin territories in different parts of the country.

The mission of the organization, then called The Spastics Society of India, was to influence and change public policy and opinion in order to create an inclusive, caring, disability-friendly India and to reach out across the country and help in the spread of services to the huge numbers of much neglected children with CP and their families. Forty-five years have passed. Was this mission achieved? I was keen to look back with a critical eye and engage with scientists, researchers and medical practitioners to enquire whether it did and if it did, how it really contributed to the nation. I was also keen to hear the voices of parents and the children who had passed through our school and become adults.

Ethical issues required neutral professionals to review in detail the methods we developed. Research makes an immensely important contribution towards achieving and establishing full human rights and social justice for people with disabilities (UN 1993). I constituted two committees: the Institutional Review Board (IRB) and the Research Action Committee (RAC). The IRB was to examine the existing body of work and give its advice on how the interventions developed by the team could be documented and how the data could be validated so that the work would rate as a scientific research study. Their function was to oversee and monitor any clinical research study, both qualitative and quantitative, ensuring adherence to scientific, ethical and legal guidelines. The IRB consists of eminent people, doctors and experts, parents and disabled activists. Its panel is chaired by Dr Samiran Nundy and co-chaired by Dr Farokh Udwadia. Others in the team were the late Dr Hiralal Desai, Dr Surajit Nundy, Professor I.C. Verma, Dr Armida Fernandez, Dr Anaita Hegde, Professor Zenobia Nadirshaw, Professor J.C. Sharma, Dr Anuradha Sovani, Dr Urvashi Shah, Dr Maria Baretto, Ms Malini Chib, while the practitioners include Mrs Varsha Hooja, Dr Shabnam Rangwala, Mrs Ami Gumastha, Mrs Manju Chatterjee, Dr Maneeta Sawhney, Mrs Reshma Tanna, Dr Sharmila Donde, Mr Sudeep Pagedar, Ms Sangeeta Jagtiani, Mrs Deepshika Mathur, Mrs Shobha Sachdev, Mrs Gulab Sayed, Dr Kurian Kuriakose, and disabled activists, and also parents of persons with disability. The earlier director of research, Dr Madhuri Pai joined us later.

While the IRB provided direction and guidance to the study, the practitioners or the RAC were responsible for carrying out the collection of data and research. This exercise was done over a period of five years. The IRB scrutinized research protocols and after several meetings passed the research study of the New Model of Care. The historical research was to go backwards and systematically examine past events to give an account of what had happened over the four decades; the practitioners would then compile the data and give their own views based on their experiences. I was to write the account itself. The study would also narrate stories and include anecdotes of the countless silent people who contributed to the movement.

Rationale for the Research

The primary aim of the work is to find ways to alleviate the suffering of the child and family; the main objective of the analysis is to study the gaps that existed and examine the effectiveness of the model that had been created. However, although these new and innovative services have borne encouraging results, there are gaps that still need crucial attention. The model and its outcomes have not been documented nor scaled out into district and rural areas, resulting in millions of families with disabled children still excluded from services and still facing extreme and severe hardships. Some of the gaps were a result of the fact that the census did not include disability as a demographic category till 2011. Robust data is still not available about the location of these children and about their needs. Most of them, especially in remote districts and rural areas, still do not receive any service and are at a high risk of becoming permanently deformed (World Bank 2007). It becomes imperative to prevent and alleviate this situation, keeping in mind that they are 'the forgotten millions of impoverished and disadvantaged people who still remain in a wilderness of neglect, forgotten and out of any service' (Barton and Armstrong 2007). After demonstrating how children with CP could be educated and treated in a special school setting, the organization shifted its policy from segregated education to inclusive education, demonstrating how children with disability could be included into regular schools, leading to a major outcome of legislative reform through the Right to Education Act. Today, education has become a constitutional right and the term 'all' includes children with disability. From a special school, the organization moved to become an institution and later to a movement for disabled people (Alur 2010a).

Yet we know that 60 per cent of the children do not get any services in the far-flung rural areas and districts. It now remains critical to ensure on humanitarian grounds that *scalability* take place and that the *unreached get reached*. Therefore, it was decided, in 2009, to study in a scientific manner with guidance from the IRB, whether the first model of treatment and management, which begun in 1972, brought about any change at all into the lives of the children and their families which they were meant to serve and whether it could give an important message to the people in rural areas about how they could teach and manage their child with some direction and support.

Methodology

Much of the discussions in the IRB meetings focused around methodology. What was going to be the best approach? Research can be categorized as being qualitative or quantitative. Qualitative research had not been considered 'scientifically robust' earlier but now perceptions in the area of disability have changed and qualitative research has attained credibility. The

arguments in favour of qualitative research are that it involves the use of a variety of empirical tools such as ethnography, field methods, qualitative inquiry, participant observation, case
study, naturalistic inquiry, unstructured and semi-structured interviews, focus groups and
documentation analysis. Would it be possible to be systematic and explicit in laying out the
methods used, analyze the findings and arrive at conclusions which are credible and reliable,
ensuring that the research is not biased or skewed?

The study spanning two worlds—one in the ivory tower domain of medical science and
universities and the other at the grass-root levels of stakeholders like parents and disabled
children in the community—it was agreed that both qualitative and quantitative methodology
were important. In the study of human affairs, broken families, parents, disabled youth and
traumatized children, qualitative data provided rich insight. I believe that qualitative research
is very much a science and has as much value as quantitative research.

It was therefore decided that a retrospective historical research of the four decades would
be done; that the research study would be a combination of two methodologies: quantitative
and qualitative.

It was also important to constantly keep an eye on the applicability of the research findings, and how they could benefit society and community welfare and well-being further, keeping in mind the cost-effectiveness of the study. Through the answers in this book, our aim
would be to disseminate truth; to establish a code of practice for the country that could reach
people with disability in every region of the country, giving them hope; to help practitioners,
policy-makers, medical and paramedical personnel; and finally to move to replicability and
scalability through the state machinery.

The book will also introduce the new philosophy known as the social model. The social
model is different from the old medical model which focused on persons with disability as
pathologized and dysfunctional. The social model focuses not on anything within people with
disability, but without, in their environment, surroundings and attitudes (Wedell 1982). The
social model has now moved on to becoming a rights and entitlements model. Current Acts
of Parliament and international declarations state that it is environment and societal attitudes
that should be changed and adapted to the disabled person, rather than the disabled person
having to be 'normalized' to fit into society.

Based on such a premise it is also about people … people who have suffered years of
neglect in this country … people who were made invisible before. It relates stories of how
children with a slight modification in the curriculum and examination systems, with the help
of skilled teachers and therapists, and a close partnership with parents (hitherto not included
in decision making), passed examinations with flying colours, thus demonstrating that it was
perfectly possible for them to appear in board examinations. It also talks about people who
have supported us and believed in our work and events that have been milestones along the
way and have become an integral part of our collective memory. Students, teachers, staff, parents, volunteers, visitors, patrons and well-wishers have all been co-travellers on this journey.
The rich tapestries of the past and present are woven together through photographs, articles
and press releases, keeping within the research protocol.

The book begins with the birth of Malini Chib, then moves on to another birth: that of SSI.
The narration has been put into a scientific, historical research case study methodology, looking

at the 10 domains of the organization's functioning: education, treatment, child and parents in partnership, training, capacity building, skills development, policy and spread of awareness, economics and sustainability, transformation of ideology and results and outcomes.

These domains are used to describe the methods that were used to create the revolutionary model of care, enabling children with CP to pass examinations, move on to universities and then to employment. Woven into this is the expansion of services having a pan-Indian presence, the first model having a ripple effect spreading to 28 states of the nation. In this study, we examine the work of six major organizations in the six locations of Mumbai, Kolkata, Bengaluru, Delhi, Chennai and Jaipur.

The book then moves on to the shift in ideology *from special education to inclusive education*, encompassing the radical transformation from a school to an institution and finally to a movement, leading to changes in legislation, policy framework and reformative action, thus paving the way to future expansion to far-flung districts and rural areas, where the majority of disabled children live forgotten and neglected.

It was not easy to capture the essence of these 45 years of challenge, the highs, the lows, the ups, the downs and the tears and smiles; despite all, it has been immensely fulfilling for all of us.

Acknowledgements

A historical research study like this, comprising an overview of 40 years of relentless work, is a long journey and a seriously difficult one to undertake. To organize the framework of the book and to search for the data took five years. I would not have had the courage to take it on but for the support and help I have received. I gratefully acknowledge the guidance given in making this book a scientific account by the IRB. Without their utmost diligence and encouragement, concern and guidance, this study would not have seen the light of day. The IRB consists of eminent doctors, scientists, academics, and other professionals and practitioners, who have been in the field of service for many years.

I am hugely grateful to Dr Samiran Nundy, chairman of the IRB, whose passion it was for this 'autobiography of an institution' to be written up and who steered us through this difficult terrain; to the co-chair, Dr Farokh Udwadia who, being such an eminent physician and author himself, showed immense tolerance and patience and insisted that the narrative should be interspersed with human interest stories; to Dr Surajit Nundy who right from the beginning gave us a very clear, transparent, forthright idea of what research is about—how we should not waste too much time talking about ourselves—and who really helped us to develop our critical faculties, leading us to establish the scientific parameters of this study; to Dr Anaita Hegde whose idea it was initially to do retrospective and prospective research and who frequently read the research findings and gave her guidance; to the late Dr Hiralal Desai, a friend and reputed researcher who spurred us along even when other members were shunning the thought of qualitative research; to Dr Armida Fernandez, my friend, who had worked with us before in Dharavi as Dean of Sion Hospital and who, through her organization called Sneha, encouraged us all along; to Dr Urvashi Shah and Dr Anuradha Sovani, both of whom had also worked as researchers in a UNICEF Project and knew our work well and trained the team for many years now; to Professor Zenobia Nadirshaw, Dr Maria Baretto and Professor J.C. Sharma, all of whom spent many days training and guiding members of the RAC. Most importantly, I acknowledge the motivation of my valuable team of professionals and practitioners who helped to compile some of the data, which helped in making this book a reality. The RAC had worked diligently for the last five years and had full faith that I would be able to deliver the goods; their faith in me which I value immensely, spurred me on. The RAC included Mrs Varsha Hooja, Ms Malini Chib, Dr Shabnam Rangwalla, Dr Anita Prabhu,

Dr Sulochini Pather, Mrs Ami Gumashta, Ms Theresa D'Costa, Mr Lucas Baretto, Ms June D'Sousa, Mrs Arati Siram, Ms Sujata Verma, Dr Kurian Kuriakose, Mrs Manju Chatterjee, Dr Maneeta Sawhney, Mrs Reshma Tanna, Dr Sharmila Dhonde, Mr Sudeep Pagedar, Ms Sangeeta Jagtiani, Mrs Deepshika Mathur, Mrs Shobha Sachdev, Mrs Gulab Sayed and later Dr Madhuri Pai. To the many parents and disabled activists, our students and our volunteers who have sent in their thoughts and whose voices will be heard in the book, I am truly grateful.

I am also immensely appreciative of my fellow pioneers and partners in this journey, who have set up excellent services all over the country, making SSI a dynamic phenomenon, leading to a movement. They responded generously in contributing to the book. I have taken important excerpts from articles written by the founder of the Delhi Spastics Society, the late Mrs Mita Nundy; contributions have also come from Delhi from co-founder, Mrs Divya Jalan, from Miss Gloria Burrett, Miss Shyamala Gidigu and Miss Vandana Bedi; from Jaipur, from the founder of the organization Umang, Mrs Deepak Kalra; from Vidyasagar, Chennai, founders Mrs Poonam Natarajan, Mrs Usha Ramakrishnan and Mrs Rajul Padmanabhan; from Kolkata, founder member Sudha Kaul and excerpts from co-founder member, the late Junie Bose, and from founder member of Reach, Purobie Bose.

I take this opportunity to acknowledge and thank all the members of the board of trustees and governing body for all their support and work round the year. Mr Kamal Bakshi, former Indian ambassador and vice chairperson; Professor Sitanshu Mehta, a parent, poet, critic and scholar; Malini Chib, author, researcher now working as diversity officer in TCS, London; Mrs Priya Dutt Roncon, honourable Member of Parliament; Mr Nikhil Chib, economist, restaurateur and trustee; Mrs Varsha Hooja, CEO and trustee ADAPT; Mr Sathi Alur, member governing Body and honorary financial advisor; Mrs Ami Gumashta, honorary director, finance and member of governing board; Mr Jayabrato Chatterjee, writer, film-maker, corporate communicator and member of governing body; Mrs Deepak Kalra, eminent professional, practitioner parent and founder of UMANG services in Jaipur; Ms Asleshla Gowarikar, senior partner, Desai and Deewanji; and Vishal Bakshi, managing director, Goldman Sachs.

Our board of advisors include: Mr Shyam Benegal, renowned film-maker and activist for social change; Mr V. Ranganathan, former chief secretary, Government of Maharashtra; Mrs Vera Udwadia, committed to the cause of disability; Mr Arup Patnaik, former director general police; Mr Nagesh Kukunoor, award-winning film-maker; Ms Dia Mirza, actor and producer; Mr Satyen Bordoloi, journalist and film-maker and Ms Shonali Bose, film-maker of international renown.

Most importantly, I thank my colleagues, volunteers, parents, disabled activists, each and every one of them, who have supported us with earnest diligence, sincere passion and commitment, making this journey a truly meaningful one. I should also like to acknowledge my friend Pervin Mahoney, an ex-editor of Pan Books, who very kindly and with due diligence did an excellent job of copy editing at very short notice.

Lastly to Vivek Mehra and his team at SAGE Publications, who have always put their belief and trust in me and my work and for making this publication possible for the many who will benefit.

This has been an East-West project created within the context of India. There were many who contributed and built up the knowledge base, sensitive to India's needs from outside India too. These alliances and collaborations were much needed in a country with little or no knowledge base on this subject. I hope this study helps generations of workers, researchers and policy-makers to improve the quality of life of the children and people who we have worked with and from whom we have learnt so much. Their grit, fortitude, courage, determination to succeed, and their shining smiling faces despite being caught up in an indifferent environment will always remain with us, while we ask the question 'Who is disabled, is it them or us?'

Mithu Alur
Mumbai, 2015

Where the mind is without fear and the head is held high;
Where knowledge is free;
Where the world has not been broken up into fragments by narrow domestic walls;
Where words come out from the depth of truth;
Where tireless striving stretches its arms towards perfection;
Where the clear stream of reason has not lost its
way into the dreary desert sand of dead habit;
Where the mind is led forward by Thee into ever-widening thought and action—
Into that heaven of freedom, my Father, let my country awake.

Rabindranath Tagore
ADAPT's School Poem
celebrates differences on the Nobel Laureate's
150th birth anniversary

Executive Summary

As already mentioned in the Preface, this book begins with a personal recollection of my own interest in disability, which occurred because of my daughter Malini, who was born with CP and who, without knowing it, became my greatest teacher.

The book will also introduce the new philosophy known as the social model. The social model is different from the old medical model which focused on persons with disability as pathologized and dysfunctional. The social model focuses not on anything within people with disability, but without, on their environment, surroundings and attitudes (Wedell 1982). The social model has now moved into a rights and entitlements model. Current acts of parliament and international declarations state that it is environment and societal attitudes that should be changed and adapted to the disabled person, rather than the disabled person having to be 'normalized' to fit into society.

Most importantly, the book is focused on human aspects of being disabled in India. It is about people who have suffered years of neglect in this country ... people who were made invisible before. It relates stories of how children with a slight modification in the curriculum and examination systems, with the help of skilled teachers and therapists, and a close partnership with parents (hitherto not included in decision making), passed examinations with flying colours, thus demonstrating that it was perfectly possible to appear for board examinations.

The book also talks about people who have supported us and believed in our work and events that have been milestones along the way and have become an integral part of our collective memory. Students, teachers, staff, parents, volunteers, visitors, patrons and well-wishers have all been co-travellers on this journey. The rich tapestry of the past and present are woven together through photographs, articles and press releases, keeping within the research protocol.

The book begins with the birth of Malini Chib, then moves on to another birth: that of the SSI. The narration has been put into a scientific, historical research case study methodology, looking at 10 domains of the organization's functioning: education, treatment, child and parents in partnership, training, capacity building, skills development, policy research and spread of awareness, economics and sustainability, transformation of ideology, and results and outcomes.

Domain I. Education: *to fill the gaps where there was no school;* it gives the background of the first special school which began in 1972 and addresses educational problems and methods used to overcome barriers in the classroom.

Domain II. Treatment and Rehabilitation Unit: covers the holistic management of CP and manpower training—therapists—and talks about assessments, screening and intervention, geared to each child's needs and discusses how to manage the child's rehabilitation.

Domain III. Child and Parents in Partnership: transforming the approach and empowering the parents as professionals; this section goes on to the next approach to parents. It talks about how parents are empowered through various programmes to gain knowledge about their child's challenges and encouraged to go on to become professionals in partnerships.

Domain IV. Training: to fill the gaps where there were no teachers or therapists or appropriate human resources; it discusses how courses were laid.

Domain V. Capacity Building in the Community: Dharavi and Karuna Sadan—strengthening the community; discusses how to empower people in the community to be multitasking workers.

Domain VI. Work Training Unit and the Skills Development Centre: discusses various methods used to get youth with disabilities placed in work situations and employment.

Domain VII. (i) Expansion of Services on the National Level: From schools to institution building. Discusses how the organization spread to 28 states of the nation, focusing on the work of six major organizations in the six locations of Mumbai, Kolkata, Bengaluru, Delhi, Chennai and Jaipur, (ii) moves on to expansion of services on the international level involving four international governments, (iii) Economics and Sustainability: discusses a new approach involving all the stakeholders moving from charity to entitlement and also discusses the multifarious activities of fundraising that took place to make the organization sustainable.

Domain VIII. Research and Transformation of Ideology: is about inclusive education. It discusses the various researches which led to the shift of ideology from special schooling to inclusive education.

Domain IX. Policy and Macro Level Change: Legislation and Policy. It discusses about legal and reformative action implemented for changing policy on a macro level.

Domain X. Results and Outcomes and the Way Forward: talks about the results, outcomes and the way forward … also touches on some of the disabled people who were impacted as well as the staff, parents and volunteers who were impacted and discusses how the organization became a movement.

These domains are used to describe the methods that were used to create the revolutionary model of care, enabling children with CP to pass examinations, move to university and then to employment and inclusiveness. Running through it on a parallel level is the story of Malini and her family's contribution.

1

The First Birth: Malini Chib

It was a stormy evening in Kolkata on the 16th of July, 1966. I was being rushed to Woodlands Nursing Home by my family for the birth of my first child. After what seemed an interminably long and very painful labour of 40 hours, the baby was born: unfortunately, blue in the face, suffocating and gasping for breath. I was told that the umbilical cord had been around her neck and she was suffering from asphyxia and lack of oxygen. It had had to be a high forceps delivery. A traumatic birth, the first few hours of her life were critical. The gynaecologist kept saying 'I have made a mistake; I should have done a caesarian.' The baby was put into an oxygen tent or an incubator; doctors had given up hope and said, 'she would not survive for more than 72 hours'.

She did survive. We called her Malini.

Very little was known at that time about damage to a baby infant's brain and its impact on her and parents. In India's premier institute in Delhi, a doctor examined Malini and brusquely said, 'Your daughter has cerebral palsy. Brain damage is irrevers-

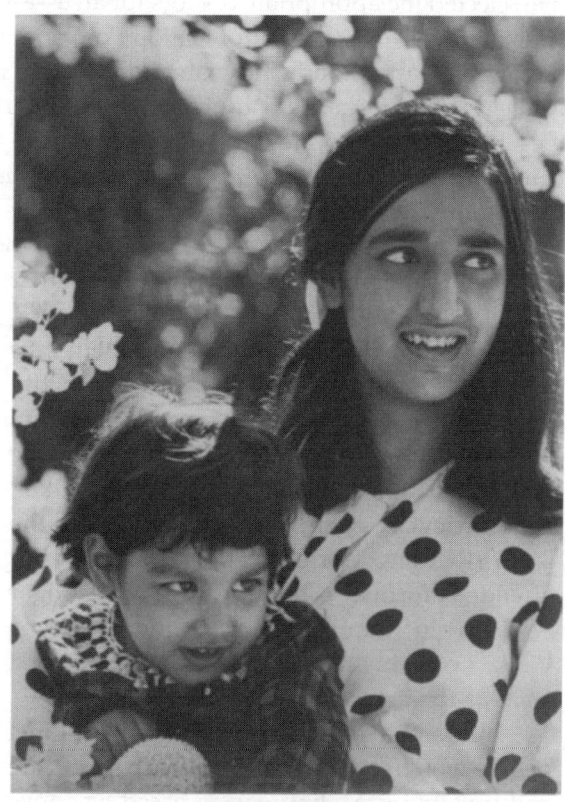

Malini and Mithu

ible. Once the brain is damaged, it's damaged for life. Nothing can be done about it.' Again they said, 'She will not be able to achieve much over five years as her brain is damaged. She will remain "a vegetable".'

Then came the tears. I was 23, my husband 25. The finality of the statement 'nothing can be done about it' devastated us as young parents. Neither I nor my husband had any idea of what cerebral palsy (CP) was. The good thing is we did not *accept* what the doctors said. My husband and I ran from pillar to post in desperation, trying to understand what had happened to our baby.

We went from doctor to doctor. Malini hated these examinations. They pulled and pushed her limbs, silently, not talking to her and Malini would shriek with fright. But they would remain cold, silent, not speaking to the baby, strange, unsmiling in their white coats and their professionalism. Malini would cling to me crying hopelessly and as her sobs would die down slowly, we would cry within us.

Finding nobody who understood her, we decided to go to England in search of treatment for Malini who was then one and a half.

Then began a long battle, a journey which took us mercifully away from this situation of negativity and ignorance in India to one of freedom and happiness—to Cambridge, England, where my brother-in-law Samiran Nundy and sister Mita Nundy lived. Samiran was the registrar at the Addenbrookes Hospital, Cambridge. He master-minded the early care of baby Malini. He selected the appropriate doctors for an assessment and prognosis, and my ex-husband Ranjit Chib (at that time, director of Gallop Poll) and myself implemented the programme drawn up. Ranjit had earlier made a dynamic decision to move us to London: as a student in Emmanuel College, Cambridge, he had observed the superior medical care in England and thought it was best for us all to relocate to London. It was very quick thinking of him as it settled the traumatic situation we were caught in India. However, his career went for a toss as he had to leave the prestigious Tata Administrative Service and his beloved Tatas and move to London. We didn't have enough funds to relocate to London and the Tatas paid for everything, flying us to England for Malini's treatment. We will never forget that. It was in London too that I gave birth to my son Nikhil, who is today a successful restaurateur.

In London, Malini received excellent care and blossomed. We, too, as parents, badly needing a healing touch, recovered. Malini became a different individual with all this care and incubation: she walked with a walker, rode a tricycle, swam with a tyre, cracked the 3 R's (Reading, Writing and Numbers) and attended formal schooling—first at Roger Ascham in Cambridge and then Cheyne Walk, London. At both places, she received state-of-the-art treatment and education.

For us, the time in England was key. I met people who treated her and me with great care and sensitivity. Malini was assessed as above average in her intelligence (so much for being called a vegetable!). Their whole approach to us and her changed our lives.

Both Malini and I progressed and I decided to study more on the subject and enrolled at the Institute of Education in London to study and became a professional special educator. The first question that rose

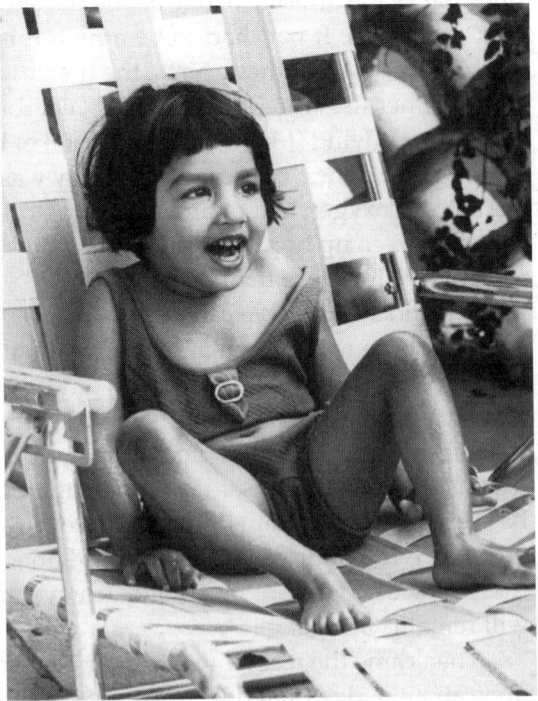

Malini in London

in my mind was: What about other Malinis? What was happening to them and how to educate other children like her? They should get the same kind of services as Malini, who was privileged enough to go to England.

However, it was easier said than done. After six years, we returned. The situation was the same! We were asked, 'What is a spastic? Are you talking about plastics?' The first question I was confronted with was 'Why educate them?' An eminent citizen in Mumbai said, 'Why bother Mithu, there are hundreds of normal children needing education.'

What a difference from the cocoon of services in England we had left behind ... the love, the care, the kindness and the compassion. It was like being thrown into a turbulent merciless ocean and not knowing how to swim.

We were again cast into a situation of despair. I wanted to run back to Engand, but there was no going back this time. My marriage was also coming to an end. The family put their strength behind me to support me any which way they could. I came from one of those privileged *bhadrolok* families of Kolkata, where there was a strong combination of British and Indian influences. My parents were staunch nationalists. The oft-repeated phrase one heard was 'you must serve India' and 'service must go beyond self'. The entire family came forward determined to be with me in this struggle.

Against such a backdrop, a new holistic model of a special centre was conceived to provide education and treatment under one roof to children affected by CP, similar to the model of Cheyne Centre but in the context of India and most importantly to introduce a large dose of love, care and kindness combined with technical expertise. The little centre by the Arabian Sea with just three students fulfilled the need of the hour and the second birth in our lives took place—the birth of The Spastics Society of India (SSI).

2

The Second Birth: The Spastics Society of India[1]

This chapter describes a case study: the first model of a centre combining education and treatment of CP under the roof of a special school rather than a hospital setting. The model demonstrates how children with this complex neurological condition of CP can be effectively managed in a holistic and integrated manner. This case study covers new methods of treatment management in the classrooms, modifications and concessions in the examinations and much needed reforms on a macro level which were introduced, enabling hundreds of children to pass officially recognized school board examinations and move onto university and employment. The Institutional Review Board (IRB) approved a historical, retrospective research study of this model to be documented through a carefully selected scientific methodology, investigating and examining the management of CP done over 40 years.

The Methodology

Aim

- To investigate whether children with CP can be educated.
- To critically examine the past records of the organization through a record of the archives, the perception and opinion of the stakeholders, including parents and disabled activists, and to provide a historical account of SSI in developing policy and practices for focusing on children with disability (CP, multiple and motor disability) in India.
- To recommend what must be done to improve care and to plan scalability.

Research Question

The research question was: 'How has the SSI's new interdisciplinary/multidisciplinary approach impacted the lives of children with CP, motor and multiple disabilities and their parents?'

[1] The Institutional Review Board (IRB) of SSI comprised Dr Mithu Alur, Professor Zenobia Nadirshaw, Professor J. C. Sharma, Mrs Varsha Hooja, Dr Shabnam Rangwala, Ms Sangeeta Jagtiani, Ms Heena Sharma, Dr Sharmila Donde, Mrs Deepshikha Mathur, Mrs Gulab Sayed, Mrs Shobha Sachdev, Ms Malini Chib, Nilesh Singit, Dr Maneeta Sawhney, Mr Kurien Kuriakose, Sujata Varma, Arati Siram, Lucas Baretto, Theresa D'Costa, June D'Souza and Sudeep Pagedar.

Subsidiary Questions

The subsidiary questions were: 'Have variables such as education, treatment, partnership with parents, training and pedagogical shifts, and macro level policy reforms, contributed to any outcomes?'

- Hypothesis 1. SSI's psycho-socio medical model has led to positive outcomes for children with CP/motor and multiple disabilities and their families.
- Hypothesis 2. The organization's shift in policy from segregated education to inclusive education has led to mainstreaming of children with disability into regular schools, leading to the major outcome of legislative reform through the Right to Education (RTE) Act.

Discussion

The approach to the study and the methods to be used was decided by the IRB. A combination of qualitative and quantitative methodology was selected. Qualitative data is usually in the form of words rather than numbers, attempting to describe people's feelings, beliefs and attitudes in their natural settings. Qualitative data provides rich insight into human behaviour (Denzin and Lincoln 1994: 106). Human behaviour cannot be understood without reference to the meanings and purposes attached by the human actors and their activities (Ibid. 1994:106). Qualitative research strategies referring to a broad approach, encompassing different blends, have considerable potential for contributing to the study of processes, and divergence between policy and practice by providing analyses which are strongly related to the cultural context and in identifying appropriate questions (Vulliamy 1990: 25). For the study of human affairs, encompassing misunderstood and sometimes traumatized children, the anxieties and varied griefs of parents and the hazard of broken families, qualitative data provides rich insight.

The weaknesses of qualitative research are also worth noting. These are researcher bias, the reliability and validity of data, ethical constructs and the difficulties relating to micro-macro theories. However, these weaknesses can also apply to quantitative research. The craft of qualitative analysis has advanced and matrix and network displays are now common. Therefore, it was agreed that while using qualitative techniques it is possible to be systematic to arrive at conclusions in establishing credibility and reliability. The IRB members agreed that this being a study of human beings, disabled people and their families, it was important to understand their perceptions, beliefs, anxieties, grief and suffering. Again, being a chronic disorder that lasted a lifetime, it needed to be dealt with a mixture of professionalism and sensitivity, love and emotion. It was then agreed that the study would be a mix of quantitative and qualitative methodology.

The organization had provided a new approach, combining specialization and professionalism with affectionate care. It was decided that a qualitative approach examining the organization's contribution, if any, under 10 domains was best suited to this context. A case study approach was selected with inter-rater reliability and triangulation to check the validity of the data.

Triangulation

Triangulation is a powerful technique that facilitates validation of data through cross-verification from more than two sources. In particular, it refers to the application and combination of several research methodologies in the study of the same phenomenon. By combining multiple observers, theories, methods and empirical materials, researchers can hope to over-come the weakness or intrinsic biases and the problems that may arise from single method, single observer and single theory studies.

Inter-rater Reliability

Verifying one's own thinking in the analytic process against two others was important to get a degree of rigour into the analysis. A combination of various methods was approved in a series of meetings.

It was also agreed that a quantitative element could be added with an experienced statistician.

The study is therefore a mixture of qualitative and quantitative research, a combination of desk and field research. Desk research involved using common qualitative methodology of literature review, historical research, document analyses, while field research used oral history techniques, focus group discussions, questionnaires and tape-recorded interviews with past students and parents. The quantitative study consists of analysing a sample of 1,445 files. Table 1 shows a combination of methods used for the investigation.

Table 1
Methodology: A Combination of Qualitative and Quantitative Research

Methodology	Data Collection
I. Desk Research a. Literature Review b. Document Analyses	**External: (i.a) Online research (i.b) Government published data on disability (i.c) Books from Tata Institute of Social Sciences (TISS) and British Council Libraray (BCL)** **Internal: (ii) Archival Department, Colaba Centre and Library Resource and Media Centre, Bandra** • Documents of the early stages of organization and staff (correspondence with respect to children with parents, professionals, organizations and government; assessment files of students; and documents of 1,445 files of children studied. • Photographs of early events and activities, brochures, leaflets and booklets of SSI, newspaper clippings, annual reports, souvenirs, speeches, papers presented, published articles, students' information registers, year-wise database of alumni of SSI • Research and publications: Booklets on facts about CP: What everyone should know about CP • Guidelines for the management of CP • Medical problems associated with CP • Employment opportunities • Reach of services of SSI, its affiliates and branches in 1988. **(iii) Greenstone Digital Library** • Uploaded digitized materials on the library server available for the research team. • New versions of IBM-SPSS Statistics-21 have been introduced to the research team for both quantitative and qualitative analysis. • Training Programmes on research methodology and SPSS conducted by Prof J.C. Sharma and Dr Anuradha Sovani on focus groups.
II. Field Research a. Case study of the organization b. A detailed sub-study of 100 cases.	10 domains examined: 1) Education, 2) Treatment and rehabilitation unit, 3) Child and parents in partnership, 4) Training and capacity building, 5) Work Training Unit and Skills Development Centre, 6) Expansion of services, 7) Economics and Sustainability, 8) Research and transformation of ideology, 9) Policy and macro level change, 10) Results, outcomes and conclusions. • Interview schedule. • Focus group discussion guide. • Tape recording of stakeholders, parents, alumni and so on responses. • Questionnaire to other organizations for the disabled.

Source: Author.

The data collection was extensive, drawing on multiple sources of information such as obser-vations, interviews, documents, audio-visual materials, triangulation and inter-rater reliability.

Professor J.C. Sharma, Fellow of TISS, was invited to support the researchers. IBM SPSS Statistics 21 was brought in and the researchers began using the same in their respective researches.[2] Dr Anuradha Sovani conducted workshops on focus group methods.

An action research approach, based on the idea that the practitioners in a service delivery pro-gramme take on the role of researchers in order to monitor, evaluate and adapt their interventions on an ongoing basis, was selected. Action research enables the actors to undertake an ongoing process of documentation and do a critical reflection to improve the effectiveness and to develop the organizations, providing an ongoing learning situation (Armstrong and Moore 2004).

This is graphically shown in the following figure.

The IRB approved the methodology which includes personal stories of children and their families within a single case study of the organization. Each area has been examined through a qualitative methodology using multiple methods of focus group discussion, semi-structured questionnaires, records of documentation available and assessing the organization's develop-ment through four decades.

Interspersed are first-hand stories by parents whose children have CP, young adults who attended the first centre in Bombay, teachers, therapists and volunteers.

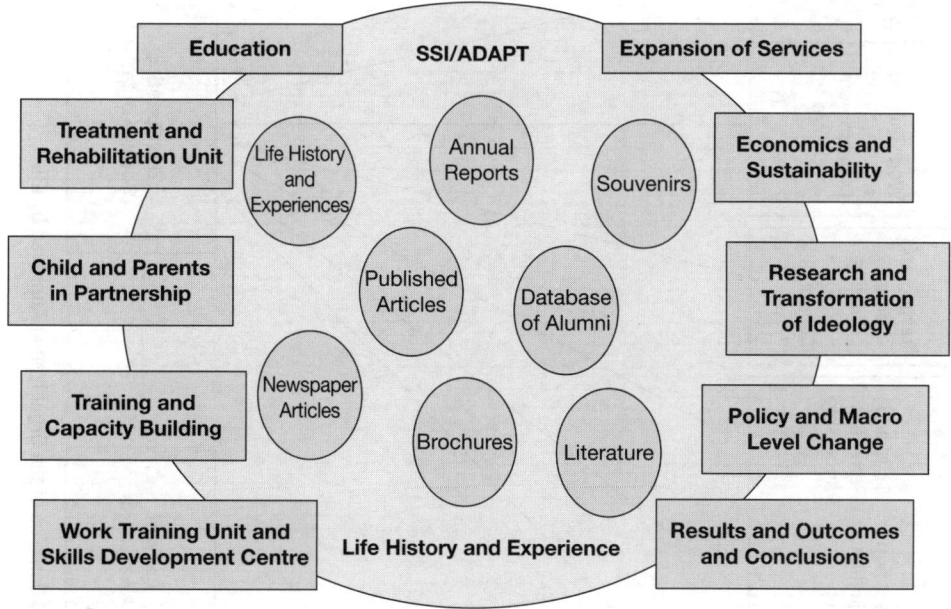

Figure 1. Showing Data Collection Using a Case Study Approach[3]
Source: Author.

[2] Training programmes on 'Research Methodology' have been introduced to data analysis using SPSS by Professor J.C. Sharma.

[3] The Case Study Methodology based on an examination of 10 domains was a method introduced by Dr Sulochini Pather which again was based on her own doctoral research. Dr Pather was one of the Members of the Research Action Committee.

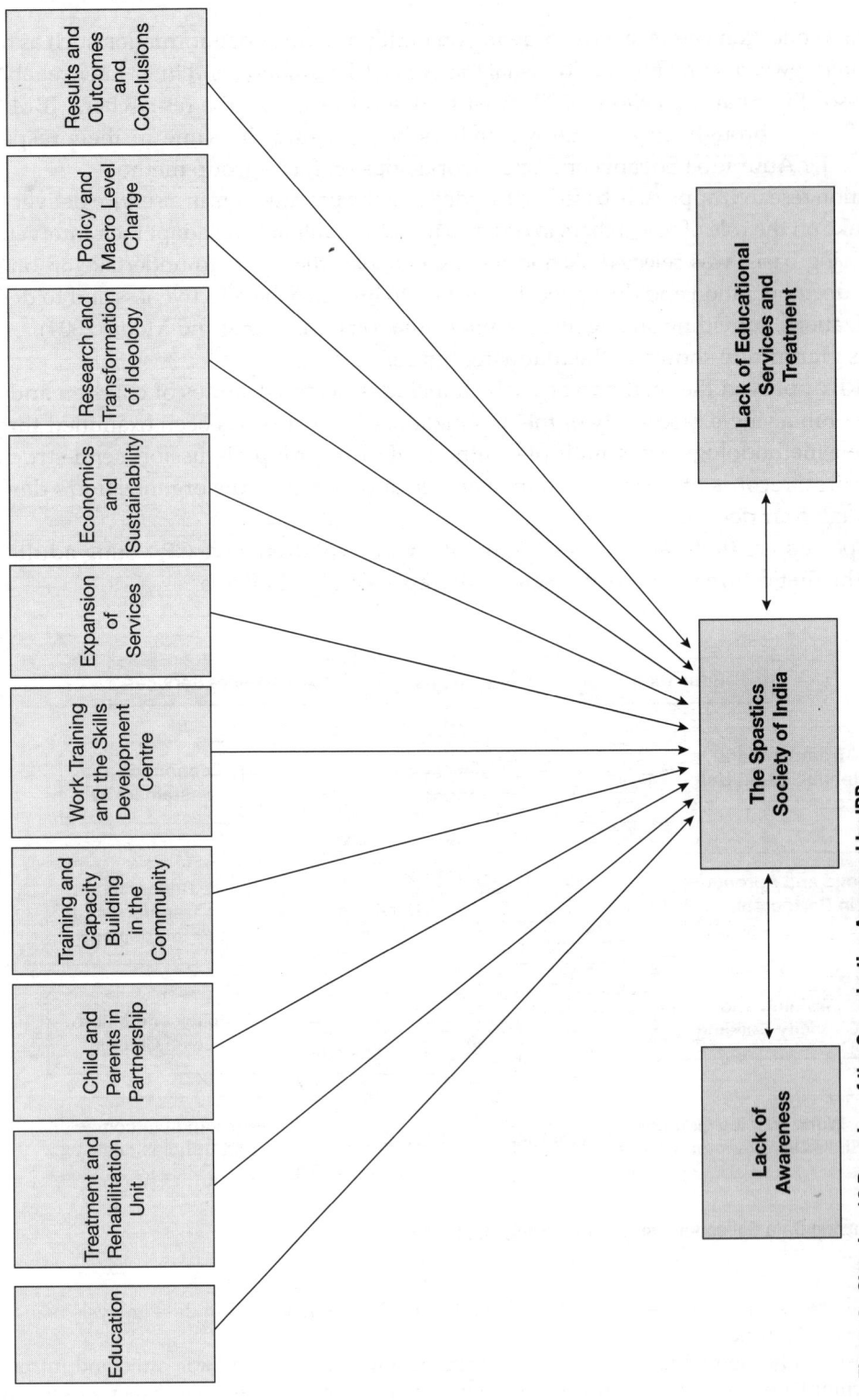

Figure 2. Showing 10 Domains of the Organization Approved by IRB

Source: Author.

3

Contextual Analyses: Cerebral Palsy

Moving firstly to a literature review, this chapter looks at definition, census and prevalence of cerebral palsy and disability policy in India.

Desk Research

In 1862 in England, CP was first described as 'Little's Disease' after Dr William John Little; later it came to be known as CP. Dr Little's hypothesis was that orthopaedic deformity (and other neurological consequences) were the result of neonatal brain injury. Neurology has always played an enormously important role, especially in the early years.

CP is caused by a brain lesion which is non-progressive and leads to impairment of functions in various areas. It presents a series of problems far more complicated than those typical of most other types of physical disabilities. According to Perlstein (1949),

Cerebral Palsy is a condition characterized by paralysis, weakness, incoordination or any other aberration of motor function due to pathology of the motor aberration of motor control centres of the brain.

Dekhoff (1957) talks of CP as a

condition which interferes with the control of the motor system arising as a result of lesions arising from birth trauma.

According to him, CP encompasses a broader brain damage syndrome comprising of neuromotor dysfunction, psychological dysfunction, convulsions and behaviour disorders of an organic type. Closely related to this definition is that of Swarts (1951) and his associates who believe that CP should be defined as an

aggregate of handicaps: emotional, neuro-muscular, special sensory and peripheral sensory caused by damaged or undeveloped or absent brain structures.

While its main characteristic is a disorder of movement and posture, there are a variety of associated problems, making a CP child multiply handicapped. Classification of the type of CP can be done by the neurologist or paediatrician based upon the characteristics manifested of the disordered movement:

There are three major types of CP:

- Ataxic in which voluntary muscle movements are not well coordinated.
- Athetosis which is marked by involuntary, slow, writhing movements.
- Spastic: the most common type of cerebral palsy; reflexes are exaggerated and muscle movement is stiff.

The degree of severity varies and can be mild, moderate or severe. According to William Cruickshank:

- Mild—would mean impairment of only fine precision of movement.
- Moderate—gross and fine movements and speech clarity is impaired, but performance of usual activities of living is functional.
- Severe—an inability to perform adequately usual activities of daily living such as walking, using speech and communication. The associated dysfunctions of CP can be as follows:
  - ♦ Sensory—vision, hearing proprioceptive
  - ♦ Convulsion—type, degree
  - ♦ Intellectual—type, degree
  - ♦ Perceptual—visual, auditory
  - ♦ Behavioural—hyperkinetic, neurotic, anxiety, withdrawal, psychosomatic, emotionally labile and vulnerable.
  - ♦ Learning—specific learning disorders

CP, therefore, presents a multiple disorder as a result of brain damage, causing abnormal pattern of movements, imbalance and incoordination. It presents a diversity of forms and many degrees of impairment. There may be associated intellectual retardation and sensory defects as well as speech and communication difficulties. It is not a disease but a condition. CP is non-fatal, non-curable, but most frequently amenable to therapy and training.

What emerges from a literature review in the international sphere is that CP is the most common motor disability in childhood. Population-based studies from around the world report prevalence estimates of CP ranging from 1.5 to more than 4 per 1,000 live births or children of a defined age range.

Grace Woods says, 'The movement handicaps divide themselves fairly distinctly into different types with varying etiology, movement defect and different degrees of additional handicaps.' Due to this, physically, CP presents a series of disorders far more complicated than those typical of most other types of physical disabilities. Each and every cerebrally palsied individual differs and unless the CP person is considered in all his or her totality, the rehabilitation programme cannot be an effective one.

Unfortunately, the physical, occupational and speech therapies are specializations with rigid boundaries, known only to the experts concerned. Discussions and conversation with parents are virtually non-existent. Often an aura of professionalization prevails and it is not kept in mind that *a humane approach is needed* for a long-term chronic disorder. *The parent is not told what activity was being carried out and why.* The child was more of a 'diagnosis' than anything else, to be discussed among colleagues. A leading doctor treating CP in India said, 'Parents are patients and you cannot share their file with them' (reported a parent from Kolkata when she asked for her child's file).

Regarding intellectual disability, however, it is interesting that CP was until the 1930s commonly thought to be associated with mental defect; it was believed that brain damage was necessarily widespread and that the intellect as well as the motor control areas of the brain were impaired. *We now know that these assumptions were incorrect.* Since treatment and education were largely unknown until the 1940s, the earlier assumptions about the low mental levels of children and adults with CP were based on observations of largely untreated and uneducated cases. Today we know that *if a severely handicapped child is left untreated, he or she will deteriorate and remain physically and intellectually underdeveloped.*

Census and Prevalence

In the subcontinent, no proper statistics regarding the prevalence and incidence of disability exists. A proper census has not been conducted by the National Census Board. Different figures have been quoted by different people. UN specialists have given some projections to the effect that 10 per cent to 15 per cent of the population of India constitutes the number of disabled people in the country. The highest numbers of disabled people are the blind, the deaf and the mentally retarded. It has been estimated that about 8–13 million people are physically handicapped. A very conservative estimate shows that there are one million spastics in India.

The first comprehensive survey on physical disability was carried out in the National Sample Survey Organisation's (NSSO) 36th round (July–December, 1981) and its follow-up survey in NSSO's 47th round (July–December, 1991). Beginning with the 36th round, the concepts, definitions and survey procedures for capturing the physical disability were retained unchanged in all the surveys on disability including the 58th round. The NSSO's 58th round (July–December, 2002) survey reported that 1.8 per cent of the population (18.5 million) had a disability. While 18–22 million people with disabilities is a large number, *this is still arguably a gross underestimation,* especially *when one considers World Health Organization (WHO) estimates of a global prevalence rate of 10 per cent* (Singal 2009).

NSSO, in its endeavour to provide information on the magnitude and other characteristics of disabled persons, conducted the third survey of disabled persons in the country during July–December, 2002. Among the physical disabilities covered during the survey and the results presented in the report were visual, hearing, speech and locomotor disabilities. Children and people with cerebral palsy were not counted (Ray 2003).

The 2001 Census ignored the disabled on grounds of inability and claimed that such a survey was beyond the scope and capacity of its operations. Frequently asked questions and statements made were: 'We don't even know the number of disabled in this country', 'we haven't had a proper survey and our entire census figures are completely insensitive as far as the disabled are concerned', 'what do you mean by disabled?' Statements such as 'being considered a non-person', 'did not come into the purview of the masses', 'did not figure at all' reinforced the invisibility factor. The call for inclusion of disability in the 2001 Census became SSI's primary policy strategy and the first major effort in policy reform.

Subsequent disability statistics were either based on sample surveys or on micro research studies carried out mainly by NGOs. Even after the passing of an equal rights and anti-discrimination law—the Persons with Disabilities Act—the government continued to exclude disability as a category in the census.

As of Census 2011, information on eight types of disability was collected, designed to cover most of the disabilities listed in the 'Persons with Disabilities Act, 1995' and 'The National Trust Act, 1999'. For the first time, a *new category of 'Multiple Disability' was introduced in Census 2011*. The question was designed to record as many as three types of disabilities from which the individual was reported to be suffering.

However, the latest census figures on disabilities have shown only a marginal increase in the number of disabled people in the country, with the figure rising from 21.9 million in 2001 to 26.8 million, of the country's current 1.2 billion population, in 10 years. In percentage terms, it has risen from 2.13 per cent to 2.21 per cent, as per the 2011 Census figures released by the Registrar General of India (2013).

The Registrar General of India (2001) agrees that the Indian data on disability is unreliable, due to a dearth of well-trained field investigators and issues of social stigma. Under-reporting due to stigma and a range of other socio-cultural variables has also been noted by Erb and Harriss-White (2002); Kuruvilla and Joseph (1999); and the World Bank (2007).

Current survey methods are unable to minimise and/or account for these factors. They are not only unsuccessful in providing a reliable picture of prevalence of rates of disability, but there is also a greater likelihood of the identification and reporting of some easily identifiable impairments while others remain hidden.

According to a World Bank report (2009), in countries which ask a simple yes/no question, disability statistics range from 0.5 per cent of the total population (Nigeria) to 3.8 per cent (Ethiopia). Lack of awareness on the part of respondents also results in low reporting. In the absence of any reliable data, it is impossible to estimate what would be the cost of making adequate provision for the handicapped in India.

According to experts and researchers the world over, asking the right question has proven the key to getting accurate disability figures.

Disability Policy in India—The National Scene
(Policy Research: 'Invisible Children: A Study of Policy Exclusion')

A policy is not made in vacuum. Policy reflects a wider, broader socio-economic, socio-cultural, historical, political and ideological framework in which it gets embedded. It involves the whole educational system as well as professionals working within the system, rather than simply the needs of individual children (Barton and Tomlinson 1984; 65–80). With this in mind, a particular policy of the Government of India called the Integrated Child Development Scheme (ICDS) was examined through a doctoral programme from 1993 to 1999, beginning at the London School of Economics and ending at the Institute of Education, University of London (Alur 2000). It is reported that although the ICDS targets disadvantaged sections of society, children with disabilities are not included within that group. Although meant to be for 'all' children from the same disadvantaged impoverished areas as the normal child, on the ground level, a child with disability is not eligible, even for the basic nutrition scheme. The result is a massive exclusion, leaving 4 to 5 million disabled children, in the age group of 0–5 at a critical stage of development, out of existing services (Alur 1998). A Government of India source reveals that only 10 per cent of people with disabilities are being covered (MHRD 1989). On a larger level, according to the 2007 World Bank study, nearly 60 million families are affected.

In the wider context, it was investigated how this had happened and what were the historical, socio-cultural and political underpinnings to explain why disabled children have not been included in mainstream services.

Historically, the issue of education of children with disability was addressed by John Sargent, British education commissioner in 1944, who recommended that provisions for the handicapped should be administered by the education department. The Kothari Commission, in the 1964 Plan of Action, also recommended including children with disabilities into ordinary schools (Gupta 1984; Jangira 1995).

However, the Government of India made it a policy to develop services through voluntary agencies (Planning Commission 1961: 598). In 1966, the education of disabled children became a part of the ministry of social welfare (now called the ministry of social justice). This move resulted in millions of children out of the safety net of education (Taylor and Taylor 1970; Miles 1994). Contradictions and ambiguities in administration blur the roles of different ministries as do the government's statements on the subject, not helping in legitimizing services as a matter of state provisions, entitlements and rights.

As a result, only 10 per cent of people with disabilities were being provided coverage (MHRD 1989). Historically, what becomes clear is that although the government's statement of intent about the need to integrate children with disability into the existing system of education exists, the practice to follow such intent is at best patchy. A subsequent doctoral study found that there was a lack of a cohesive inclusive policy in the country (Alur 2003).

The findings showed that there were many factors that had caused this marginalization to take place from the policy framework. The outcome of the findings and the common linkages that emerged is illustrated in Figure 3.

Dichotomy Between Policy and Practice

On a broader level, when the disabled group was being transferred from the ministry of education (now human resources development) to that of welfare, during the policy formulation stages, the issue of education lost focus. The special needs of disabled children were not considered. The objectives of the ministry of welfare became centred on 'rehabilitate' rather than 'educate'. The ministry was meant to act 'as a nodal agency in coordinating services for the disabled'. A lack of specifying the target of educating disabled children resulted in the absence of setting up the mechanism for implementation.

Today, in India, a majority of the services for the disabled child is delivered through the voluntary sector. This has become official state social policy. The continuance of state supported special schools brings into sharp focus the contradictory government approaches in maintaining special schools, as well as in attempting to integrate the disabled child into the regular school system in a piecemeal fashion. Work for the handicapped is still considered

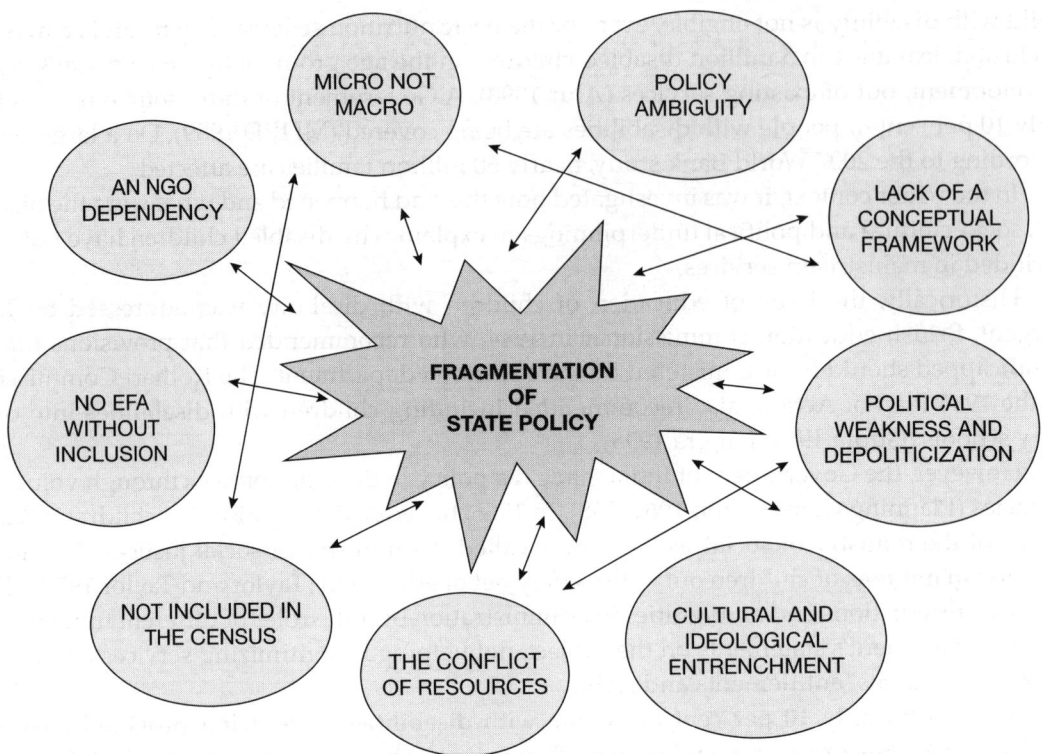

Figure 3. Distortion of Policy, Resulting in the Non-inclusion of Disabled Children Due to Wider Ideological, Political and Structural Fragmentation.

Source: Alur, M. 2002. 'Status of Disabled People in India—Policy and Inclusion'. *Exceptionality Education Canada*, 12(2–3): 137–168.

'good' and humanitarian acts of charity (Tomlinson 1982). *Such an approach has resulted in a systems failure and exclusion from programmes.*

Micro Not Macro

Today, the vast majority of people with disability, nearly 98 per cent (GOI 1994), remain outside the ambit of any service from the state.

Non-governmental Organizations

The voluntary sector has no doubt played a very active and vigorous role in introducing new concepts of education and services, but it has been grounded on a micro level, contributing to a mere 2 per cent coverage due to discontinuous funding and inadequate infrastructural support.

Today, because of the state's lack of involvement, the service delivery approach of the NGOs, the negative attitudinal barriers restricting the disabled people from being a part of our lives, 98% of the disabled population of our country remain without any services at all, trapped within a framework of faulty beliefs and isolated … with their needs not recognized.

Depoliticization

The reliance on NGOs makes the work isolated and piecemeal, moving away from the issue of provision, entitlements and rights; from a macro level policy spread to segregation and marginalization from mainstream society. Concentrating only on the technical needs of disabled children and segregating them in special school situations removes the issue from the public arena, absolving the state of responsibility (Barton and Tomlinson 1984; Kirp 1982; Oliver 1988; Vincent et al. 1996).

The disabled have been classified with other vulnerable and weaker sections of the population such as women and children, the scheduled castes and scheduled tribes. These other groups have had powerful political lobbies, while the disabled have been left behind and segregated. The work for the handicapped is still considered to be a humanitarian act of charity. This has not helped the issue to become a matter of rights either. The result is that the issue has been depoliticized, removed from the public domain and the state absolved of its responsibility (Alur 2002).

Cultural Mindset

'Society's attitudes are a greater disability than having a disability itself' is a view point that has been expressed by many writers and quite often articulated by disabled people themselves. Underpinning the exclusion of disabled children are stereotypical cultural and social values dominating the minds of people.

The findings indicate that the national policy concerning disabled children lacks cohesion and does not give clear directives for the implementation of inclusion to take place. *The majority of disabled people and their families are buried deep within traditional institutionalized discrimination, stereotypical thinking and systemic bias.*

As we see also in this review, there is a huge awareness gap regarding the numbers of people affected by CP, no knowledge about them and also where they are and what their needs are.

Today, the RTE, a historic legislation, has been passed and the education of all disabled children has become statutory and a constitutional right. Acts of Parliament have been passed, entrusting the responsibility for providing services for handicapped people to the state. Legislation backed with fiscal support in India has empowered the disabled child and their families to seek legal redress if they find statutory services not complying with the law or discriminating against them.

Today, the question is not whether disabled children should or should not be educated but exactly how should they be educated. It is most critical to work out how to operationalize the RTE.

In the following sections, we undertake the case study of SSI that helped to put disability on the map through a study of 10 domains as explained in the methodology. Although a professional and technical body, the care was translated into action through love, feeling and compassion. The next section examines this *new model of care: of professionalism combined with a large dose of humanism.*

Domain I

Education

Background: The First Special School:
1972–98 — To Fill the Gap Where There Was No School

Moving onto the case study of The Spastics Society of India (SSI), the 10 domains, as detailed in the methodology, will be examined in the following sections.

In 1972, when my husband and I returned to India, I found that during the six years we were away, nothing had changed. There were still no schools for children with cerebral palsy (CP). It was not even included in the government's Ministry of Welfare's (the sole Ministry responsible for children with disabilities in India) classification, on the basis of which funds are allocated to various services throughout the country. It was then that that I resolved to provide for India's children with CP the same levels of care and stimuli Malini had received in England but within the Indian context and within a framework of love and care. I called it professionalism with care. Again, I was fortunate to have good contacts. So the organization started out, as things usually do in India, at the top. My entire family and many friends came forward to help me in spreading the service.

A friend arranged a meeting with Indira Gandhi, the prime minister of India at the time. During that meeting, I showed her a few slides about my daughter. She asked me her name and her age. She got very interested in what had happened to Malini and she wanted to know what CP was. Her reaction was very humane and she asked what Malini was doing now that we were back from England. I told her that she could read, she knew her numbers and she had done well in school in England, but it was shocking to know that there was no school for her to attend in India. As one mother to another, she reached out and told me that if there was anything I thought she could do, I should let her know. I told her that I would be in touch and that for now I only needed her blessings (something my aunt, Lotika Sarkar, had briefed me to say!). This was to be the first of many meetings with Indira Gandhi.

She was very kind and recommended me names of 12 eminent citizens of Mumbai who might help me. Amongst the names were two famous actors and active workers, Sunil Dutt and the late Nargis Dutt. Mrs Dutt became the first patron, and a very active one, of the society. After her death, Sunil Dutt took up the mantle. Both were members of the Rajya Sabha (the Upper House) and served our society to their last days (Alur and Bach 2010).

Nargisji, as we called her, was a remarkable person. She was India's most celebrated, most popular and most glamorous actress. To have on board the first lady of the Indian screen was a tremendous help for the newly born society: it glamourized an area that was always thought of as gloomy and dreary! When I approached Mrs Dutt, she was eager to take up the duties and responsibilities as a patron. She said, 'I always wanted to be a doctor.' Nargisji also said, 'I don't want to be a figurehead, I want to do administration and attend office'. She even selected the board room which she said she would use as her office! Unfortunately it was not to be. She died of cancer and never saw the national centre. With her death, we lost a powerful figure.

On 2nd October, 1972, or Gandhi Jayanti, SSI was born. We started the first special school for the education of children with CP and other physical disabilities. It combined education and treatment under a special school rather than a hospital setting. It was difficult to find an appropriately large place in a crowded city like Bombay. Mrs Indira Gandhi remained true to her word as she intervened and helped by writing to the then chief minister of Maharashtra, Shri Vasantrao Naik, to find an appropriate bungalow in which the first centre could be set up.

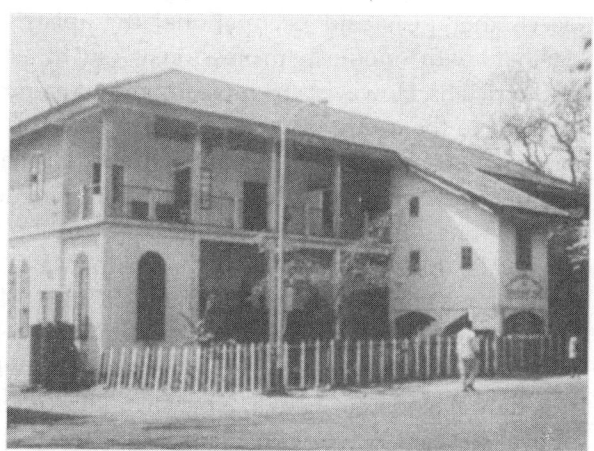

1972, The Spastics Society of India, Colaba

With the help of the Indian Army, we found one in Colaba, Mumbai. It was an idyllic setting within the protected army territory overlooking the Arabian Sea. The organization began with three children but evolved rapidly, increasing the numbers and adding services for their early identification, assessment, education and treatment.

The first professional for the centre was myself, Mithu Chib (nee Bose, now Alur), a qualified special educationist from London. Mrs Nargis Dutt became the first patron of the society and after her death Shri Sunil Dutt took up the mantle. Two professionals who joined the society through the British Council and the Overseas Development Agency (ODA), now called Department For International Development (DFID), were Pamela Stretch, a physiotherapist and Leslie Gardner, principal psychologist of the UK Spastics Society. A third professional who joined us was a speech and language therapist, Asha Kumar. A technical exchange programme was set

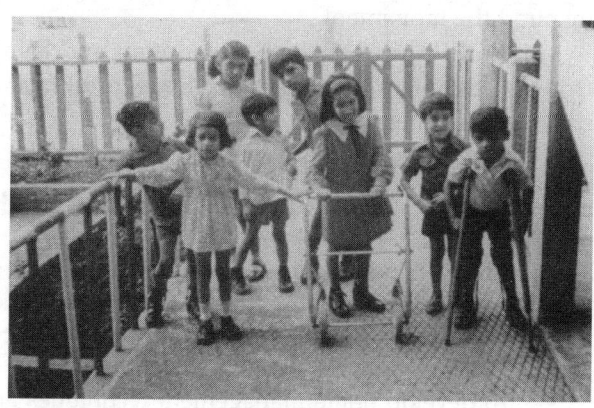

First batch of children

up and a team of professionals from the UK regularly worked with us. Many other professionals and non-professionals came forward to contribute to the fledgling school.

No one specialist has the answer to a condition presented by diffused damage like CP. It is classified according to its type and severity. The degree of disability and its impact in each case may differ from mild to moderate to severe. Therefore the management requires a team of professionals, allowing analysis of each individual client, to create a programme suited to his/her needs (including parents). There was a large team of specialists who came forward to make the organization technically strong.

A team of specialized professionals comprising of special educationists, physiotherapists, speech therapists and occupational therapists, psychologists and social workers worked together with medical professionals such as neurologists, orthopaedic surgeons and paediatricians. However, the most important members of the team were the parents. The doctors affiliated to the centre in the early days were Drs Eddie and Pilloo Bharucha and neurologist and paediatrician Dr Raj Anand. Dr P.K. Mullaferoze was the orthopaedic surgeon, later Dr Praveena Shah, neurologist, Dr Anaita Hegde, paediatric neurologist, Dr Urvashi Shah, and Dr Anuradha Sovani joined the organization to help in any way they could. Mrs Nergesh Palkhivala, Mrs Radhika Roy, Mr Arun Maira, Mr Hadi Kizilbash, Mr Yezdi Malegam, Mr Noshir Khurody, Mr Ranjit Chib, Mr Sathi Alur, Mr Kamal Bakshi, Mrs Junie Bose, Miss Pamela Stretch, Professor Sitanshu Mehta and Dr Manek Bharucha also joined later.

Mr Kamal Bakshi, vice chairperson of SSI, who also served as the Indian ambassador to Iraq, Italy, Austria, Sri Lanka, Norway and Sweden, has been associated with the organization for over 30 years. Advisor on all important matters and virtually a member of the Able Disabled All People Together (ADAPT) family, he has been immensely inspirational and supportive of all colleagues, addressing all national and international events, conferences and issues affecting the society's national presence, as well as playing an integral role in the daily governance of the organization.

Professor Sitanshu Mehta has been a part of SSI almost from the beginning and has given it strong support as a father figure. An academic and father of a disabled person, he has chaired sessions and presented papers at many national and international conferences. His humour and kindness towards his colleagues, above all, has given us the courage to move on and inspired the movement.

Mr Sathi Alur, chartered accountant and legal advisor, helped to develop the institution from a fledgling organization to a huge, multifaceted professional institution, functioning on a national and international levels.

Goals and Objectives of the New Organization

- To ensure that children with multiple disability such as CP are provided education.
- To introduce a new model of treatment which looks after the holistic development of the child.
- To develop an assessment and early intervention procedure for at-risk children.
- To develop interdisciplinary rapport.
- To develop home management techniques and to empower and train parents to carry on effective programmes at home and work with other parents in cooperation.

Process of Change

Assessment and Early Intervention for At-Risk Children

Substantial research has shown how critical the first five years of the child's cognitive, social and emotional development are, and we have found that whatever experiences the child is exposed to in the early years, good or bad, rich or impoverished, will mould its personality for the rest of its life. An enriched environment is essential for the child's healthy growth and this includes both home and school. Parents as well as teachers, who are the supervisors of the child's development, need training and a systematic build-up of knowledge concerning the needs of the growing child. It is now an accepted fact that just as the body needs food as nutrition and nourishment, so does the mind for its own growth and development. Remembering the tortuous clinical examination to which Malini had been subjected in various hospitals in India, I decided that one of the first areas I would focus on would be the assessment of the disability and that the new organization should develop 'care and assessment'.

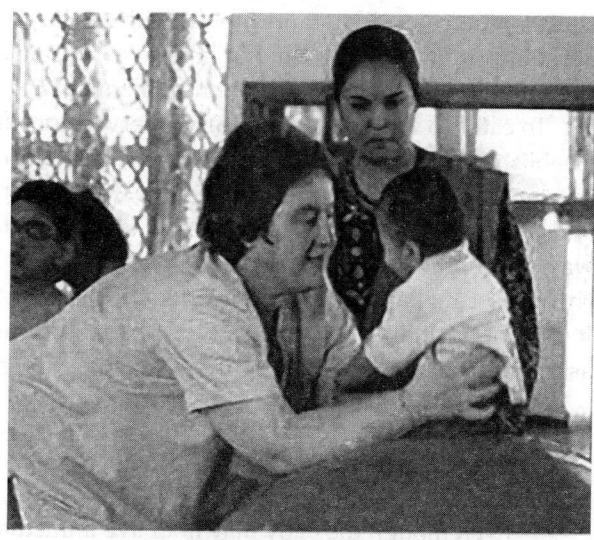

Pam Stretch* with a baby of 6 months

*We were fortunate to have Pamela Stretch who came through the British Government and stayed on for 23 years. She pioneered treatment and management of cerebral palsy in India. A unique personality, she was also one of the pioneers of the organization and helped develop skills all over the country. She loved her parents and the disabled infant and adults. We were very fortunate to have her right from the outset making this an East-West project, to introduce what was termed then as 'professionalism with care'.

Malini's Assessment in India

'Your daughter has cerebral palsy. Brain damage is irreversible. Once the brain is damaged, it's damaged for life. Nothing can be done about it.'
I was 23, my husband, Ranjit was 25. The finality of the statement 'nothing can be done about it' devastated us as young parents of our first child. Then began a long battle, a journey which took us away from this situation of negativity and ignorance to England, where my brother-in-law (Samiran Nundy) and sister (Mita Nundy) lived. (There, Malini received excellent care and blossomed. We, too, as parents, badly needed the healing touch. After 6 years, we returned. The situation was the same! We were asked, 'What is a spastic? Are you talking about plastics?')

– Dr Mithu Alur

The Need for Early Detection: Early Infant Clinics

Infant clinics were set up for high-risk babies. I had also learnt that it is not possible to assess children with multiple disorders such as CP in a single examination. It requires a team of specialists who can understand the difficulties the child and the parents face after the diagnosis. Most importantly, it is a time of immense trauma and crisis for the mother which calls for the full attention of doctors and other members of the team.

To cater to such needs, an early intervention clinic—for babies only a few weeks old—was established. The medical team worked very closely with the parents who after a thorough examination of their baby were taught the correct techniques for carrying, changing napkins and feeding the baby. During the early stages of life, while the baby with CP suffers in its own way, the mother encounters unique problems too. She feels inadequate and 'disabled' because she cannot make her baby happy, feed it properly, change the napkins or hold it as required. It is not a normal experience. Once a distressed mother, after her son was diagnosed with CP, asked the doctor, 'Do I feed him?' (Of course, she meant breastfeed!)

The following strategies were introduced:

- Early in infancy, the baby was helped to feel her body, play with her feet and legs, put her fingers in her mouth, move the hands and observe them, and move her feet and legs.
- Even though the baby may not have immediately been able to clasp, hold and feel toys, he/she was provided with toys of various textures, colours and shapes. This helped in increasing the eye-hand coordination, communication, intellectual development and correlating speech.
- Therapists 'talked' to the babies, thus indirectly encouraging and teaching parents to do the same. In our experience, we found that over a period of time the feelings of chronic sorrow, depression, grief, anger, loss and guilt experienced by the parents of an infant unable to reach his or her milestones on time were reduced.
- Following the despairing revelation about her baby, the mother was taught how to love and care for her new-born with a lot of cuddling. With this kind of nurturing, the baby soon started responding and thriving.
- The parents were taught that the disabled child had the same needs as a normal child and must be treated as normally as possible. (Of course, the baby must be breastfed!)

Outcome

- The best judge is a parent! Parents began to know that their child was responding and learning to appreciate and adjust to the situation around him or her. Once the mother developed the bond with the physical contact, she felt much happier and rarely considered her baby 'different' than other so-called 'normal' ones and so the process of acceptance began.
- By bringing in a high-risk infant to an early intervention clinic or infant stimulation clinic, the physio-, occupational and speech therapists were able to help in different areas such as sensory-motor, early speech development as well as bringing normality in the life of the family (this was pretty much like what baby Malini received at the Hospital for Sick Children at the Cheyne Centre in London during the mid-1960s).

Interdisciplinary Rapport

Being a condition which lasts for life, CP needs a regime which is ideally continuous and longitudinal. Management requires a holistic approach where the child is looked at as a whole person by every professional. Sometimes there are invisible barriers between various disciplines. The aim is to break these walls with regular informal and formal meetings. Contrary to popular traditional methods of therapy, a child is not 'broken into pieces' for different professionals to work on. For example, a physiotherapist looking at the legs and an occupational therapist looking at the hands. *A team approach* was designed to take best care of the child. Each professional's intervention was designed around the goals of the whole team. So a speech therapist looked at *seating requirements* facilitating the child to vocalize better, an occupational therapist *worked on walking* with the goal of reaching a washroom or a classroom, and a physiotherapist worked on improving hand functions so that a child could push his/her own wheelchair (Prabhu 2004). A child's rehabilitation programme included inputs from all concerned disciplines. The team members talked to each other in arriving at a consensus on a common goal. Then each team member worked towards this goal for the treatment. This we called an interdisciplinary team approach.

Venues of treatment were changed and were not always in one designated treatment room. Therapy was provided in classrooms, in the corridors, in the playground and continued at home in a less formal atmosphere than a hospital.

Role of the Parent: Home Management

When we started in 1972, physiotherapy, occupational therapy or speech therapy were specializations known only to those experts. *Discussion and conversation with the parents was non-existent.* The concept of explaining to the parent what was being done and why it was being done was missing. A medical approach to the child's examination existed. I remember when Malini was being examined, the therapist kept ticking off the checklist and continued to read the list aloud. 'She doesn't know how to hold a pencil' and ticked the appropriate box. 'She doesn't know how to put her shoes on' and ticked another box. On and on it would go like this until the list was exhausted and every item checked off. Eventually, Malini would start crying.

Being a parent, I put a strong focus on parents *as an important member of the*

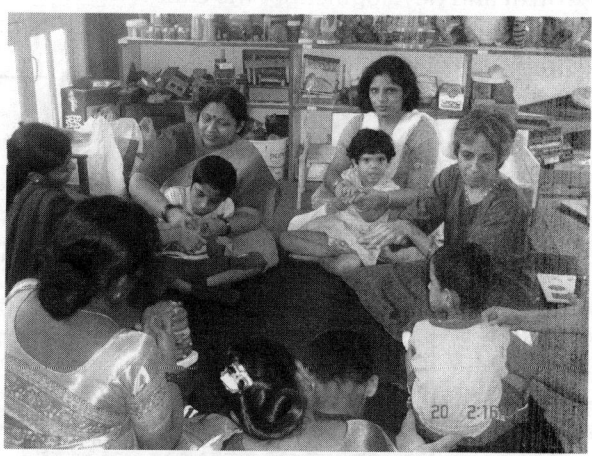

Home Management: Amena Latif* conducting a session

*Amena Latif viewed in the picture has tremendous passion and energy for parents and students. She is on call 24 hours a day and has begun the Home Management and Vocational Section. Amena is the Deputy Head of Education at the Bandra Centre where she focuses on young adults who need vocational training and has been with The Spastics Society/ADAPT for over three decades, having contributed to the formal and non-formal education of children with special needs.

assessment team and spent a great deal of time with them in establishing a rapport. The interdisciplinary team kept in mind that, in the early days, our patient who was an infant was not aware of what had happened to him or her. It was the parents who were caught in a quagmire of trauma. *Their grief, their bewilderment and confusion about what was going to happen to their child, became our primary concern.*

Home Management Became a Critical Programme

Families, especially the parents, had to compensate for this lack by providing necessary inputs through an alternative, modified environment. Working closely with the therapy team, parents learnt to create a sustainable nurturing environment at home.

Parents were counselled regularly by the team of professionals. Besides, following exercise routines, creation of self-help groups as well as other supportive services began to build up. We found that coordinated effort of parents, paediatricians and paramedics helped in the growth and development of the child.

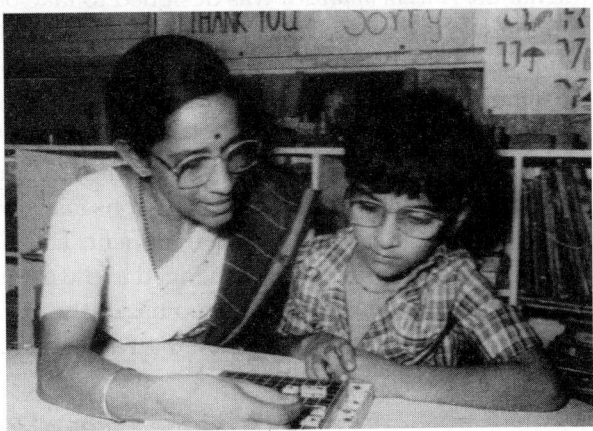

Mrs Maya Muddaya, Principal, doing an individual session

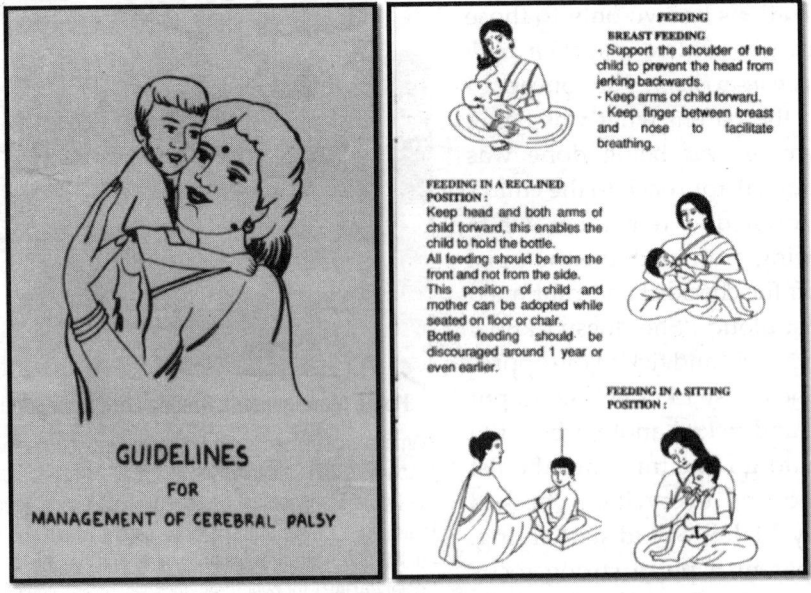

An early publication of The Spastics Society of India

Role of Therapists

Therapists were careful and tactful while talking to parents as there was a high risk of alienating them. At the early stage, the physiotherapist or occupational therapist gave practical advice to the parents about

- How to carry their child
- How to feed their child
- Importance of proper seating and posture
- Self-help skills
- How to build on language and communication

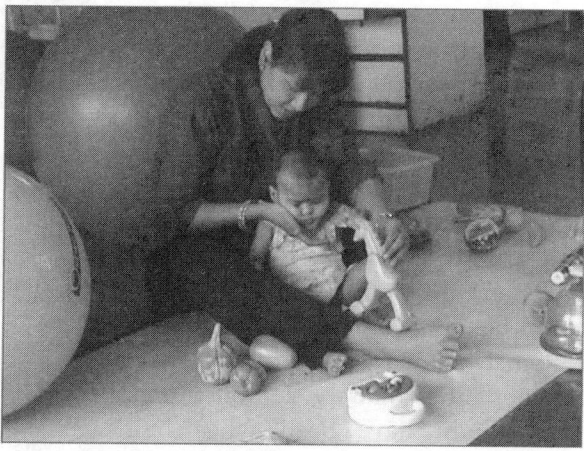

Dr Anita Prabhu with an infant of 8 months

Dr Anita Prabhu was one of the professionals who took over when Pam left. Very fond of her student she gave generously to her students showed she had great leadership and management qualities; she pioneered with Malini Chib, the ARG Rights Group, becoming the first Co-Chair.

Research studies on CP have also shown that because of the difficulties in childhood, a baby's *learning opportunities are limited*. For example, due to gross motor problems, movements like creeping, crawling and rolling are restricted, so exploring the environment like a normal child does not happen. Lack of fine motor coordination, such as restricted grasping and poor holding capacity, limit the learning experiences through touch. Due to 'rigidity' of muscles, the baby cannot really 'feel' his own body. Thus, an infant with CP receives only very limited sensory stimuli. If there are associated problems of hearing and sight, the situation is, naturally, even more complicated.

Role of Teachers

Classroom Modification: Diagnosis in the Classroom

It was a general belief that physical damage meant mental damage as well. A person with a distorted body could not really

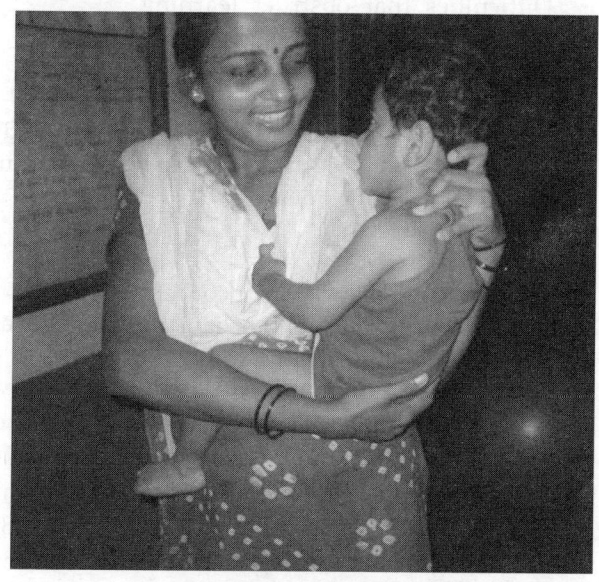

A parent carrying a child correctly

be thinking and must be a vegetable or something! This of course we know was erroneous thinking and not at all true. There was substantial evidence which had accumulated to indicate that children with CP suffer from damage to that area of the brain which controls movement or the motor area. However, 50 per cent of children with CP are normal in intelligence. The areas that control our thought processes are often intact. Their powers of retention, observation, memory and logical reasoning function normally and if taught the three R's, they could benefit substantially from education. This then was one of the main functionalities that we demonstrated. They might have been wheelchair bound, grossly deformed, physically unable to verbalise their thoughts, but their minds were functioning. They remained what has been graphically defined as 'intelligent minds caught in disobedient bodies'.

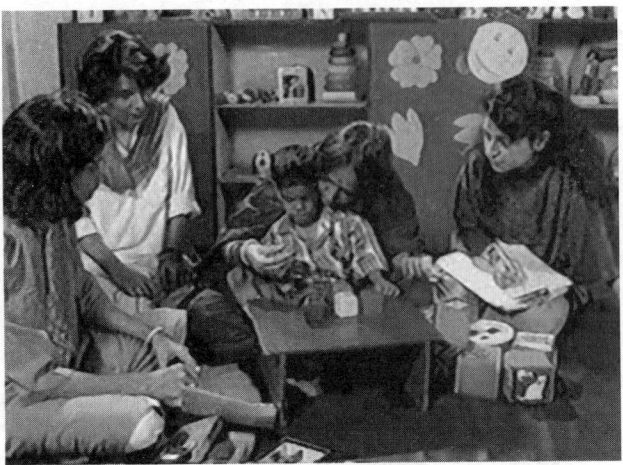

Dr Mithu Alur assessing Toshan Chatterjee while Varsha Hooja*, Zomerote Irani and Sherezade Khambata learn how to make it enjoyable

*Varsha joined the organization when she was only 22 and has been with the organization for 33 years! An educationist she was initially a teacher of the deaf, she qualified to become a special educationist for cerebral palsy earlier. Principal of the Centre she is now Chief Executive of the organization, and a Trustee in the Governing Body.

Difficulties that obstruct learning in the classroom would be:

1   Problem of locomotion or mobility;
2.   Poor hand function and inability to write holding a pen or pencil;
3.   Possibly poor speech or the lack of speech, causing a breakdown in communication;
4.   Perceptual difficulties;
5.   Sensory defects;
6.   Hyperactivity;
7.   Limited attention span or concentration;
8.   Emotional liability and behaviour disturbances.

It cannot be too strongly emphasized that the greatest danger lies in misdiagnosis, mislabelling and in setting inappropriate academic goals, resulting in erroneous instructions and great wastage of the child's time, which he or she can ill afford. In fact, the damage being diffused rather than specific, the child faces multiple combinations of problems, indicating multiple handicaps which it is critical to address (Alur 1978).

Therefore, accurate diagnosis and careful analysis of a child's profile became the first essential tool in planning intervention. Careful diagnosis also predicted the rate at which new learning would occur, consistent with the child's capabilities and the level of performance a child was expected to maintain. This ultimately ensured progress and the possibility of alleviating learning disabilities.

Individualized Educational Programmes (IEPs)

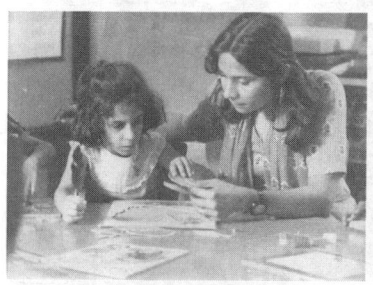 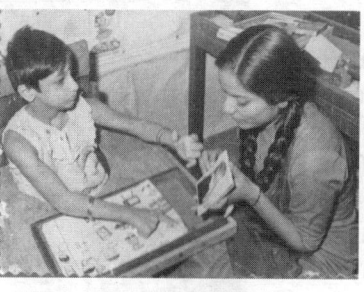 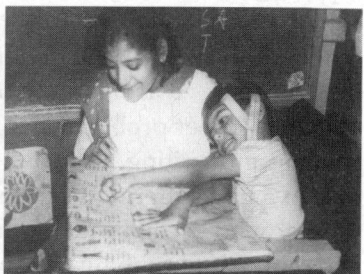

| Yasmin Asur takes an individual session in reading | Picture matching | Learning to use the communication board |

Every plan that was created had to be child-specific and highly individualized. This was called an Individualized Education Programme (IEP). Activities were differentiated as per the needs of each child.

To increase mobility, walking aids like a rollator or crutches were given to each child. Children were also made to move around in crawlers or chairs fitted with castors to encourage mobility. The fact that they could not move was not important, but the fact that they wanted to and must move, enjoy and feel the thrill of locomotion despite their disability was the crucial factor.

Postural management in the classroom needed to be implemented by providing appropriate seating aids. The physiotherapist provided grab handles for extending the hand that was most affected; a backrest to give proper support and a footrest to prevent the foot from dropping or pointing in the typical spastic position.

Other physical alterations to the building such as ramps, lifts, easily manoeuvrable doors, suitably adjusted toilet seats and special desks and chairs were necessary.

A vast range of manipulatory skills were introduced through early play activities, involving bilateral coordination for working on the hands. Aids developing good visuo-motor skills as well as developing the thumb/index finger or the pincer grip were part of the programme.

To remediate problems such as perceptual deficits and hyperactivity, proper remedial programmes based on gross motor coordination were planned.

One of the most important considerations was that the child's sensory impressions were impoverished due to gross limitations in the quantity and quality of experiences. In a normal classroom situation, accurate visuo-spatial and visual perceptual abilities enabled a child to learn to read and write correctly and to undertake any academic work that required recognition, recall and reproduction. For example, map work in geography, spelling, identifying words in dictionaries and so on. On the other hand, the child with visual perceptual disorders would have difficulty in identifying, discriminating and copying simple shapes and patterns. He or she would have a poor concept of their own body, would suffer from

confusion about left and right, concepts of directionality would be inadequate and later on this lack of discrimination would lead to difficulty
in identifying 'b' from 'd', 'p' from 'q'
and many other problems in drawing,
spelling and writing. There is a famous
case of a boy suffering from these disorders, who recognized his mistakes
and said, 'Mummy, why can't my hand
do what my eye can see?'

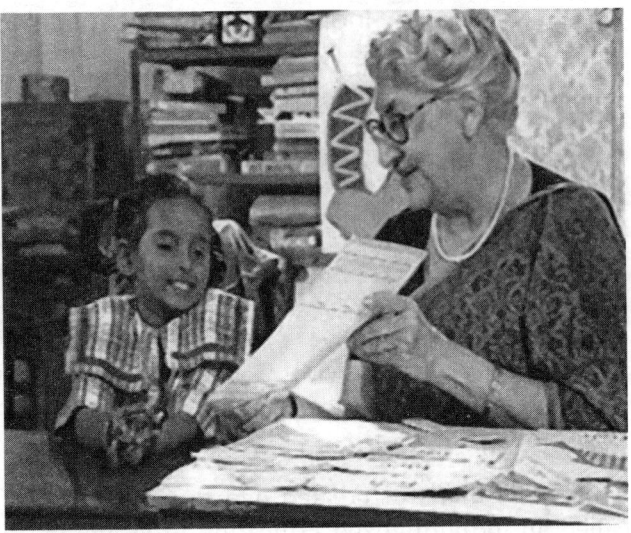

Uma Bannerjee using flash cards to teach Meena English

In the classroom, therefore, this
would impede educational progress.
Corrective action had to be introduced.

Many of the children came to us
from poor, socially-deprived homes.
They had received little or no stimulation and this, together with their
disability, further handicapped them. We began to design a curriculum which included
early stimulation from one to two and a half years, a rich primary experience combined with
corrective exercises.

These corrective training exercises in the classroom were based on research already conducted by well-known remediators. To name a few of the experts, the training provided by
Brereton of the Mosman Centre in New South Wales, Frostig at the the Marianne Frostig Center
of Educational Therapy and Kephart, Cruickshank and Tansley to concentrate on details, discrimination and movement in space, which were incorporated into the curriculum. Klaus
Wedell and his principles of good pedagogic training and task analyses were also part of the
training of the teachers. Simultaneously, this training was supplemented by good teaching. In
addition to this, the child also tended to suffer from emotional difficulties. Often he was aware
of his puzzling inability to match the performance of his peer group and of the disappointment
of his teachers and parents and he tended to become frustrated and confused.

The syllabus was the same that a regular school adopted. By the age of 5–6 years, the
children were ready for a formal, academic syllabus. Eminent educationists, such as Uma
Bannerjee, principal, infant section, Cathedral School, brought in state-of-the-art preschool and
primary school curriculum, teaching methods and best practices from regular school; Spenta
Madan, head of Fort Convent, senior section, did the same for the secondary stream.

To encourage success in other areas, extracurricular activities such as music, painting, art
and crafts, drama, sports, yoga and PT were introduced for the first time. Focus was placed on
those areas, where the child could enjoy and excel, building up on their strengths rather than
falling for their weaknesses. Exhibitions, annual concerts, participatory sports with regular
schools helped in the process of demystifying disability, thereby contributing to a growth in
the child's self-esteem and confidence. A week of activities were created showcasing children's

talents in painting, art and crafts sports and drama where they showed their prowess in singing and dancing. The week was called the `I CAN' week and was developed to spread awareness about their abilities.

We also found that the child sometimes lacked in confidence, could not work on his own, was over-reliant in a one-to-one situation, had poor attention span, low tolerance for frustration, low self-esteem when confronted by a task and other psychological problems which led to disorganization and confusion. Art, drama, dance, sports and music gave the opportunity to the students to express themselves, depending on their aptitudes, differently.

Some Lessons Learnt

Non-verbal Communication Related to Academic Feedback

As mentioned earlier, often the main tools of communication (i.e., speech and writing) affecting educational progress, are damaged in some cases of CP. In such situations, non-verbal communication with a variety of aids had to be substituted. Fortunately, over the years, a wide range of mechanical and electronic aids have been developed so that a child can keep up with the studies and the syllabus.

Inexpensive technologies to break barriers in the classroom were:

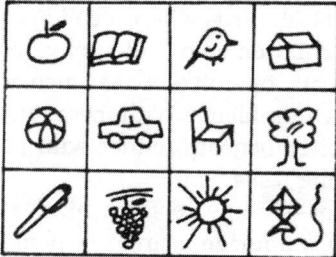

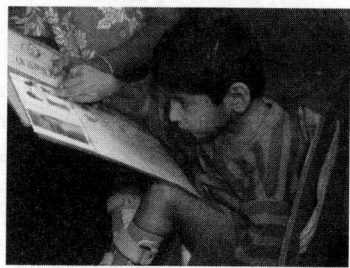

Ojas being trained to use the Communication Board

- Communication boards and picture boards— Individual, tailor-made communication and picture boards for simple recognition of common objects and discrimination exercises in the early years.

- Flash cards or magnetised numbers, letters and words—The simplest and cheapest aids used were letters, word boards and flash cards which we used extensively for reading, numbers, construction of sentences and grammar, where a child simply touched, pointed or looked at the right answer to a question.

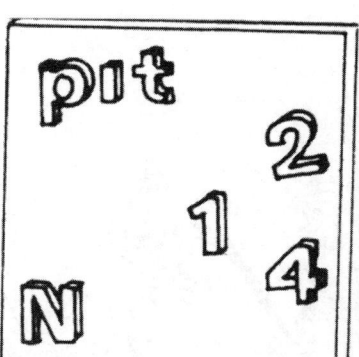

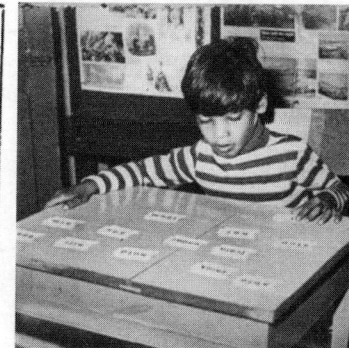

Learning to communicate through flash cards—Imtiaz later went onto becoming a Librarian

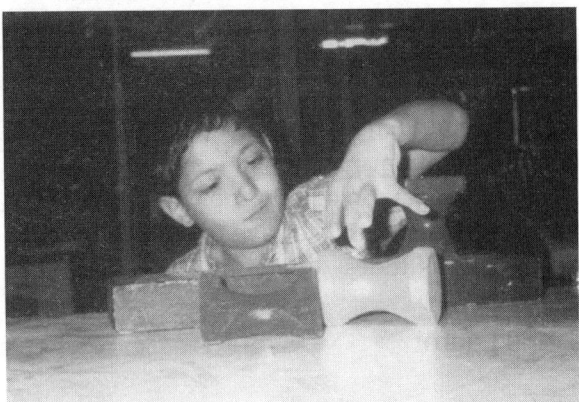 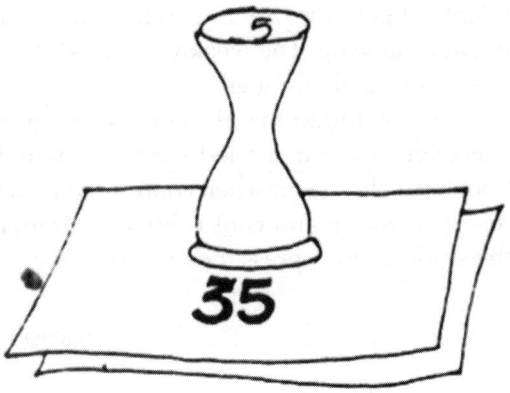

Rubber stamp

- Rubber stamps—A very cost-effective aid used for solving arithmetical problems was the rubber stamp which could be used easily by a student with severe speech problems and inability to write.
- Bliss charts—These charts used a system of symbols for words and all the different parts of speech. Children communicating through Bliss symbols had boards catering to their own needs and level of ability. Flash cards where a child gestured or pointed to the answer were used for severely affected children who could not verbalize their thoughts.
- Rotary pointer—Electronically operated boards such as the rotary pointer were made available to children with speech problems. With these, the child merely touched a microswitch or panel (with a microswitch beneath) either with his foot, hand or elbow to do simple matching and discriminating tasks.
- Meldreth A4 Touch Tutor—A low-cost teaching aid, designed by Malcolm Jones at Meldreth Manor School, Cambridge, using inexpensive home-made programmes. It was for perceptual or visuo-spatial discrimination in matching pictures, numbers, shapes and alphabets to test comprehension for children with problems of communication. The aid was gifted to us.

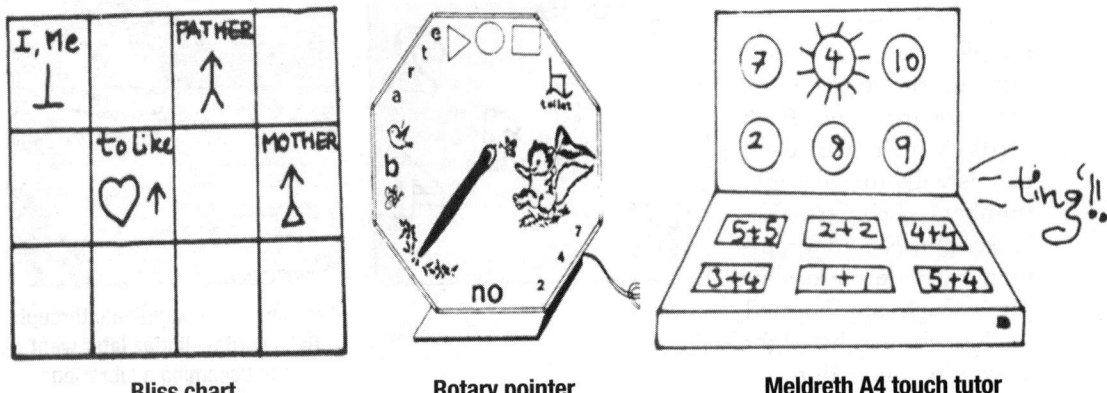

Bliss chart   **Rotary pointer**   **Meldreth A4 touch tutor**

- Language master—This was really a tape recorder with a quick feedback used for higher level students with problems of speech and comprehension.
- Typewriters—After the age of seven or eight, we would move children onto more adult forms of communication aids such as typewriters. There were various kinds—manual and electronic—which could be fitted with key guards, if necessary, to prevent the child's finger slipping from one key to another.
- Expanded keyboard—This was the largest keyboard which could be attached to any electronic typewriter. We used it for a very severe athetoid student who went on to attend college.
- Canon communicator—This was the smallest 'typewriter' in the world and was produced by the Japanese. It was portable and could be fitted onto a wrist or a wheelchair. It provided print outs on thermo-sensitive paper.[1]

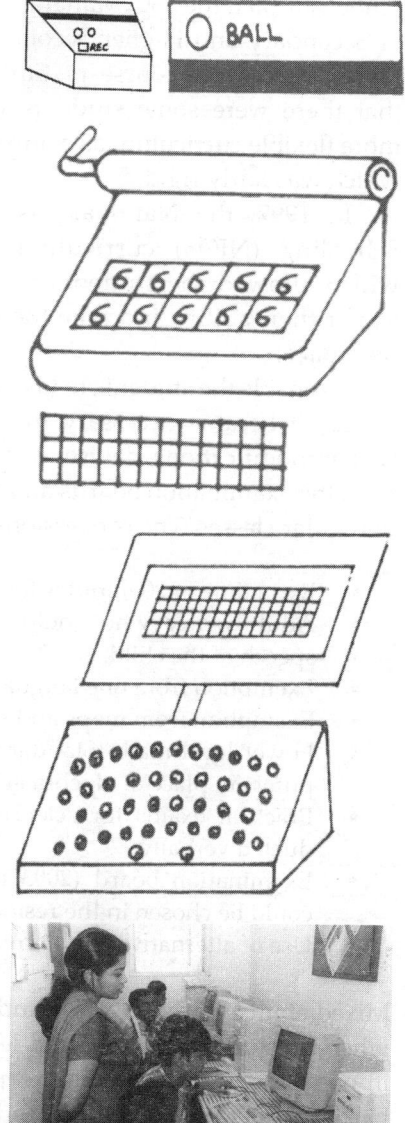

With the use of the hand-held Canon communicators, which produced two-way visual 'speech' on a small panel and also had speech synthesizers, a person with a severe speech disorder could efficiently carry on conversations and, more than that, hold a regular job.

Vipasha, who was very severely disabled with serious speech/communication problems, used a Canon to communicate her needs. She used it in the lecture hall, library or canteen, whenever someone could not understand her (see photo on the next page). Vipasha passed her Secondary School Certificate (SSC) with 74.14 per cent and was later one of the few who actually earned a PhD on Michel Foucault and Jacques Derrida.

The most commonly used aid in the school was of course the electric typewriter. A special guard was usually provided for this.

Computer – a form of communication

Curriculum Modification and Public Examination

It was observed that to overcome barriers to learning, some modifications in the curriculum were needed. The

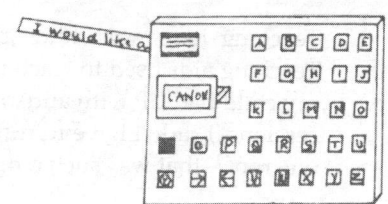

---

[1] Many of these aids were introduced by Leslie Gardner, principal psychologist, of the UK Spastics Society, who set up the Psychology Department for SSI.

school adopted the SSC, Maharashtra State Board of Secondary and Higher Secondary Education, Pune. During the course of time it was noted that there were some students who needed a more flexible curriculum as compared to the SSC which was fairly rigid.

In 1997, the National Institute of Open Schooling (NIOS) curriculum was adopted which allowed the students to select subjects as per their ability and take the exams at their own pace.

To enable the students to take their state level exams, it became necessary to implement curricular modifications, devise specific concessions from the examination boards and apply the same in regular classes. The concessions granted were:

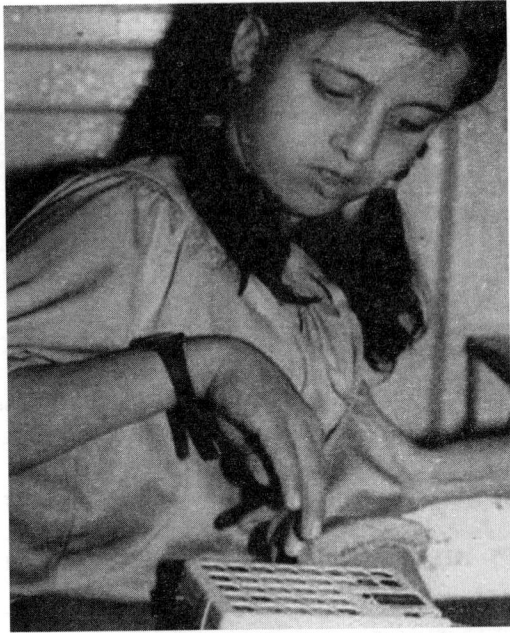

Vipasha exhibiting her skills of communication using a typewriter

- Extra time of 20 minutes for every hour.
- Adult writer who could understand the speech of the child.
- Exemption from one language
- Exemption from maps and diagrams
- Lower level math (Standard VII) and computers in place of algebra and geometry
- Practical exams for science could be conducted verbally.
- Examination board (2003 onwards) centre could be chosen in the residential vicinity
- Use of alternative communication

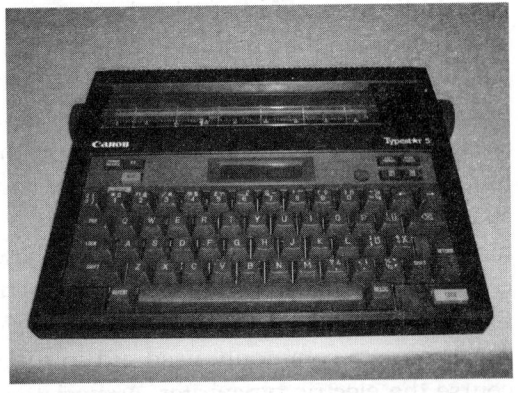

Mixed ability teaching was found to be effective, whereby students with varied levels are taught in one class with each child keeping a different pace. Cooperative learning and collaboration,

Sharmila Bhagtani, parent of Barun Bhagtani (trainee of WSU)

Teaching here was child specific and the lessons taught were well consolidated. Teaching aids used to teach my child were a combination of visual and auditory since my child had CP with autism. He was also given lower level Maths besides other concessions. I didn't have to run from one place to another, all facilities were here under one roof—that was such a relief.

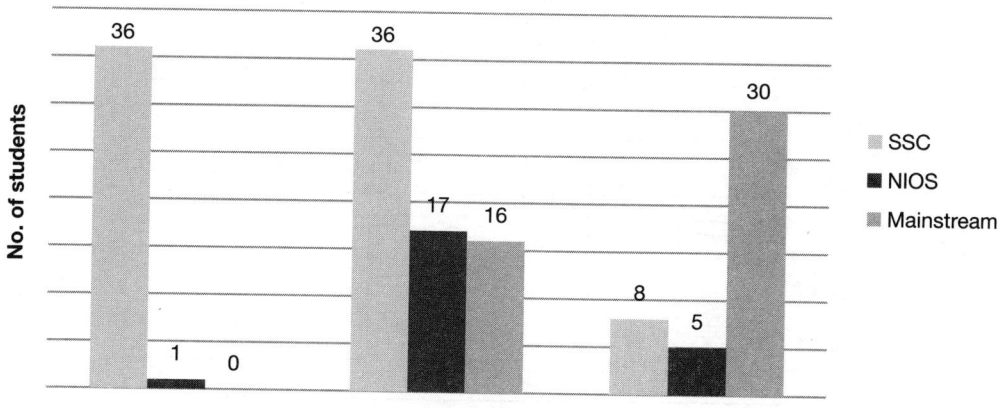

Figure 1.1. The Number of Students Who Passed Public Exams (SSC, National Institute of Open Schooling [NIOS] and Regular Schools)

Source: Research Action Committee for the IRB meeting.

use of effective teaching aids, educational field trips, picnics, celebration of festivals, participation in interschool activities such as debates, sports, musical events, were instrumental in enhancing the social and emotional development of the students.

Since there were no schools for children with CP, formal education for them began from the year 1972, starting from standard 1. It took 10 years to prepare the first batch to take their first, formal state-level examinations in the year 1983.

Figure 1.1 depicts the number of students who passed various public examinations for the period of 1982–2012.

In the first two decades, the focus was on demonstrating that with focused intervention children with neurological problems can pass examinations and excel in schools. With the idea of inclusive education being introduced in the third decade, mainstreaming had begun. Also, children who could not cope with regular SSC curriculum started appearing for the softer option of NIOS. In the fourth decade, there was a clear shift towards mainstreaming.

(The number of students taking public exams peaked during 1998–2002. For the last two decades, however, the organization promoted inclusive education and included students with disabilities in mainstream schools. Thus, from the year 2003 onwards students took their SSC public examinations from mainstream schools and NIOS examinations from SSI.)

Results and Outcome

- With simple modifications in class, we demonstrated that children with disabilities could be educated. Children excelled in academics with the help of concessions granted by the state board of Maharashtra. These concessions were then permitted by most of the examination boards across the country as well as by universities.

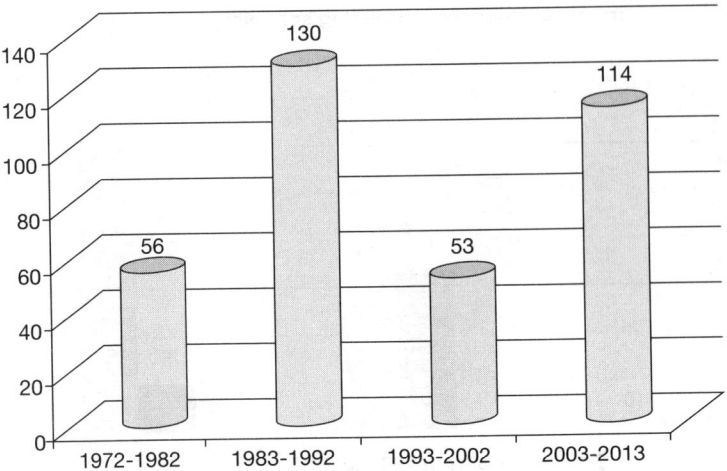

Figure 1.2. Number of Therapists Trained over the Years

Source: Research Action Committee for the IRB meeting.

- Diagnosis as early as one month began with the mother. Holistic programmes, combining education and treatment were demonstrated under one roof. Early infant clinics, where high-risk babies were assessed, helped to create awareness that children with CP must have early detection and continuous management.
- This kind of holistic treatment where doctors, paramedics, special educators, social workers and psychologists worked together with parents took root and began to show results. Regular and continuous treatment trained the child to be independent.
- Figure 1.2 shows the number of therapists trained from 1972 to 2013.
- SSI made a technical contribution, providing a very strong base for children, youth with CP and other physical disabilities.
- A major achievement of SSI was that neurological disability and CP, which had previously not been recognized amongst the government's classifications, was recognized as one of the 11 official classifications accepted by the Government of India's ministry of social justice and empowerment.

Voices of Parents and Students

Shobha Sachdev	Toshan Chatterjee	Nilesh Singit
With Special Education here my daughter Deepa's remedial educational programme included Perceptual training to help her read better which was of utmost importance for her. Here education was a part of the multi-disciplinary	I didn't have any problem in education as the teachers were very cooperative. If I didn't understand any topic they would repeat it for me and clarify all my doubts. This didn't happen in college. In school I was involved	When I joined this school, for me it was like any other school. I came here because the school in my neighborhood didn't take me. I did not know anything about special education or regular education. Once in school, I

approach that worked for my child, something that was not available outside. Furthermore, auditory learning methods wherein all her class notes were tape-recorded for her to memorise the subject matter thus making it specific to suit her specific learning issues. The main advantage of education here was that Deepa was given the flexibility in the curriculum and she could move from SSC to NIOS and learnt at her own pace.

in all co-curricular activities like drama, games, independent living camps. Alternate days I had therapy, this was included in my time table to improve my physical condition. All these activities helped me tremendously once I went out into colleges. I gained a lot of knowledge during the school years.

realized that this school was different as all children here had a disability. School was fun, my teachers were very good. As I grew up and interacted with children of my age group I realized that I had learnt much more than they had in their schools. My teachers had definitely done something better than theirs.

Janmejay Bhati (JJ)

Watching a television programme on special children, JJ's mother realized her son was similar to those on screen. The family from Kota visited Bombay two years later and brought JJ to SSI.

At three and a half, JJ wasn't walking yet. He was put on a home management programme, covering speech, physiotherapy and education and was to visit Bombay every three months.

The parents learnt Vojta-style physiotherapy. Within a month, JJ was standing and walking. The delighted parents agreed to follow SSI's every suggestion.

In 1989, JJ's father got transferred to Bombay. JJ joined the Colaba school. His father would accompany him from Vashi to Colaba by train. With constant support from ADAPT's sensitive staff, JJ completed his 10th and 12th from NIOS, proceeding to do a B.Sc. in IT from Kota.

Today, an independent JJ runs his own telemarketing company.

His mother, empowered by bringing him up, counsels special children's parents, often referring them to SSI.

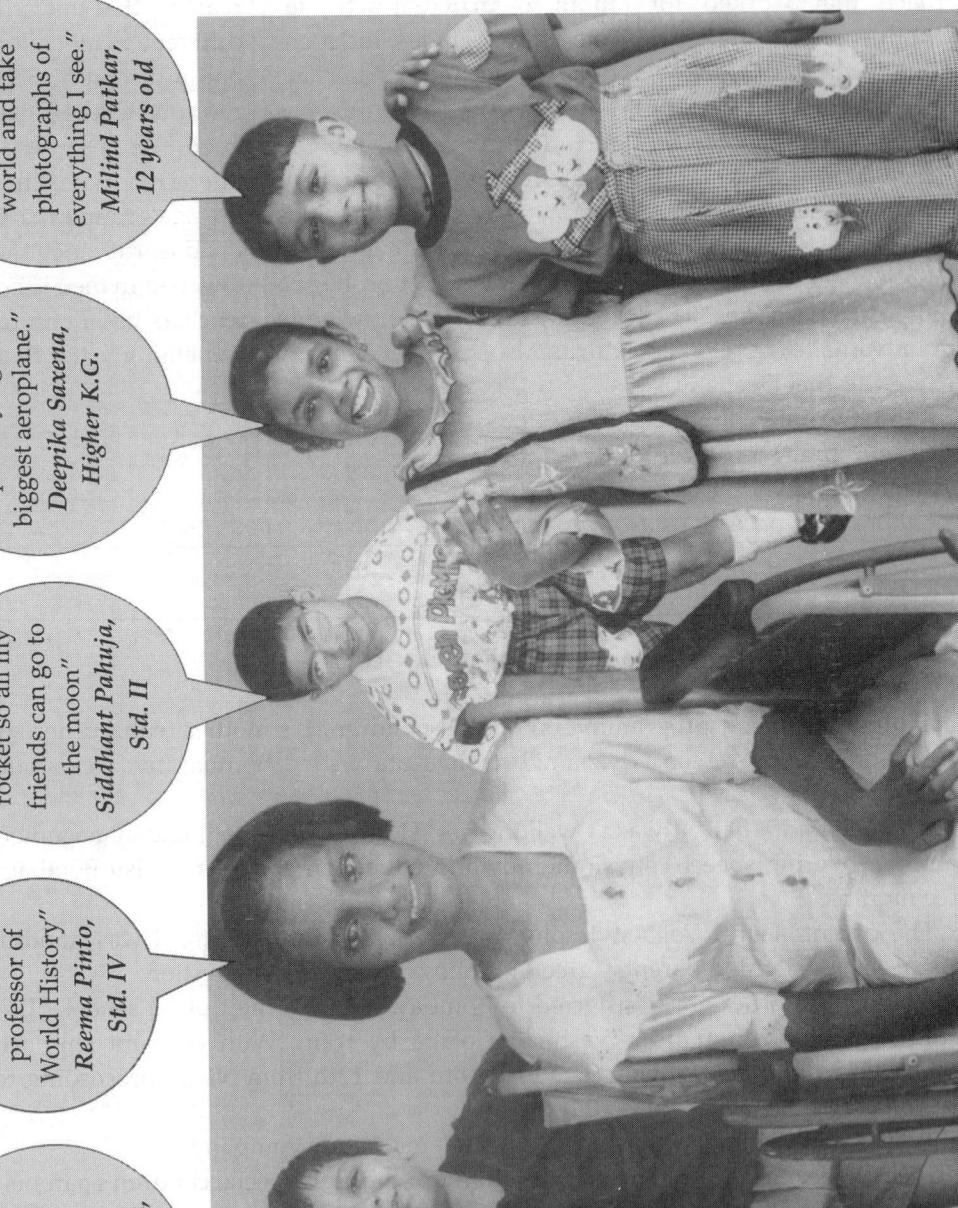

Domain II

Treatment and Rehabilitation Unit

Background: To Fill the Gap Where There Was No Multidisciplinary Approach to Treatment and Management

In 1972, therapy was a domain for experts only. Discussion and conversation with the parents was non-existent; while focusing on therapy and education for the child, services of counselling and empowering and involving parents and the family were virtually unknown. The concept of explaining to the parent what activity was being done and why or for what purpose was missing. Children were more of a 'diagnosis' to be discussed amongst colleagues. A leading doctor of cerebral palsy (CP) in fact said, 'Parents are patients and you cannot share their file with them—they do not understand.' *This had to be changed. It was clearly embedded in an antiquated medical approach and so the change began.*

A unique, transdisciplinary approach to provide services like physio, occupational and speech therapy, social and psychological counselling and remedial education was developed under one roof. This approach became the hallmark of the organization, breaking the barrier between education and therapy and cutting down the 'walls' that exist between departments.

To begin treatment services for CP, a very experienced physiotherapist specialized in the treatment of the condition,

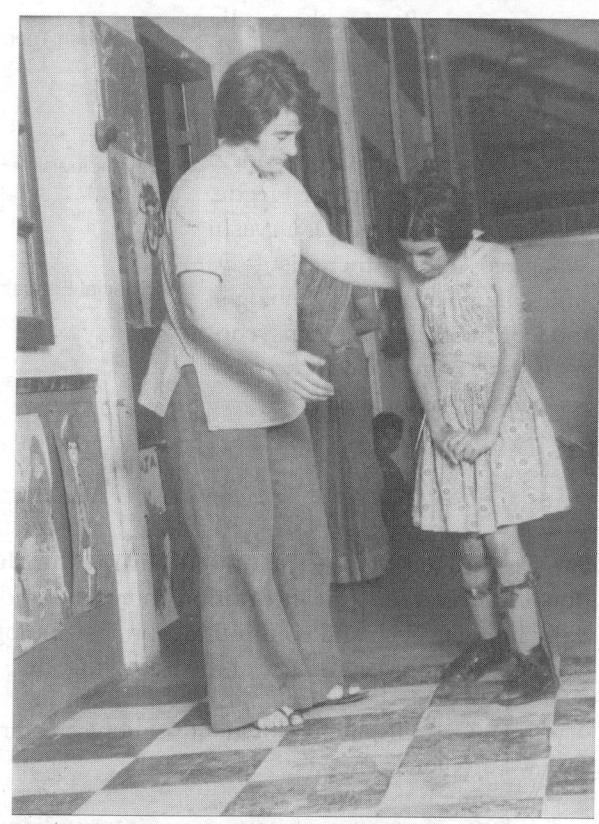

Pamela Stretch conducting an individual therapy session with Malini Chib

Pamela Stretch, came from the UK through the British High Commission and the Overseas Development Agency (ODA), later known as the Department for International Development (DFID). She was instrumental in *pioneering the treatment of CP in India* with a holistic approach, making it culture and context specific to Indian needs, with Mithu Chib (Bose, now Alur), a professional special educator qualified from the University of London and returned from the UK with her family. Together with leading educators from regular schools, Uma Banerjee from The John Cannon and Cathedral School and Spenta Madon from the Fort Convent, they set up the first model of *special education combined with regular education. This was the first Centre for Special Education set up in Colaba.*

All of them worked closely with doctors. Dr Eddie Bharucha, leading neurologist, who had set up the neurology departments of several hospitals such as the King Edward Memorial (KEM) Hospital, Bombay Hospital and was one of the founder members of the Children's Orthopedic Hospital; Dr Pravina Shah neurologist and Dean of KEM, a founder member of the Epilepsy Foundation India, were the neurologists; Dr P.K. Mullaferoze, director of the Children's Orthopedic Hospital, was our consultant orthopaedic surgeon, Dr Raj Anand and Dr R. Khubchandani were the visiting paediatricians. Later we were joined by Dr Armida Fernandez, neonatologist, Dr Anaita Hegde, paediatric neurologist, Dr Urvashi Shah, cognitive therapist, Dr Anuradha Sovani, psychologist and Dr Manek Bharucha, psycho-analyst, to name a few who have been closely associated.

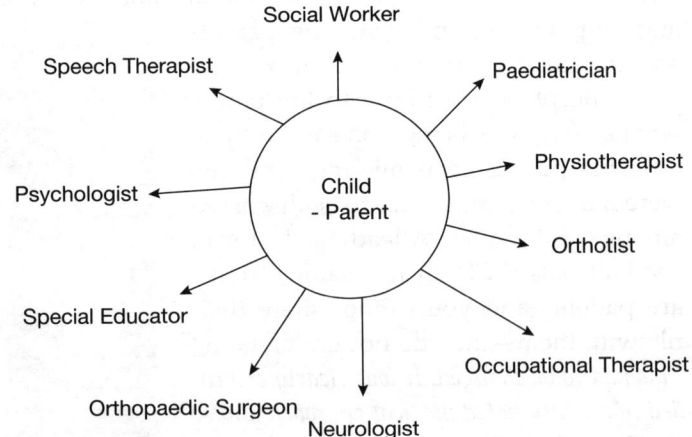

Interdisciplinary Rapport

Methods

Services offered by the Therapy Department included assessment, physical therapy, occupational therapy, sensory integration therapy, hand function training and training in skills of daily living speech and communication, psychology and social work.

The treatment consisted of the following:

- Different techniques of identification/screening/assessment
- Early intervention
- Communication
- Different treatment strategies of intervention: Psychosocial Aspects
- Human resource development: Training

- Individualized therapy inputs as well as group therapy: Therapy and treatment principles were woven in with the extracurricular activities such as music, painting, drama, sports and so on.

Different Techniques of Identification/Screening/Assessment

Identification of the child's needs and developing a suitable treatment plan is a very specialized and crucial area. Parents needed to appreciate this so that it could be focused on at home. By understanding therapy programme, they would be able to appreciate the outcomes. We found that many parents had completely misunderstood the condition and kept thinking for the first few years that given regular therapy their child would soon begin to sit, walk and talk. It was only after a few years that they realized the long-term nature of CP. In fact, most parents stated that it was only after the love, patience and care shown to them, that they gradually began to understand their child's abilities and potential. Arnav's (student) mother said that when her son was born she had a difficult labour and her son had to be admitted to the neonatal unit. For the first couple of months, they did not know that anything was wrong with their son. It was only when he turned seven months old and he did not begin to sit, that they started visiting different doctors. Finally, they were told that their son had CP and they should begin therapy. This is what she said, 'We didn't know what CP was and were not explained about the condition, we were confused and thought that once we started therapy he would be OK within a couple of months and soon learn to walk and talk.' It was only as the years passed by did they eventually understand the long-term nature of the disability and it was after Arnav's enrolment for therapy at The Spastics Society of India (SSI) that she said, 'With the love and commitment shown by the therapist at SSI we began to understand our son.'

How did we do this?

During the assessment period, a long time was spent with parents; sensitivity, understanding and kindness were vital ingredients to be added to specialization. The aura of professionalism had to be discarded when one was face to face with suffering. In the early 1970s, this attitude to parents was completely new. While observing and assessing the needs of the family, we never forgot that parents were in a state of shock about their child; it was a time of acute crisis when they learnt that their child was handicapped for life. As a well-known paediatrician has said, 'They were our "primary patients". They needed immediate care and attention' (ICPS 1976).

We needed to know about family dynamics, the socio-economic level of the household and the number of family members living together. In India, there are large joint families. Parents-in-law, uncles, aunts, grandparents, all live together. In a typical home, the mother-in-law usually dominates. The son would have to show complete obeisance to his mother—her word is law! It was always the daughter-in-law's fault. We could never change age-old traditions that have existed in India for centuries. Rehabilitation could only be worked out within the system and considered within this cultural set-up (Alur 2010b). Therefore, work began training all members of the joint family, mothers-in-law, uncles, great-aunts, siblings and so on. On a personal level, my own family members, as I mentioned earlier, also stepped in to help in some way.

After battling for over a decade, we managed to get very young babies. This was for us indicative of success. Doctors began to refer infants to us of around one or two years. The children then went through an intensive early stimulation and home management programme and, later, a preschool programme after which they got admitted to a regular nursery class.

Early Intervention

The importance of early detection cannot be stressed enough. The post-war era brought an increasing awareness of the need for rehabilitation, leading to a burgeoning of interest in all aspects of rehabilitation. By the early 1950s, a variety of treatment approaches specifically designed to address neurological disability came into being, most of which had a theoretical basis in neurophysiology.

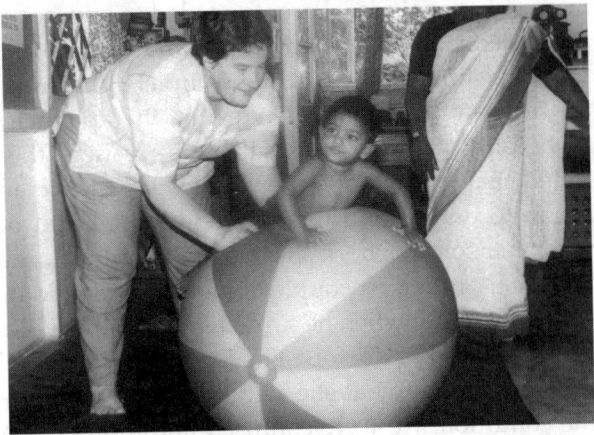

Pamela Stretch demonstrating Vojta therapy to parent

The Bobath Concept was one of these approaches, its founders being Berta Bobath, a physiotherapist, and her husband Dr Karel Bobath.[1] The Bobaths had the ability to learn from experience and to adapt their concept with the changing needs of the patients. The Bobath treatment was introduced, which stressed the inhibition of abnormal movement patterns to facilitate normal movement patterns, a treatment concept and approach that is relevant today and is one of the most widely used approaches.

For us, early detection began as early as when the infant was 10 days old. We used a technique called the Vojta technique of evaluation, started by a Czech neurologist to detect if a baby had what was known as a central coordination disturbance by testing its postural and primitive reflexes. Dr Vojta[2] and his team from Munich visited the organization and trained our therapist to diagnose developmental delay at a very early age using kinaesiological examination, consisting of seven postural reactions which were tested in seven different positions and based on the responses seen, a developmental age was determined. This enabled the therapist to prepare an

---

[1] Together, they developed the Bobath Concept for the treatment of children with CP and adults with neurological conditions. In their lifetime, they travelled extensively, teaching and training tutors throughout the world. They both received many honours for their pioneering and innovative work. They died in 1991.

[2] Professor Vaclav Vojta was from the Czech Republic. He got his PhD in neurology and paediatric neurology in 1947. Professor Hellbrugge from Kinderzentrum. Munich, invited Professor Vojta to join his medical team in Munich in 1975. Dr Vojta then became social paediatric consultant at the Kinderzentrum. Dr Vojta set up his treatment approach all over Europe, UK, Japan and India, to name a few countries. Both Professor Hellbrugge and Dr Vojta worked with the therapists of SSI, Bombay.

appropriate programme for the baby based on his/her needs. 'Intrinsic Development', a modification of the Vojta technique, was developed by Pamela Stretch.

Treatment principles of other proponents, such as the Peto method of treatment in groups, started by Professor Peto of Hungary, were also very suitable to India where there was a lack of manpower. Research in the area of therapy was explored in the initial years with Dr Margaret Yekutiel, director, Recanati School for Health Professionals, Israel, joining us in the treatment and guiding us as a researcher.

A very new concept of 'eclectic approach' was established. The aim was to get the children early and begin management with an eclectic approach, involving various techniques suited to each individual child and involving parents at home and a large team at the centre. In the following section, I expand this a little.

A Multidisciplinary Team Approach Towards the Child

The multivariate dimension of CP necessitated the need of a team of specialists who combined their knowledge in their respective disciplines to plan for an effective intervention plan for each individual child. Prominent neurologists, orthopaedic surgeons and paediatricians became a part of the panel of doctors who supported these new concepts. The concept of treatment for children with CP underwent a radical change.

The team consisted of medical doctors, paramedical staff of physiotherapists, occupational therapists, speech therapists, social workers, special educa-

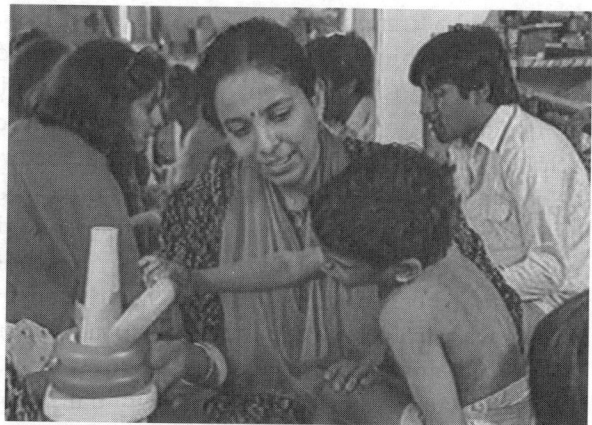
Judith Vaz and Mallika Jariwalla in the background working on strengthening the upper limbs

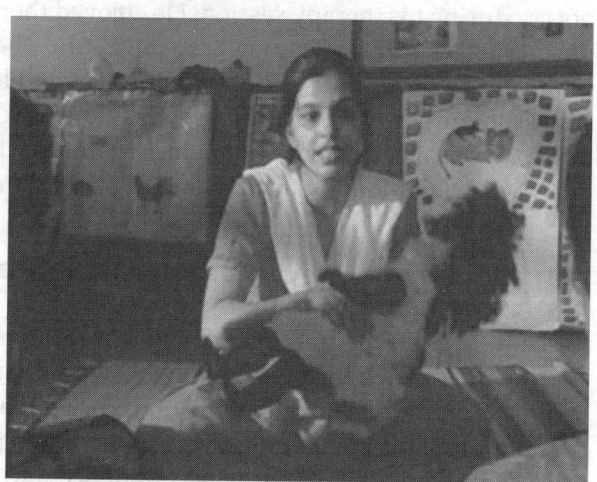
Dr Shabnam Rangwala* demonstrates how to manage a child with cerebral palsy

*Shabnam like all of us in the organization has worn many hats. She is an Occupational Therapist, who has been the Head of Therapy for 19 years. She too has an excellent relationship with the students and parents. Passion for her areas of work drives her. She is also the Director of Community Services and has pioneered services in Dharavi and Pelhar, doing international projects. A researcher and lecturer, with her multi-faceted talents she started new activities for the disabled, like sports for disabled children and wheelchair paragliding!

tors, psychologists and, of course, the parents who were the most important members of the team. The social model rather than the medical model was developed. For the first time, instead of words like 'treatment' and 'cure', a word like 'management' was introduced. The 'walls' that orthodox thinking had erected between the different therapy departments were broken down and 'de-hospitalization' of therapists took place. The concept of the whole child—physical, intellectual, emotional and social—was introduced, resulting in a series of assessments, including intellectual, functional and social factors, administered over a period of time to all the students. A case conference was held on a weekly basis to discuss the needs of each child in order to determine the best intervention and education plan. The child and family was the central point of all interventions. Therapy for children was introduced as being fun and play, with a greater emphasis on the interest and motivation of the child, which led to cooperation. A balance was struck between the medical, therapeutic, social and educational needs of the child.

The organization managed to set up a new model of care that cut across professional boundaries and established multidisciplinary teams of medical, paramedical and the parents working in cohesion to treat the chronic disorder of CP. It was the approach to the child that was of consequence, a little bit of kindness with a large dose of expertise.

Omar's mother said: 'When our child was admitted to SSI, it was the first time that he did not cry during his therapy session. He enjoyed therapy and always wanted to go to the therapy department as therapy was made so much fun! The group therapies provided to our child also gave us an opportunity to de-stress ourselves and learn from other parents who had challenges similar to ours. We made good friends and learnt simple tips on how to manage our child at home. We also learnt about home management which, when I think about it today, helped us plan for the long-term management of our child's needs.'

a. Parents in Partnerships

Realizing the need to understand and support parents emotionally, the vital step to empower them with knowledge about treatment was initiated. We changed the rules here and parents became important members of the multidisciplinary team. Assessment did not mean only filling up forms; assessment times were transformed into occasions where rapport could be established with parents to gain their confidence and to start educating them about their child's needs. The therapeutic approaches used were in line with the current international theories, but adjusted to be culture- and context-specific. Most importantly, because it was a parent who began the services, the new approach emphasized *reaching out to parents both professionally and emotionally with love and care.*

The acceptance and understanding of basic therapy concepts by the parents was considered of prime importance. Parents were part of the handling and management programmes for their children as it became clear that no programme would be effective without a home management programme.

A home management programme was explained to the parents in simple terms, with a demonstration that helped them to understand how they could conduct therapy at home for their child. Training included how to carry their child, how to feed their child, importance of proper seating and posture, self-help skills and how to build on language and communication. We should not get so wrapped up in our specializations that we lose sight of the fact that we are treating a child who is 'special' but has the same needs as a normal child and has a family who will need guidance in order for the child to achieve his/her full potential. Specialists were trained not to lose their compassion while assessing families and the child and we began the new humane approach of treatment, which combined professionalism with care.

These techniques were also taken up by the other spastics societies. The late Mrs Mita Nundy, who was one of the founder members of SSI, Delhi, writes: 'Parents need to be in touch regularly, if possible once a week through Home Management Programme. A group of parents and their children spend five hours together every week throughout the year. They have made friends. All the staff have been trained in counselling techniques. We have sometimes told parents that they need not return next week but should carry out the home programme and return after a longer period. They have invariably requested that they come back weekly. One mother said, "I know there is time reserved for me by all the staff every week and I need it to discuss my problems and ask my questions." Another explained, "The only friends I have are in the centre." For others, we think it is the support they give each other.'

b. Manpower Training: Therapists

Training of manpower was initiated. Medical students from Mumbai started visiting the organization to learn about the new model. The first formal six-week course titled 'Management in Cerebral Palsy' began in India in 1978. With a national spread, it aimed to spread awareness on practical aspects of management with a hands-on practical approach. The course was begun with support from the British Council and two renowned figures in aspects of management of children with CP, Sophie Levitt and Noreen Hare conducted the course. Levitt did so in 1981 and Hare after that. The main thrust of the course was to teach ways and means of becoming a multitherapist, or in other words, a transdisciplinary worker. Pamela Stretch and her Indian team conducted the courses. The medical profession joined us: people like Dr Eddie Bharucha, Dr Mullaferoze, Dr Pilloo Bharucha and Dr Praveena Shah.

The new courses helped in creating awareness about CP among doctors and therapists and were therefore able to break new ground, creating much needed knowledge and manpower to treat this very complicated condition. This effort was aimed nationwide and the knowledge base helped spread awareness all over India.

Pragya, a speech therapist, who attended one of the management in cerebral palsy (MCP) courses in the earlier years, said that it had opened a new area of learning for her. Her passion for working with children with CP got ignited and she has continued to work in this field for over 35 years…. She said that it was only through the sound learning that she received through the intensive MCP course that she was able to find her calling!

Dr Urvashi Shah, a highly skilled medical professional and one of the founder members of the Epilepsy Foundation India, came in to support the faculty.

c. Aids and Appliances

Research into low-cost and indigenous aids had been initiated. This was done in close partnership with engineers and technical institutes from across the country. In the year 1979, a new Aids & Appliances Department was created by Ranjana Sen to provide indigenous aids and appliances for the handicapped, specifically spastic children around India. This department published a book containing innovative aids and appliances for people with disability called *Upkaran*. This handbook was a milestone in its time and in the area of rehabilitation literature in the country.

For the first time a course on 'Adapted sports for children with physical disabilities' was introduced by faculty from Israel, initiated by Dr Margaret Yekutiel, Dr Anita Prabhu and Dr Shabnam Rangwala.

Later Phase: 1993–2012

The organization in the later years moved away from segregated special education to inclusive education, establishing an inclusive community model of rehabilitation and care. In that second phase, treatment was further demystified, building capacity and awareness amongst parents and the community; deprofessionalization and humanization of the professional away from the sterile ambiance of institutions and hospitals to the community was initiated and the concept of inclusive therapy was introduced, which included the concept of three 'R's' for the professional: retraining, relocation and redeployment of time. Again, indicative of success was the fact that medical professionals accepted the potential of children with CP and began to advocate inclusive education for the children.

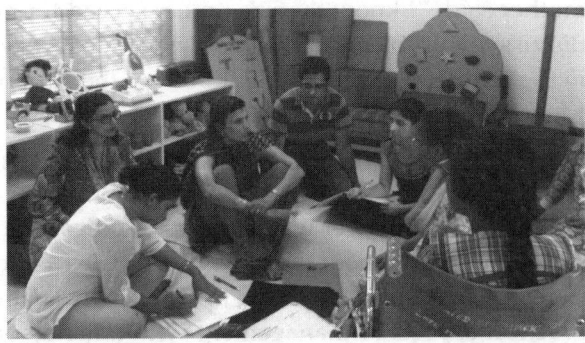

Dr Anaita Hegde* at a case conference at ADAPT

*Dr Anaita Hegde is a leading paediatric neurologist. She has herself lived with disability and feels very close to her patients. She has been involved in many services around the city with the Spastics Society as a consultant paediatric neurologist and with the Children In Need of Special Care and has been associated with SSI for many years.

To impart further knowledge to the parents, numerous simple publications in the area of therapy were developed. These publications gave, in a simple and easy-to-understand manner, information to parents on the different types of CP and their causes. Some of the publications included basic medical aspects of CP, management of epilepsy, gross motor development and its role in therapy, need of therapy in the life of a child with CP, surgical interventions in CP and so on. Parents were always imparted information on the latest techniques available in the area of management of CP and were given the support to select the best for their child.

Communication

Department of Psychology

The child's psychological, emotional and mental states play a vital role in his or her growth and development. During their growing years, children may manifest various behavioural problems and undergo emotional problems, which affect their ability to develop. The aim of the psychology department was to help students reach their maximum potential through a holistic approach which included medical intervention, counselling sessions and behaviour modification programmes (which may manifest due to their physical condition).

Department of Speech and Language

'Communication' is the means we use for social interaction, which is essential for personal development. Communication means the conveying of desires, feelings and ideas from one person to another through the use of symbols. In CP, of all the problems of severe handicap those of communication are the most serious. A child with a communication problem can be condemned to emotional solitude, an intellectual silence too distressing to imagine and the prospect of remaining crippled in mind and personality. The interdisciplinary approach introduced included speech and language therapists. Again, therapists used a holistic approach when planning the intervention. The motor ability for speech, language ability and communication levels were all areas assessed carefully. The speech therapist worked closely with the teacher, the parent and other therapists. Existing practices of speech therapy focused mainly on the overt features of speech, mainly voice production and articulation.

Communication Damage in Cerebral Palsy

We were confronted with children with CP who were extremely intelligent with *a mind that works but a body that doesn't* (an oft-quoted phrase) and unable to provide feedback. Both their abilities of speech and hand function get damaged, preventing them from using traditional means of communication such as a pen or pencil for writing, or speaking, causing major academic barriers in a classroom. One of the urgent tasks before a teacher and a speech therapist was how to get the outside world to understand the speech disorders of this very intelligent person. The traditional means of recording work, receiving an output or feedback, or regurgitation of knowledge imparted, became impossible. Non-verbal means of communication was used in conjunction with an individual's residual/existing abilities to speak or to write. This was technically referred to as augmentative communication. It supplemented, augmented or increased the ability of a person to meet his or her communication needs. Two modes were used: (a) Gestural mode: This involved no instrumentation but required some slight control of movement on the part of the person, such as head nodding, eye blinking, hand movements and so on. (b) Gestural-assisted mode: This involved instrumentation and some body movement to achieve communication. For example, a Bliss board, wherein the user points (gestures) to the symbols (instrument) on the board in order to communicate.

Criteria for Selecting an Augmentative Communication Aid

Bearing in mind the aim of augmentative communication, it was important to assess an individual's skills and potentials which would help in the selection of a suitable augmentative communication strategy. The following aspects were considered: motor control, intellectual level, sensory functions (hearing, vision, tactile and kinaesthetic), language status and communication needs of the person.

The optimum aid for a person was the one that came closest to allowing him to effectively meet his communication needs and was:

- Acceptable to him and those in his environment
- Well understood by others who are minimally trained to interpret messages transmitted by the aid
- Portable
- Easy to learn to use
- Cost-effective
- Efficient and interferes as little as possible, if at all, with the ongoing activity

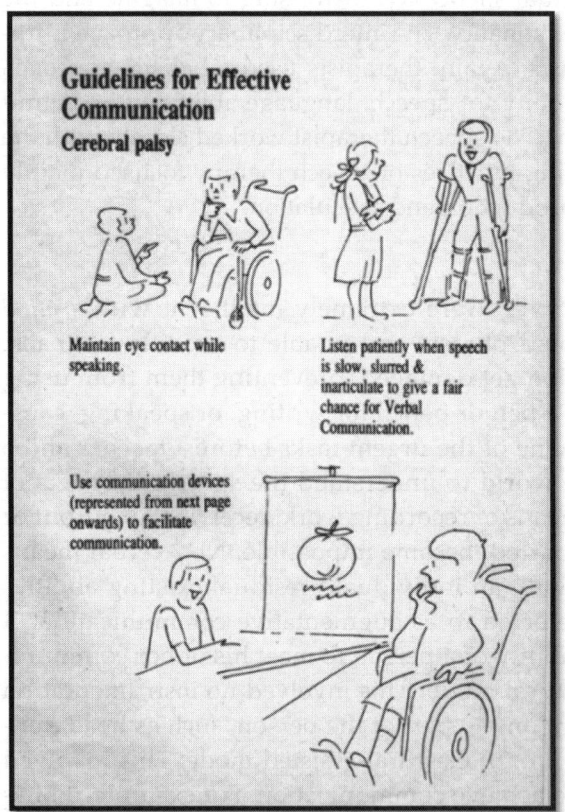

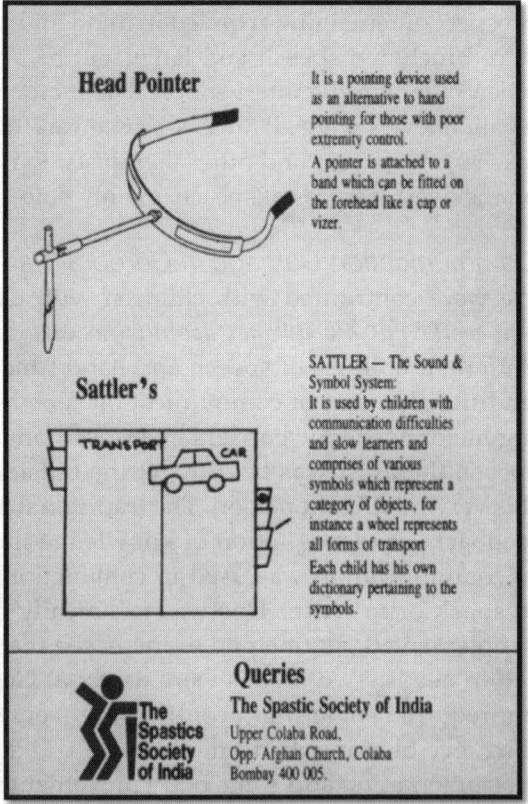

'Bridging the Communication Gap'

The impact of augmentative communication on users and others was found to be highly desirable and the users showed decreased frustration, increased confidence, increased attention span, independence and improved performance. Another important aspect of an augmentative communication strategy was its impact on speech. Our experiences revealed that augmentative communication did not reduce the individual's motivation to communicate. In fact, it was found to facilitate speech in some children and adults.

Classroom intervention by all therapists: In the early years itself, due importance was given to the need to demystify and simplify the treatment programmes for parents and caregivers. The speech therapist was not only supposed to provide a single treatment session but she also worked closely with the teacher, the parent and other therapists.

Methods Used

- During meal times, maintaining posture, developing good patterns of vegetative functions (which refers to swallowing and basic functions of coordination of lip, tongue and jaw) and using adaptive devices were demonstrated and practised. Training parents and caregivers through home visits were frequent. Outpatient services also undertook the intervention programme for infants. Emphasis was on communication in any form—speech, gesture and sounds. Speech therapy was not restricted to the session alone.
- Developing and strengthening the prerequisites of speech production: relaxation, breathing exercises, development of vegetative functions (biting, chewing and swallowing) and oral motor exercises.
- Students were assessed and trained to use various devices like the 'Big Red Switch', 'Joysticks', 'Camera Mouse' and modified keyboard with communication software such as the 'Interactive Communication Board'.
- Various Internet games were utilized to help students understand the functions of the devices. Tangible devices such as picture books and spelling boards continued to be used within the classroom to assist effective communication. The goal was now to procure a digital communication aid which could be used personally by every student to speed up the communication process to the level of verbal conversation.

Lessons Learnt

- Information technology brought with it immense benefits.
- Breaking barriers of communication through augmentative and alternative communication (AAC) was a major goal.
- Adapted switches: cost-effective devices to access existing programmes for education needed to be developed.
- The development of language and vocabulary was given due importance through the use of electronic aids like the Language Master and Touch Tutor: for persons who had difficulty in having their speech understood, the use of certain aids such as Sattler symbols and Bliss symbols facilitated communication. These aids were also used for examinations.

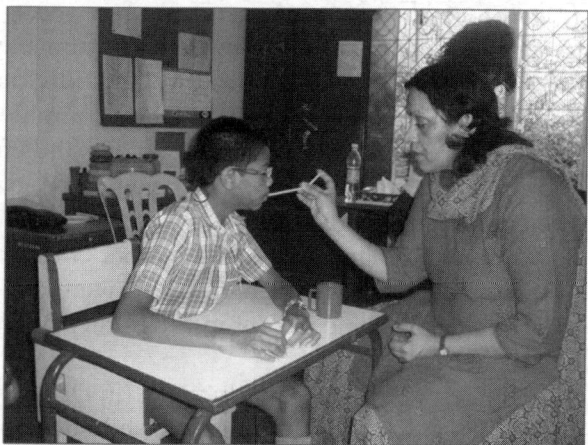

Dr Asha Kumar* demonstrates correct feeding techniques

*Dr Asha Kumar, who began Speech and Audiology had a special skill of approaching disabled people as equal friends, establishing a strong rapport with them.

- It was important to train in an adjusted, modified environment, appropriate to the needs of the person.
- The Speech and Communication Department had, over the years, striven to keep itself informed on new developments by attending and presenting papers at seminars conducted by training colleges, medical institutions and other organizations in related fields.

The late Mrs Mita Nundy wrote about the ways in which we differed from hospitals. 'The services we offer may seem to be similar to what is offered at rehabilitation outpatient departments of hospitals. There are differences, some of which substantially raise the costs, but are crucial to the effectiveness of this kind of treatment of a chronic handicap.'

Psychosocial Aspects

At the centre itself, there is an atmosphere of leisure—magazines, tea, comfortable mattresses to sit or lie on. Relationships are further strengthened at social gatherings organized for families by home management during the year. Aspects of work in home management provide a crucial support system which seems to be a psychological necessity for many of the mothers. The encouragement and enthusiasm of the staff is also a necessary boost to the will of the mother to continue her training programme when rewards can be so slow with such severely handicapped children.

Human Resource Development: Training

Training and Equipment

In our experience, another way we differ from a typical outpatient programme in a hospital is the training aspect. This is done through individual demonstrations, lectures and workshops; cyclostyled literature and printed Hindi pamphlets explaining facts about CP. The publication of printed material was a response to demands from individual and group sessions. All aids and equipment recommended in the home programme are loaned from an equipment library. The equipment ranges from books, educational toys, and training equipment, to accelerate development of hand function, to infant crawlers, rollators, buggies and wheelchairs. Many of these aids that have been designed were not available in the market. Educational equipment that is available is kept in the library because many families do not have the funds to buy them easily.

The Centre for Special Education (in Delhi) has been a training ground for teachers from regular schools as well as students of child development wishing to learn about integration for disabled children. Physio and occupational therapy students are attached to the centre for their practical training. Specialization in this aspect of development medicine and dissemination of useful information through conferences and workshops has started because this special school exists (Alur 1982).

Transport is another area that had to be provided. Attendance was most irregular till transport was provided by us. Not even one per cent of the population of a city like Delhi has access to means of private transport apart from a bicycle. The overcrowded public transport system is not suitable for transporting handicapped children. The lack of free transport could well be a prohibitive factor in families using hospital services for physically handicapped children.

Results and Outcome

- Towards the later years, new courses focusing on the specific needs of younger therapists were planned. International agencies and faculty were invited to address the therapist and spread knowledge through these courses.
- The latest treatment protocols of Neurodevelopmental Therapy (NDT) and Sensory Integration (SI) therapy were introduced for the first time at SSI within the framework of the social model used by Pamela Stretch and supported by Judith Vaz. This course aims at shifting the focus of the professionals to a combination of skills to look at the child's social independence along with functional abilities and educational performance. The changing role of the therapist was stressed and the key principles of inclusive education taught.
- Courses by senior, international occupational therapists to develop new strategies for promoting independence and self-reliance for the disabled within the context of the Indian lifestyle and available resources were also conducted. This led to more and more therapists learning about the social model approach which they had never been exposed to within their curriculum of medical schools.
- The 'eclectic approach' was maintained with introduction to latest therapy techniques through training courses organized by senior faculty from The Bobath Institute, London, as well as NDT and SI-trained therapists. Therapists were encouraged to attend training courses throughout the country to learn about newer models of therapy and incorporate the knowledge gained into the treatment protocols of the organization.
- Interdisciplinary team approach combining medical, paramedical, educational and socio-emotional services were set up under one roof. Due to the fact that all services were offered comprehensively under one roof, large number of children came from different parts of the country.
- New concepts, such as Bobath and Vojta, unknown in the country were introduced. Group therapy and conductive education started by Hungarian neurologist Peto were also introduced. Neuromotor sensory integration programme was created. The importance of the use of the 'eclectic approach' was established.
- Parent partnerships were strengthened and parents thus empowered started taking up lead roles around the country. Parents started taking up the responsibility of therapy and due to their empowerment were equal decision makers in the treatment for their child. Parental involvement kept the work on the ground level with a bottom-up approach.
- The 'Management of cerebral palsy and other physical disabilities' course established the much needed therapy training in the country. Therapists came from various parts of the country like Baroda, Bhuj, Cuttack, Bangalore, Mumbai and some came from neighbouring

countries like Pakistan and Bangladesh. Through the training of therapists the organization was indirectly impacting the lives of large number of parents and children with CP throughout the country.

- Therapy for children was first of all introduced as being fun and play, with greater emphasis on the interest and motivation of the child, leading to cooperation. It was important to be able to strike a balance between the medical, therapeutic, social and educational needs of the child.

Domain III

Child and Parents in Partnership

Background: Transforming the Approach and Empowering the Parents as Professionals

One of the major contributions made by the organization was its endeavour to reach out to the parents and the community. Till then, the prevailing attitude was that parents were not allowed to look at the files, they were treated as people who could not think and were merely relatives of the patient and not everything could be revealed to such people! With the birth of The Spastics Society of India (SSI), a strong focus was given to parents, rich or poor.

We said that parents are in a state of severe shock about their child. It is a time of acute crisis when they learn that their child is handicapped for life. As a well-known paediatrician has said, they are our 'primary patients' and need immediate care and attention. I had received such sensitive care and attention when I was with Malini in England but suffered dreadfully in India for, among other causes of suffering, the way Malini was examined here was often rough.

Doctors and parents became key partners. A new partnership with parents was launched. They were not treated only as parents, but made to understand, thereby empowering them to contribute as important members of the team.

Early detection and a link-up with the family in the first two years are crucial. We found that sometimes parents 'shop around' endlessly for a 'cure'. They believe in faith healing, advice from gurus or strong medication as a quick panacea. All this plays a powerful part in delaying the start of proper management. We changed this and made it a mandate to stick to the training being given. Once the child was taken away, she or he could not be readmitted.

Methods

How did we do this? During the assessment period, we spent a long time with parents, getting to know about family dynamics, the socio-economic level of the household and the number of family members living together. In India, we have large joint families where the mother-in-law dominates. We could not change age-old traditions: rehabilitation could only be worked out within the system and considered within this set-up: in the Indian cultural context, it is not enough only to train parents as there are large joint families consisting of parents-in-law, aunts and grandparents.

We began training parents and their extended families. The aim was to involve parents and the extended family of aunts and mothers-in-law in the management of their child: to empower them to make their own decisions about the welfare of their child (similar to what happened to me when I was trained in London); to give them effective home management programmes and transform parents into resource people.

Parents were empowered in three areas:

- Parents' support system
- Home management
- Parents as leaders

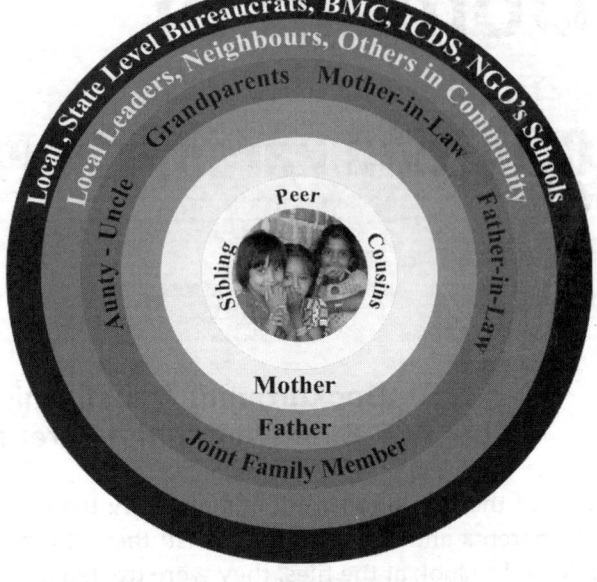

Figure 3.1. The Whole Community Approach

Source: Mithu Alur, Principal Investigator, UNICEF Project 2003.

Parents' Support System: Home Management

Parents were trained in techniques of management of their child at home through a new programme called Home Management. Parents were explained the rationale behind any therapy or educational activity. A home programme was designed by a multidisciplinary team for each child. This programme was explained in simple terms along with a demonstration on how they could conduct therapy at home. The therapists observed the parent perform therapy to ensure proper handling. The programme was then followed by the parents with their child at home. The programme was reviewed and modified at regular intervals based on the developmental changes. In Dharavi, often labelled as Asia's largest slum, children and parents visited the centre twice a week and were taught techniques in the areas of feeding and dressing, therapy and intellectual stimulation.

The approach changed. Therapists were careful and tactful while talking to parents so as not to alienate them. In the initial stages, the physiotherapist or occupational therapist gave practical advice.

Parents were trained to follow the Portage checklist of activities. Each week they chose a particular activity and worked on it with their children, keeping a daily written record of the child's progress on an activity chart. They received regular feedback and gradually they moved up to the next level and to different activities. Other strategies included:

Mother and Child Playgroup

This service was introduced in 1984. A playgroup was formed of children along with their mothers and met once a week for therapy sessions and group activities such as singing, painting and learning through play. Mothers learnt about the management of their children's disability at home.

Workshops for Parents

Various programmes were conducted over the years for parents, addressing various issues with the aim of educating and empowering them.

Teacher Training Courses

Many parents enrolled in the courses conducted by the organization to gain more knowledge to help them manage their child's disability.

Parents' Action Forum

A need was felt for greater parental involvement in awareness raising and advocacy campaigns. A parents' action forum was formed to work towards sensitizing individuals and governmental agencies to address the concerns of the disabled.

By including parents in the multidisciplinary team, they were made to understand the sequence of education and treatment of their children. They became aware of the step by step holistic rehabilitation of the child. This increased participation provided social and emotional support to the parents. Parents were encouraged to become professionals. They trained in areas of education and treatment. They were also encouraged to become leaders and master trainers. Those who could afford it went abroad to get trained and become professionals.

Regionally based and autonomous societies that have grown with help from SSI, based on our first model, were initiated by parents and family members such as aunts, great-aunts and grandmothers! Initially helped by us, they were then encouraged to be autonomous.

Community-based Rehabilitation

In Dharavi, the slum community was brought in, children and parents visited the centre twice a week so that home management techniques could be worked out for feeding, dressing, therapy and intellectual stimulation for those children who cannot attend full day school.

Parent Training in Portage

Portage is a system of transferring knowledge and skills from professionals to para-professionals and non-professionals.

SSI incorporated Portage as an important tool in its Home Management programme. Parents were instructed on the use of the Portage manual and given a checklist of the activities of the child. Each week they chose a particular activity and worked on it with their children and came back for more information and feedback for the social worker whenever necessary. The parents kept a daily written record of the child's progress on an activity chart.

Shift in Ideology

When the organization shifted its policy from special school to inclusive schools, parents became much-needed partners in the inclusion process. Initially, parents were apprehensive about inclusion. Parents of children, with and without disabilities, were met with. Remembering the doubts expressed, their first response was 'How will our child cope?'

Regular 'parent–teacher–therapist' meetings were held at the onset to understand parents' fears about the transition to regular schools, which were then addressed. This was done to keep a continuous pulse on parental support and needs, mainly the mothers. It took a series of meetings to convey to parents the concept of inclusion, its benefits of peer learning and social development. A great deal of preparation was needed.

Parents' support groups for inclusion was created. Parents were trained to introduce the concept of inclusion into regular schools to their children, the changing role of parents was stressed upon and their dependency on National Resource Centre for Inclusion (NRCI) gradually reduced. At some of the meetings, students who had already participated in the inclusion process were invited along with their parents to share their initial apprehensions and strategies that worked for them.

When the parents were included in the inclusion process, most of them became advocates of their own children and their disabilities, thereby acquiring leadership quality. They become partners in inclusion and they undertook the majority of initial preparatory work for inclusion. This approach resulted in a direct interaction of parents with the heads, with no intermediary coming between them and facilitated in making a relationship between parents, teachers and heads of regular schools, thus enabling these actors to take ownership of the inclusion process.

Parents soon took over and got their friends and neighbours to help. Eventually, it was they who took ownership of the inclusion process, sorting out any barriers that came in the way of their child. Over time, many became very confident ambassadors of inclusive education. They were empowered to give their children a continuum of support.

Parents as Professionals

The parents were aware of the step by step holistic rehabilitation of the child.

By being included in the multidisciplinary team, they understood the sequence and the rationale behind the education and treatment of their children. Their increased participation helped to provide social, emotional and academic support to the management.

Parents got trained at various training programmes of SSI and as a result, SSI was established in various places like Delhi, Chennai, Calcutta and Jaipur by them. Spastics Society of Northern India in 1977, Spastics Society of Karnataka in 1980, Spastics Society of Tamil Nadu in

1980, Spastics Society of India (Chennai), now Vidyasagar, in 1985, Disha in Jaipur and Reach in Kolkata were formed.

Parent Trust

A non-governmental initiative by a group of parents and rehabilitation professionals, working for the disabled, was formed by the government and it was called the Parent Trust. This became The National Trust, working in collaboration with the ministry of social justice and empowerment. The trust carried out a broad educational programme on long-term planning and care for families of disabled individuals and their caregivers. The primary effort was to make the parents conscious of the critical need to make long-term plans for their disabled child. One of our parents, Poonam Natarajan, headed this trust, making dynamic inroads across the country. As part of this endeavour, the Life Insurance Company designed a plan, Jeevan Adhar, for handicapped dependents.

Parents became a critical resource for the successful growth and sustainability of inclusive education. Seventy per cent of parents managed to secure admission for their children into the neighbourhood schools through their own efforts, coupled with the support we provided them. This transfer of leadership from professionals to parents was key to reaching a greater scale of inclusion.

Stories from Parents Who Played a Critical Role[1]

Shobha Sachdev changed her career path from being a pathologist to becoming a professional special educator. In 29 years, she has shown herself to be a skilled professional, lecturer and teacher. A part of the senior management, she is involved in the organization's resource mobilization and many of the organization's national and international events.

Deepa Sachdev and Her Mother Shobha

'When my daughter Deepa was 6-months-old, a leading paediatrician told me that she had cerebral palsy (CP) and would probably be a vegetable. Not ready to believe him, I started my run from one doctor to another, reading about CP and sending her reports to the United Cerebral Palsy Association USA. All the knowledge I gathered, increased my belief in my child and I started taking her to various hospitals for physio and speech therapy.

I was concerned about her education. Her physiotherapist told me to check SSI. At SSI,

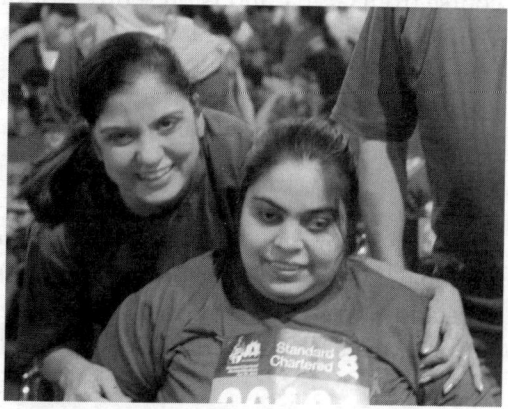

[1] Questionnaire tools designed by Professor Zenobia Nadirshaw and Dr Maria Baretto.

I was greeted by Mrs Junie Sethi who at once took Deepa from me into her arms. I knew then that this was the place where my daughter would bloom. However, seeing the older children, I realized that I was not dealing with a short-term illness but a lifelong condition.

Deepa was admitted to the first nursery class at SSI. Mithu Alur suggested I do the teachers' training course at SSI. Two mothers, Mithu and Deepak Kalra, were my teachers and gave me a lot of support, guidance, encouragement, empathy and knowledge. This was the beginning of my empowerment. After completing my course, I joined SSI as a special educator.

To remedy her visual perception problems, Deepa was put on a one-to-one remedial programme, her lessons were recorded to suit her learning style and she completed her Xth Standard through the National Institute of Open Schooling (NIOS) with good results. When she left SSI, Deepa had transformed into a caring, confident and educated young girl.

Today she runs a beauty salon and is very happy. She has been successful due to all the inputs she got from SSI. I, as a mother, have also grown from a confused parent to a confident professional.'

Toshan Chatterjee and His Mother Manju

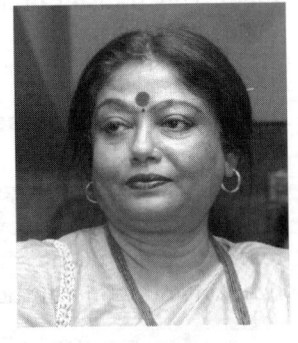

As a mother, Manju Chatterjee has shown tremendous feelings of reaching out to other parents. She has been principal of the centre and is now a director of the organization. Her organization skills and revenue generation are well known: her colleagues and donors esteem her dedication during the 15 memorable years she has spent in building up the organization.

'I am the mother of Toshan who has CP. Earlier, he could not move on his own or express his requirements. We brought him to SSI in Mumbai from Jammu. Dr Alur took him under her wings and things started happening…. Today, Toshan is completely independent. He scored 82.3 per cent in his class X board exams in 2004. After his graduation from St Xavier's College, he completed a three years' advanced level degree course from GNIIT and is presently working as a data compilation officer at Able Disabled All People Together (ADAPT).'

—Manju Chatterjee

Anoop and His Father K.C. Chakraberty

'I am the father of a disabled boy. My son, Anoop is employed by the General Post Office in Mumbai and is married. For this I am grateful. However, it has been a difficult journey to get here and I give full credit to SSI and now the NRCI for this. I have seen Dr Alur inculcating deeper values in them, encouraging them to fly higher, achieve more.'

—Mr K.C. Chakraberty

Vickram and His Mother Deepak Kalra

'Twenty-four years ago when my son was born with CP and mental challenges, the rehabilitation scene was very different. Hardly anyone knew about the condition including the medical faculty. There was one person who brought a ray of hope in our lives and gave me and my son a second life. It was Mrs Mithu Alur who set up the first centre for rehabilitation in Bombay that not only provided all services under one roof for persons with brain damage for the first time in India but also snowballed a movement in the entire country.'

—*Mrs Deepak Kalra, Umang*

Nilesh and His Father Dilip Gidwani

'My son was born "brain damaged". My family and I have been through various stages of a learning process to understand what was handed out to us by the pious Hands of God. The staff of the society under the stewardship of Mrs Mithu Alur (a mother of a similar child like ours) led us down a path of revelation, light and education that enlightened our perspective as parents of a multiply disabled child.'

—*Dilip Gidwani*

Vipasha and Her Father Professor Sitanshu Yashaschandra

'We are parents of a gifted, courageous and physically challenged daughter, Vipasha, who is also a poet. She is, so far as we know, the first and only person with spasticity to earn a doctoral degree from an Indian university. Vipasha has been guided and enabled in this through the pioneering and perfectionist work of one institution, SSI, Mumbai, and one person, Dr Mithu Alur, the founding chairperson of SSI and "mother" to the brave children with CP and their families. Dr Alur's deep and warm understanding of the huge problems and great promises which the child and the family faced, and the skills and warmth of the highly motivated group of therapists, teachers and assisting staff, which gave our daughter and us a fighting chance and led us from darkness at our dawn to a morning of hope.'

It all began because of the indomitable spirit that the two—a mother and a child, Mithu-ji and Malini—shared. The spirit, the resolution and the action, everything came from within the two and through their resolute bonding. The child, the poet Wordsworth would have said, is the mother of the woman. Malini has, through her own inner resources, shaped Mithu-ji's world, as much as the other way round. This chemistry, one might say this alchemy, characterizes not only their personal world but also the larger world of their larger family, ADAPT.

(Source: Professor Sitanshu Yashaschandra, Fulbright Scholar and Professor Emeritus, M.S. University, Baroda. Trustee of The Spastics Society of India)

Ishwar and His Mother Poonam Natarajan

Poonam Natarajan, founder chair of SSI, Madras, now Vidyasagar (Chennai), ex-chairperson, The National Trust, ministry of social justice, New Delhi.

'The wonderful services that have incubated for the past 40 years were pioneered by Padmashri Dr Mithu Alur way back in 1972. In 1980, we took our one-year-old child, Ishwar, to the Afghan Church School of SSI. This had been founded by Dr Alur. That school became my inspiration and lifelong passion. It was a happy place full of fun and laughter. I wanted my son to be in such a place and I also wanted to work and participate here and so did my mother, husband and our whole family.

It was with the training, support and inspiration from Dr Mithu Alur that I founded services in Madras (now Chennai) as a branch of SSI. The Chennai services, now known as Vidyasagar, have grown in many ways; the seeds were sown by Mithudi, Sathi and Malini. It is their love and constant interest that helped Nattoo, Ishoo and me to set down roots in south India. Mithu di became my teacher and mentor. It was with her and Sathi's support that we were able to have a building of our own. She helped to design a beautiful facility, besides raising the funds for it. A gift, the students of Vidyasagar enjoy and cherish.

It was Mithudi's passion for inclusive education that made Vidyasagar a leading organization in this area. Vidyasagar has practised inclusion as part of its vision and mission. Vidyasagar will be 30 years old on 15th of March, 2015, and as it looks back and looks forward, the golden leaf in its book will be about the pioneering support of its parent organization, SSI, Mumbai (now ADAPT). Both Mithu di and Sathi have laid the foundation and stood by solidly in tough times. I am sure Nattoo and Ishoo would also join me in remembering the beginning of this remarkable journey which today is Vidyasagar, the Chennai services.

Many people in Chennai have helped to shape these services after the foundation was laid.'

—Poonam Natarajan, Vidyasagar, 2015

Prarthana and Her Mother Prety Kutty, journalist

'She doesn't know it yet, but Dr Alur has made me fearless.

Our world, the one where special kids and their parents live, has always been a closed and protected one. It's been a world where we would take our special kids to special schools and to social gatherings that either comprised immediate family (who knew that we had a special kid) or to those parties that involved a whole bunch of special kids as guests or hosts.

Never did we venture into territories that had 'normal' set-ups, unless we could leave our special kids at home with someone. It wasn't that we were ashamed of our kids ... it's just that the thought of people staring at our kids warded off any thoughts of involving our special kids in 'normal' social situations. This was our world ... a world where we prided ourselves as 'wonderful parents to our special children'.

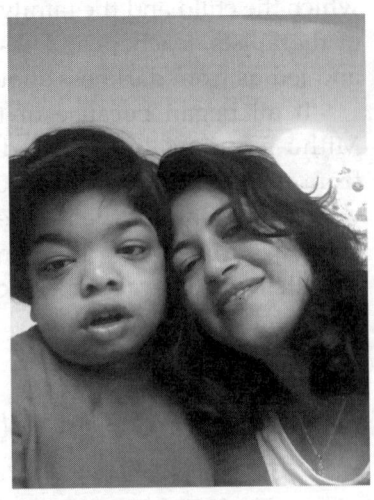

But the grotesque truth was that we had cut ourselves off from the rest of society … simply because we were afraid of answering sympathetically annoying questions posed by the people we would have to encounter. We had built our own fortresses around our families and we guarded them well.

I lived in one such fortress. I had a 10-year-old special child, Prarthana, and a 4-year-old bubbly Shivakshi, a normal child. I don't seem to remember too many instances where I had lowered the defences of my fortress and socialized with the parents of normal kids from Shivakshi's school.

It just seemed too threatening to interact with parents of normal kids, in spite of the fact that I had a normal kid myself. This was my world…. The one I had encased myself in. That's when I got an opportunity to work with Dr Alur at ADAPT. It was her absolute confidence and zeal in the whole concept of inclusion that caught me unaware. She believed in including our special kids into normal schools … Lord! That was something as frightening as the annihilation of the planet!! The very thought gave me goose bumps on my skin!!

But her conviction was so strong that every time she would mention the word 'inclusion', even in informal conversations, she would exude a sense of determination. Her brow would frown a little, her eyes would gleam and she would have this deep soulful look … every time she broached this topic. For some reason, in spite of my initial wary self, I wanted to share her optimism and determination. The more I interacted with her, the stronger my heart felt.

It was not long before I was willing to open the gates of my fortress and walk right out … baring myself and my special child to society … unashamed … unfettered.

Suddenly, it was a new me. I stopped trying to quieten my child at public places, I stopped hurrying at family dinners just because my non-verbal special child was throwing a tantrum, I stopped squeezing my special child against me in the elevator to keep her from reaching out to another person. I simply stopped being the buffer that I had been all these years. For once, I let society take responsibility for my special child.

And it felt like heaven! It felt like a ton had been removed off my shoulders. It felt like the world was whole again. It brought peace and tranquility back into my life.

Yes, this is my child, born out of me … but I will not hide her in a fortress just because she is special. She is a part of society … and she will need to be accepted as an individual. And if push comes to shove, I will not hesitate to wage war against stereotypical social norms. I don't think I will rest until society opens its heart to special needs. It's the future of our children … all our children.

Thank you Dr Alur for being so brave and for raking up the bravery in my heart. Bless you.'

Nihit and His Mother Mrinal Agarwal

'Today, I want to thank the school for giving a definite direction to Nihit's education and life. I want to thank the school for daring to think that our very special children can go through mainstream education and for making it happen too!

Thank you, school, for providing an opportunity to Nihit to grow in as normal an environment (inclusion) as is possible. Thank you for the joy of train rides, visits to temples, churches, mosques, police stations, concerts and picnics. Thank you for helping Nihit grow up to his potential.'

Abdul and His Mother Alifiya Kadir

'It has only been a year at this wonderful organization and the changes I see in Abdul are so many. He has started talking, has become more confident and academically, too, he has shown interest and progress. The teachers and volunteers are full of passion and so dedicated. With a heavy heart, we are moving residence to Madhya Pradesh. But before we leave, a very big Thank You to Dr Alur for creating and developing such a school…. It is a heaven for disabled students!'

Analysis

The new process of partnering with parents in the management of their children built up trust and made them key resource members in the continuum of support needed in the inclusive process. In addition to managing their children at home, parents were encouraged to become professionals and become teachers, therapists, principals of schools and are now in management positions (Alur 2010b).

Lessons Learnt

- Parents as professionals changed the dynamics of dealing with parents in India, giving them a status they lacked earlier.
- *Professionalism combined with care* changed the lives of families with severely disabled children and the new approach of treating parents as important voices to listen to helped to change the situation for hundreds of parents in the subcontinent.

The next decade of service shows that, given the confidence, parents and family members played a key role in expanding services.

Domain IV

Training

Background: To Fill the Gap Where There Were No Teachers

Next, we tackled manpower by way of training teachers, therapists, social workers, psychologists and so on. Earlier in India, special education teachers were trained in short-term in-service education programmes and certificate programmes or they went abroad to train in special education. National agencies of education like National Council of Educational Research and Training (NCERT), National University of Educational Planning and Administration (NUEPA), National Council for Teacher Education (NCTE) did not include special needs in their curriculum. Teacher training in teaching children with disability was under the guidance of national institutes for the handicapped and some NGOs and even so cerebral palsy (CP) was not covered in the curriculum.

To fill this gap, The Spastics Society of India (SSI) began courses in 1977.

Method

The first postgraduate diploma course in the education of the physically handicapped (name changed to Postgraduate Diploma in Special Education [Multiple Disabilities: Physical and Neurological in 2003]) was set up in the country in 1978.

The course aimed to develop the skills, abilities and knowledge of teacher trainees to meet the physical, educational, social and emotional needs of persons with physical and neurological disability. The curriculum was developed in collaboration with specialists from the British Council, Spastics Society of the UK and the Institute of Education, University of London. Many external faculties from overseas have visited the

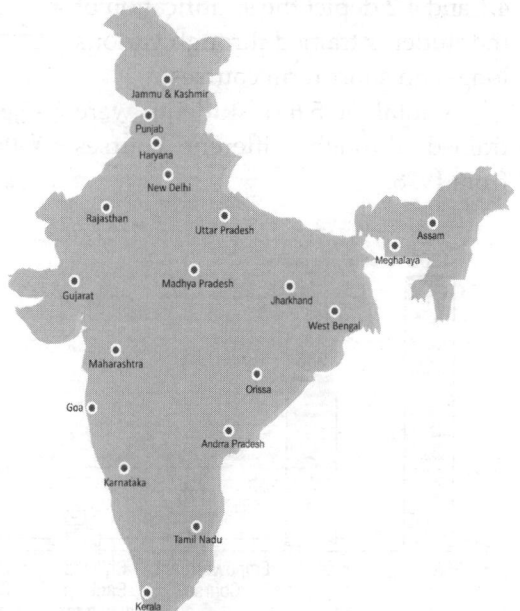

Over four hundred teachers across the nation have been trained

This figure is not to scale. It does not represent any authentic national or international boundaries and is used for illustrative purposes only.

organization and enhanced the knowledge base of the trainees, especially Mr Leslie Gardner, principal psychologist, Spastics Society of UK, and Dr Klaus Wedell, director of special education and psychological needs, Institute of Education. The course was a blend of theory and practice: extensive teaching practicum, case studies, a dissertation, a remedial kit and a range of school visits and classroom observations made it broad-based, addressing a range of classroom difficulties. In the 2000s, the course also focused on action towards the achievement of universal elementary education, one that includes children with disabilities in the mainstream education system.

The course got affiliated to the University of Mumbai in 1983 and was granted permanent recognition by the Rehabilitation Council of India (RCI), a statutory body regulating training programmes in the field of disability.

The pre-service Teacher Training Course (TTC) has, since its inception, trained 410 special educators till 2010; the Community Initiatives in Inclusion (CII) course has trained 228 master trainers from the Asia Pacific region since 2002; the short-term six-month programmes of inclusion course and Early Childhood Care and Education (ECCE) have trained 57 trainees till now. Mothers, siblings and other family members of children with CP and other multiple disabilities as well as young graduates from different disciplines constitute the alumni of the course. Figures 4.1 and 4.2 depict the stratification of the students trained through various long- and short-term courses.

A total of 5,694 students were trained through different courses from 1978.

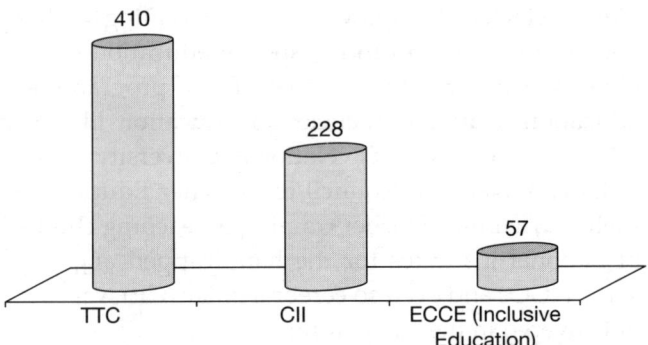

Figure 4.1. Stratification of Number of Students Trained Through Various Courses—Long-term Training Courses

Source: Research Action Committee.

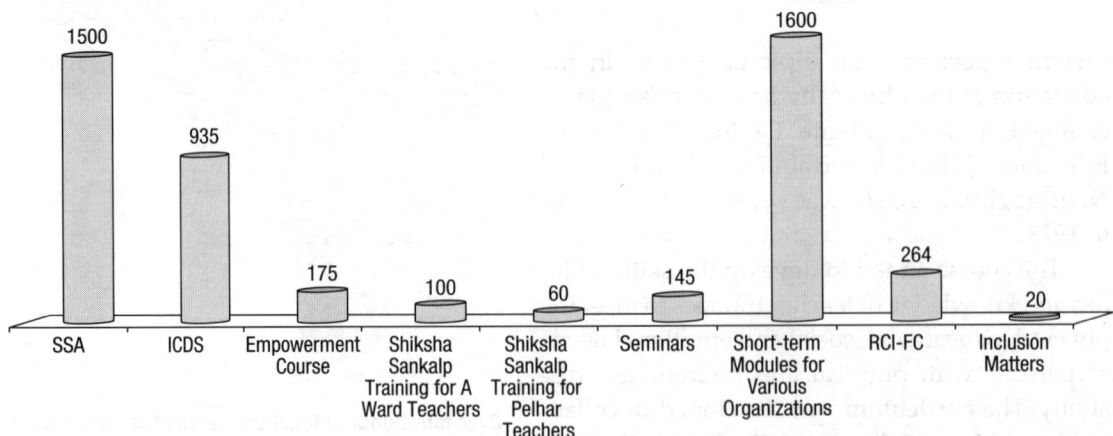

Figure 4.2. Stratification of Number of Students Trained Through Various Courses—Short-term Training Courses

Source: Research Action Committee.

Digitization of Library Services at ADAPT
(Able Disabled All People Together)

In the fourth decade, a path-breaking initiative undertaken by the library and media resource team at ADAPT has been the digitization of ADAPT's library services. No mean task, the vision behind it was to facilitate, for all, access to the rich experience and expertise gathered at ADAPT over the past four decades.

The project emerged from a series of high-level meetings between Dr Mithu Alur, founder chairperson, ADAPT, Dr Ekkerhard Henschke, former head, library services, Leipzig University, Ms Arati Sriram and Ms Malini Chib, the then head of library services, ADAPT. Taking place between Mumbai and London, the outcome of these meetings was a very fruitful one. It was decided that Dr Henschke would identify and depute two librarians from Germany who would undertake an internship of three months' duration at ADAPT, India, thus initiating the process of digitization. The Greenstone digitization software was identified as being the most suitable since it was already being used in India and there existed a support group for the same among the users.

What Is Greenstone?

Greenstone Digital Library Software is an open source software for building and distributing digital library collections. While produced by the New Zealand Digital Library Project at the University of Waikato, it is developed and distributed in cooperation with the United Nations Educational, Scientific and Cultural Organization (UNESCO) and the Human Info NGO.

Technically, Greenstone runs on all versions of Windows, Unix/Linux and Mac OS X, which gives it a wide range of application within miscellaneous conditions of given facilities within an organization. The lack of configuration necessary to get Greenstone started makes it very easy to install. Using contemporary standards such as Open Archives Protocol for Metadata Harvesting (OAI-PMH), Greenstone is highly interoperable and allows one to include harvested documents into its collection. Furthermore, Greenstone is able to export collections to METS and can ingest documents in METS form. Collections also can be exported to DSpace and any DSpace collection can be imported into Greenstone.

The software comes along with two interactive interfaces: one for the user and one for the librarian. The user interface operates within the locally installed web browser and enables the user to access the digital library and to search and browse within it. The librarian interface is a Java-based graphical interface where material for the collection can easily be gathered or even be downloaded from the web. The librarian interface is also the part where the collected material will be enriched by adding metadata. It also enables the librarian to design the searching and browsing facilities that the collection will offer the user and build and serve the collection.

Another great benefit of Greenstone Digital Library Software is its ability to handle several formats of documents such as: PDF, Word, RTF, HTML, Excel, PPT, Email (various formats), source code, any kind of images, including GIF, JIF, JPEG, TIFF formats, as well as audio formats like MP3, OGG, MPEG, MIDI and so on.

Ms Annika Fricke and Ms Meike Gran spent three months at ADAPT. Dr Alur guided them in drawing up a work breakdown structure based on the results based management system, which clearly listed the tasks that would be undertaken in the three-month period and the time frame and performance indicators for the same. Dr Alur also introduced Ms Fricke and Ms Gran to the vast archives of the organization. To create these archives, all available information was compiled together, categorized and catalogued. Appropriate themes were created to make retrieval simpler. The archival section, housed at our headquarters in Colaba, is of tremendous help in compiling a historical account of the four eventful decades, spanning the work of what was once known as SSI, eventually evolving into ADAPT. Later, Sujata Verma, as senior librarian, catalogued the archival sections in preparation for this retrospective study

The Greenstone software was installed, in 2008, in the library computers at Bandra and Colaba. A day-long workshop on the operation of Greenstone was held by Dr Shubhada Nagarkar for a core team to familiarize them with the functions of the software.

Till date, over a thousand documents consisting of speeches, published articles, newspaper reports, presentations, newsletters, brochures, literature reviews, annual reports, posters, photographs, films and fact sheets have been catalogued, scanned and uploaded. Furthermore, metadata has been added with a view to enabling users to access material on the basis of authors, topics, keywords, dates and occasions. A list of keywords has been created by Dr Henschke and is being continually updated. By the end of the first three months, the catalogue contained 10 annual reports, 24 items of audio-video material, 268 books, 18 brochures, 4 charters, 13 E-journals, 6 fact sheets, 4 flipcharts, 3 journals, 4 literature reviews, 11 newspapers, 7,881 newspaper clippings, 1 OHP slide, 69 papers presented at conferences and seminars, 35 photographs, 15 posters, 130 presentations, 55 published articles, 108 research publications, 20 seminar papers, 75 speeches and 2 theses.

Additionally, example templates for document type/format had been created, which defines which metadata to add to which type of document/material within the collection. Referring to these example entries, people would easily be able to work on further entries of documents to the collection by keeping its inner structure.

This digitization continues, and over time, will serve to permit users across the world access to the work being done at ADAPT.

Training and Capacity Building: Results and Outcomes

- A method of decentralization began and the result was that full-fledged courses were begun in other SSI's of Delhi, Kolkata, Chennai and Bangalore. On the national level, the students who had come to Mumbai for training went back to their own states/countries and started services for children with disabilities based on the Mumbai model. Thus, new services began in 18 regions of India including Kolkata, Chennai and Delhi. Our Management in Cerebral Palsy (MCP) alumni now works in hospitals, private clinics, schools and NGOs in Maharashtra, Andhra Pradesh, Karnataka, Tamil Nadu, Gujarat, Madhya Pradesh, Himachal Pradesh and Pakistan.
- Spreading awareness with Government of India agencies, the Rehabilitation Council of India (RCI) requested us to conduct short training programmes and workshops for the State

Council for Education Research and Training (SCERT), the District Institute of Education and Training (DIET), zilla parishads, the Department of Education, Brihanmumbai Municipal Corporation (BMC) and the Statewide Massive and Rigorous Training for Primary Teachers (SMART-PT). As a result, collaboration took place between DIET, District Primary Education Programme (DPEP), BMC, Maharashtra Prathamik Shikshan Parishad (Maharashtra Primary Education Council–Education Department of the State Government of Maharashtra) and SCERT.

- Orientations were also conducted for students of the various schools and colleges.
- Training was geared towards enhancing and empowering the stakeholders of other mainstream schools, parents, volunteers, community workers and disabled activists.
- Capacity building and empowerment of community teachers were carried out through short-term courses.
- At the national level, two one-month RCI bridge courses for teachers and volunteers working in special schools were also introduced.
- This engagement with the state districts and the centre slowly put CP on the map of the country.

Impact of Teacher Training by Professionals and What They Said

Chandrika Maheshwari—consultant special educator, honorary consultant and trainer for the resource support team at Muktangan

'The teachers training course at SSI was so intense that it opened up my life to special needs and disability. Today, it's my life. What I learnt at SSI as a teacher transformed my life. It made me understand my own potential as special educator, as a human being. It touched every aspect of my life. Being a professional in this field has been very fulfilling as it brings out new challenges every day and constantly keeps me motivated.'

Charanjit Kaur—senior special educator, Bombay Cambridge, Andheri East

'I did the course in 1992–93. The course was very comprehensive and touched upon all aspects of special education equally. I don't think there is any other course which addresses all disabilities. All other courses are very specific to one disability. It has equipped me to cater to all children in my mainstream school, irrespective of their ability/disability and make a difference to their lives. It would be helpful if courses like these can be extended to a Master's degree and SSI could take the lead.'

Sangeeta Jagtiani—deputy director services/head of education, ADAPT

'I joined SSI as a volunteer and interacting with the students led me to do TTC at SSI in 1992–93. The course exposed me to the different aspects of disabilities, their unique abilities and the multi-level teaching aspects that make a huge impact to the learning process of the children. It changed the way I 'think'. While putting into practice my knowledge, it was here that I later got exposure to inclusive education. As I facilitated the transfer of students from special education to mainstream education in mainstream schools, I saw them flower and bloom achieving their maximum potential. This added another dimension to me as an educator and as a professional.'

Deepshikha Mathur—deputy director training, ADAPT

'My goal to work for children with special needs was kindled during graduation when a special educator working with Action for Ability Development and Inclusion (AADI), Delhi, introduced us to special education. SSI became my ultimate goal. This was realized when I did my TTC in 2001; despite being from a psychology background, for the first time I felt that I had entered a profession that I was comfortable in. TTC taught me about all disabilities and not just one. It gave a holistic perception and made me work on difficulties and weakness of our children instead of disability. Over the years, this inclusive perspective has helped me grow professionally and personally and I am able to work with diversity and think in a wide framework.'

Sharmila Donde—deputy director, training

'When I joined the TTC course, I was like a blank slate... I did not know anything about disability.

I just had the desire to work in this field. The TTC sensitized me and made me aware of the persons with disability and their needs and rights. The course equipped me with attitude, skills and knowledge to work in the field of inclusion. It not only gave me the knowledge about disability, teaching strategies, the principles of inclusion but also helped me think laterally and creatively to find solutions to my difficulties. This course gave me the confidence and experience to teach children with disabilities and later on as a teacher-educator to transfer the attitude, knowledge and skills to other trainees.'

Voices of TTC Students

Lawrence Admont, a French citizen and a nurse by profession, completed the TTC as an internal student. Her aim was to start her own centre in Bhuj, Gujarat, that would provide all facilities under one roof for children with disabilities. There are at present very few such centres in Bhuj. Her dedication and commitment to work for disabled children helped her overcome the challenges she faced in understanding the language and context of another country. The dictionary was her constant companion in the initial months. Lawrence passed the examinations with flying colours and over the last year has started a small inclusive centre called Asha Kiran in Bhuj with seven children of different disabilities.

Aditi Shardul is a highly motivated and committed single mother of a boy with CP. She joined the course to get to better understand her child. After completing the course, she wanted to start a support group for parents of children with CP and has created a website for parents named spasticsinfo.com which she supports. Aditi has also conducted workshops and compiled a booklet for parents entitled *Parenting Differently*.

Anjum Gupta is a teacher in a school run by the Navi Mumbai Municipal Corporation. She joined the foundation course as a part of the in-service training offered by the Navi Mumbai

Municipal Corporation. With the new knowledge, she realized that her 16-year-old cousin studying in a mainstream school in Santacruz exhibited the difficulties faced by children with dyslexia. His parents and teachers regarded him as lazy and a slow learner. She immediately brought the child to us for guidance. We referred him to the learning difficulties clinic at the Sion Hospital and guided them to apply for concessions from the state board.

Mr Godbole has put in 20 years of service in a Thane Municipal Corporation School as a drawing teacher. After the contact sessions, he and his ten colleagues decided to pass the knowledge on to other teachers in their ward. They acquired a Marathi booklet on disability from the Sarva Shiksha Abhiyan (SSA) coordinator. They created an awareness generating module and, with the help of a ward officer, delivered it at a meeting of 100 teachers. The programme was a success and they are motivated to conduct similar programmes in future for different target groups.

Father Vincent Lourdoswamy came to attend the course when he was appointed director of Snehalaya, in Pune, a special centre for children with CP. After finishing the course, he introduced inclusion in his centre and sent four children from his centre to mainstream school. The centre had invited staff from ADAPT to continue conducting a training programme for all their staff.

Domain V

Capacity Building in the Community

Background: Dharavi and Karuna Sadan— Strengthening the Community

We then moved into the community and began working at Dharavi, Asia's biggest slum. The manifestation of 'raw poverty' is certainly the case in the slum of Dharavi.

Amartya Sen (1981), writing about poverty, says,

> There is indeed much that is transparent about poverty … and one does not need elaborate criteria or cunning measurement or probing analysis to recognise raw poverty (cited in Alur 1998: 27).

An endemic problem in India is heavy migration of rural population to the urban areas, as governments have not been able to provide the basic necessities of healthcare, education, employment, water and sanitation in rural areas. In India, the word 'slum' connotes absence of proper housing, lack of basic amenities such as water, drainage, sewage, unhealthy and unhygienic environment with high levels of pollution, as a result of excessive urbanization and population explosion (Alur 1988; De Souza 1978; Desai and Pillai 1970; Roy and Dasgupta 1995; Singh and Pothen 1982). Most metropolitan cities in India now have an average of 40 to 60 per cent of the population living in slums which are called *jhopadpattis*, *chawls* and *jhuggis* (Alur 2003).[1] In Mumbai alone, 50 per cent or more live in slums situated in the inner city and over 20 per cent of them in Dharavi slum alone. Seventy-five per cent of the children are further disadvantaged as they come from impoverished backgrounds. In our work with children with disability and adults and their families, we have found that majority of the people we serve are from the lower middle class.

The Spastics Society of India (SSI) had mounted a survey of 11,820 households (Billimoria and Krishnaswamy 1986), examining the prevalence and incidence of disabilities among children in the city of Mumbai. The study revealed that 63 per cent of them are from lower income

---

[1] *Jhopadpattis*: An Indian term to describe slum-like conditions and people living not in proper concrete housing but in huts or shacks in a shanty town spread. *Chawls*: An Indian term for a slum in the cities. A common characteristic of all slums is substandard housing and lack of basic amenities such as water and sewage facilities. *Jhuggis*: An Indian term for slum dwelling typically made of mud and corrugated iron.

groups (the family's total income not more than ₹1,000 per month) and the largest concentration of children with disabilities was in the areas where the slums of the city were situated.

We began working in Dharavi around 1983 when the late Junie Bose, our honorary secretary, started a clinic with an NGO in the slum. The wife of the then governor of Maharashtra[2] Mrs Bilkees Latif, a very active, socially committed person who also was working in Dharavi, invited us to start schools in Dharavi. Junie and I decided to start a new model which was going to be our community model. We met Mrs Latif and discussed about the space we would need. Space in the city of Mumbai is a precious commodity—mostly a possibility out of the reach of a common city dweller. We were, however, fortunate to have her support. She had seen and appreciated our work. We were offered two large halls and two small rooms to start our school. We began providing treatment and educational facilities, and called the project Karuna Sadan.

Thanks to Mrs Latif, the Centre for Developmental Disabilities began at the community-based hospital Urban Health Centre, Dharavi, in 1985. It had an excellent location, situated right in the heart of Dharavi. Junie Bose, Deepak Kalra, Varsha Hooja and, later, Shabnam Rangwala were the pioneers (after Junie passed away) in the community development work.

Mumbai is divided into 21 wards for administrative purposes and Dharavi is situated in ward 'G' (see Figure: Ward-wise map of Mumbai). Devoid of any greenery (playground or park) dusty and dirty, it is sprawled over 175 hectares. Dharavi is a densely populated neighbourhood and the streets and doorways are filled with people coming and going or crowding all the time. The housing in Dharavi is made up of squatter constructions and improvised shelters of pavement dwellers. The dwellings are made of a variety of materials and there are open drains between the closely packed huts called *chawls*. A typical hut is a small space of 10 by 10 feet, dark, windowless, with an average family of five to seven members living in it. Sanitary conditions are practically non-existent and potable water is scarce, available only once during the day (Alur 1988).

All the common factors which characterize slums are present in Dharavi: sub-standard housing, congestion and overcrowding, lack of drainage and sewage disposal, lack of clean water facilities, lack of access to nutrition and other basic goods and environmental

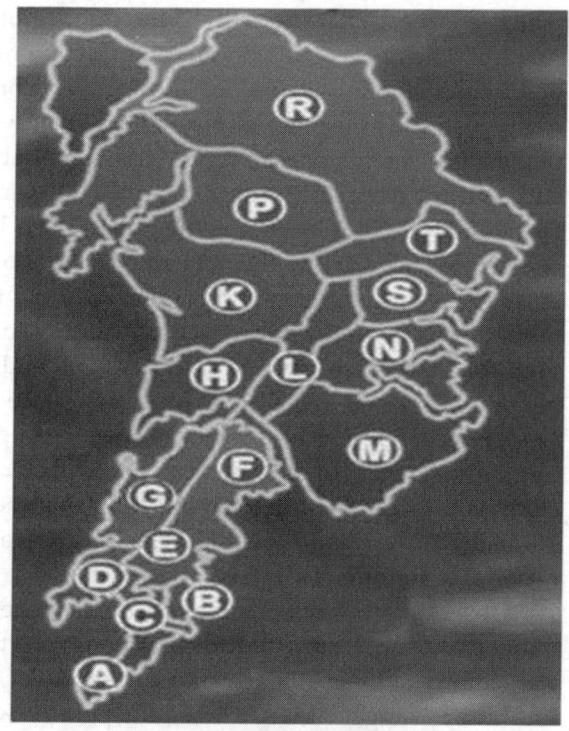

Ward-wise map of Bombay

---

[2] His Excellency Idris Latif and the governor who succeeded him was His Excellency Shri Sadiq Ali.

deterioration, all of which result in high rates of infection and disease (Ibid 1988). Inhabitants of Dharavi live in extremely overcrowded conditions, with little or no privacy.

Yet, the sense of community is quite strong. In our experience, people here have a relatively integrated, satisfying and self-sufficient culture. They receive a lot of support and strength from each other. Quite often, neighbours will accompany families to the hospital or be there for comfort in case of accidents—little gestures, performed instinctively for each other, that the rich and affluent do not have time for.

I found Dharavi an exciting place to work in. It was vibrant, multi-cultural, multi-lingual, multi-religious, actually a microcosm of India, with many common places of worship, temples, mosques and churches next to each other. It bustles with entrepreneurial activities. Small shops dot the lanes and by-lanes. We actually do not find many beggars. Majority of the work force belongs to the unorganized and informal sector, involved in unskilled or semi-skilled work. They are engaged in trades such as broom-making, rag-picking, fishing, and leatherwork. Most of the city's domestic labour comes from Dharavi. The women usually work as maids, cooks, sweepers or have menial factory jobs. Other skilled labour force includes plumbers, electricians, carpenters and drivers.

Dharavi is also home to a variety of entrepreneurial businesses (medical stores, tea stalls, tanneries, grocery shops, sweet shops, *paan-bidi* shops and ration shops. The economic traits which are most characteristic of the culture of poverty, including the constant struggle for survival, unemployment and underemployment, low wages, a miscellany of unskilled occupations, child labour, the absence of savings, a chronic shortage of cash and the absence of food reserves in the home, are all present in Dharavi. Many of Mumbai's affluent residents swear that the best leather bags and brief cases are to be found in Dharavi and the best fried fish and kababs came from Koliwada, Dharavi! The average earning in Dharavi is around ₹2,500–3,000 per month (₹1,500, now, being the poverty line in India, approximately £25 per month).

Before I began work there, I had no idea about its culture. People in these areas could speak as many as nine different languages. Running through Dharavi is an intensity of feeling and human warmth and a strong sense of individuality. I found a huge capacity for joy, gaiety, a hope for a better life, a desire to understand and to love and a readiness to share whatever little people possess; all in the midst of a great sense of trade and business.

Above all, I found resilience in the face of grinding poverty that besieges the people who live there. If you visit their homes, they will always drag up their best chair or spread their best cloth on the floor for you to sit on. After that they will proceed to make you a cup of *chai* (tea). No matter how poor they are, I have always found in them a marvellous sense of caring and hospitality for others.

Observing the children face obstacles to get educated, we found that the situation was in many ways similar to what was happening in the rest of India. Gender bias was quite strong, particularly amongst the Muslim community (Alur 2007). Girls were kept at home in order to look after younger siblings, when the parents went to work. *In such a milieu, children are at high risk of lagging behind in education and acquiring secondary difficulties. So we began tackling some of the challenges related to the children of Dharavi* (Alur and Bach 2010). Figure 5.1 shows the number of children with disabilities admitted to ADAPT (Able Disabled All People Together).

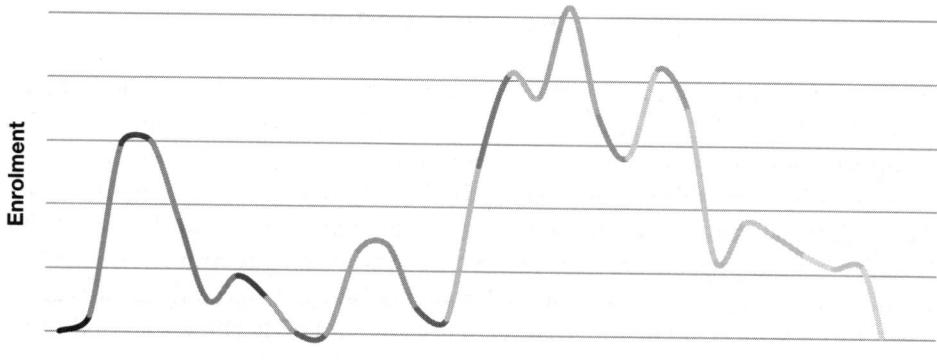

Year 1985 to 2012

Figure 5.1. Number of Children with Disabilities Admitted to ADAPT Community Services
Source: Research Action Committee.

Using the 10-point assessment scale, Rajiv Gandhi Nagar area in Dharavi was surveyed for incidence of disability. Parents were encouraged to enrol children below 5 years to ADAPT pre-schools. Since the research area was then an 'unauthorized' slum, the Integrated Child Development Scheme (ICDS) *anganwadi* was not available. Naturally, this cohort was deprived of nutrition supplements and automatic immunization. During the 30 years of functioning, 1,300 pre-schoolers were given pre-reading and pre-writing activities to help with their social and emotional development. Although randomized control trials were not conducted, qualitative data on improvement in social and communication skills was gathered through focus group discussions and personal interviews with parents. Without the pre-schools, these children would have stayed out of schools because the majority of them have no birth records, and living in 'unauthorized' areas means they have no legal rights to health, education or any service rightfully available to any citizen.

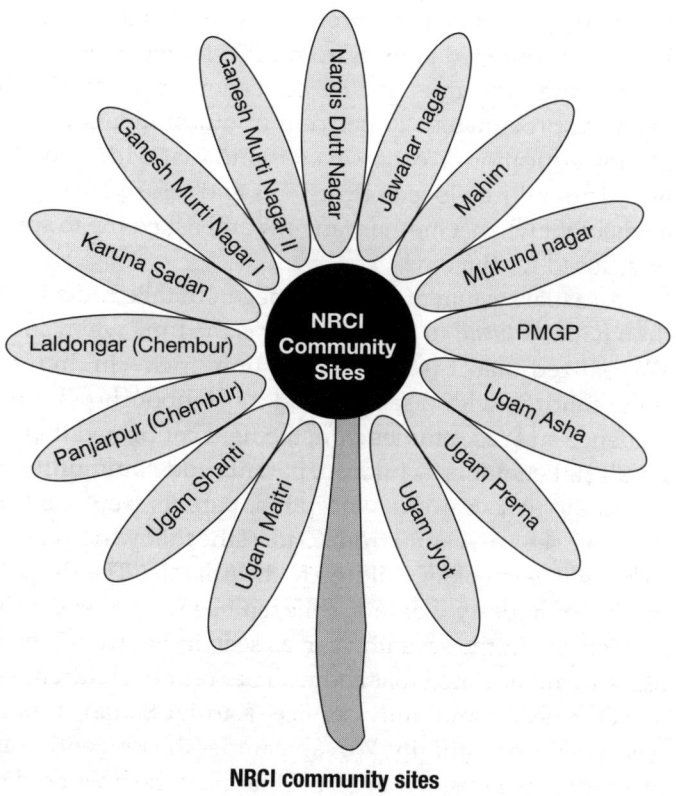

NRCI community sites

Inclusion Begins

A demonstration model of inclusion in the community called *Ugam* (The Beginning) began. Started by Dr Madhuri Pai in early 1999, five pre-school facilities called 'Ugam' were set up with support from the Canadian Development Fund. This was to be our new model of inclusion wherein disabled children as well as children without disability would study and play together. This was the source of the new National Resource Centre for Inclusion (NRCI)-I project. The idea was to provide services along the lines of the government's ICDS schemes. The ICDS operated 166 *anganwadis* in Dharavi; however, these covered only 25 per cent of the population. We located areas of Dharavi that were not covered by ICDS. We started five pre-schools following the ICDS norms of a *balwadi* for every 100 households. The target beneficiaries were all children in the age group of 2–5 years. We made sure that there was no discrimination on account of religion, caste, gender, socio-economic status or disability.

As we worked in the area not serviced by *anganwadis*, we got a spontaneous response from the community. Each Ugam pre-school enrolled between 70–90 children. A quick, easy to administer, 10-point screening and placement test was used to identify disabilities if any. All children attended Ugam nurseries for three hours. Teachers lived in the same neighbourhood and were trained by SSI. Unlike ICDS, nutrition supplements and meals were not given. Even so, we did not have any problems like low attendance or irregularity. Many children over five years of age, with disability and who had no previous access to educational services, also started attending Ugam. We also encouraged parents from ICDS target areas to have their children join the *anganwadis*.

For the first time, quality education and effective treatment services were accessible to them. Approximately 20 per cent of our students were the first generation in their family to get any education. We, however, found that with a good 'head start' programme they did very well. The children loved our schools and refused to stay at home even on holidays! I remember an incident when a mother rang me and asked me to speak to her child and tell him that school was closed for the day!

A casual system of inclusion began to take roots in the community. For the first time, children had a *balwadi* to go to! That was the time when suddenly there was a spurt in enrolment. We realized that it is a myth that only 'rich' children can learn to be educated. For the first time, children with disability had a neighbourhood *balwadi* they can go to! A lot of anecdotal evidence and case studies from the field confirmed that this inclusion experiment was working for all stakeholders—children, parents and community teachers.

In the first year of its inception, parents were a bit hesitant to send disabled children to a inclusive set-up. A jump from 63 to 92 the following year was because of the parents volunteering to bring in even older children to the *balwadis*. The drop in 2004 occurred when, with the efforts of our community workers, children began to attend neighbourhood government schools. The sudden rise in the seventh year, as seen in Figure 5.2, needs a closer look but a preliminary age assessment indicated that about 35 per cent of children were not eligible to enter formal school.

Our next community service, Karuna Sadan, was the first example of a hospital-school based in the community. We came under the Preventive and Social Medicine (PSM) Department of a municipal hospital in Sion, Dharavi, which worked on identification, early childhood education, treatment, parent training, counselling for children with disability and their families and all the services that SSI was experienced in delivering. In the beginning, to ensure enrolment, we

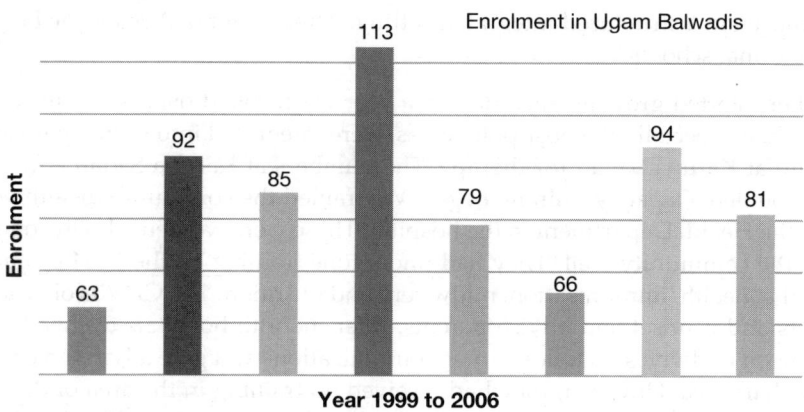

Figure 5.2. Shows Enrolments During the Project Period
Source: Research Action Committee.

ran a door-to-door campaign to identify children to be enrolled. Simple handouts were made to spread awareness about the work of the centre. The general awareness about disability and more specifically about the need for education of the disabled was abysmally low.

The first question we were asked was, 'Can my child be educated?' It is this lack of awareness that would remind me of those painful early days in my own life when such a question would be in my mind too—a question asked all too frequently in the community. Fortunately, our two site supervisors—Gulab Sayed and Ishwar Tayade—were from the community.

When we first started and used to go into the community, parents asked, '*Kya apang bachcha padh sakta hai?*' (Can a disabled child study?)

'*Mera bachcha leta hi rehta hai—woh baith hi nahi sakta, padhega aur likhega kaise?*' (My child can only lie down. He/she cannot sit, how will he/she read and write?)

'*Woh to theek se bol bhi nahin sakta, aap isko padhaoge kaise?*' (He/she cannot speak properly, how will you teach him?)

Site supervisor Sayed said, 'We encouraged parents to bring in their children and see how the other children were being taught. When they witnessed this, they began to have faith in our programme and asked other parents to come in too.'

Deepak Kalra, mother of Vikram who had CP and who had begun several services in Rajasthan, writes:

'The first service to be started was the therapy unit. Community workers reached the beneficiaries and made them aware of the services and how it would change the lives of children at home. Large numbers started coming for therapy and parents wanted more and more service for their children. I was asked to take charge and start expanding services as per needs of the children. Varsha and I started off and it was an overwhelming experience.'

'We started a play group where children could come and play with the toys (that we had collected from all the classes of the Colaba centre). This brought in a large number of children with disability along with their siblings and neighbours. It was difficult to tell any child who was out of school not to come, at the same time our resources were so meagre, we could only reach limited numbers. This was the beginning of integrating disabled and normal children in a structured integrated setting. After a stint of 3 years, we began to put them into normal schools.'

'The numbers started growing each day. In a year we enrolled over 300 children. A large number of them, specially the post-polio cases, were integrated into municipal schools and followed up at Karuna Sadan for therapy. The numbers at Karuna Sadan education programmes doubled. Capacity training began. We trained the community health volunteers (CHVs) of the Health Department in the hospital. These were women who lived in Dharavi and knew the community well. They had undergone training by the PSM Department of the hospital in health, immunisation, midwifery and nutrition. The CHV's role was to make house visits and counsel and advise parents, refer them to hospitals to give birth rather than relying on midwives, to follow up on immunizations and give advice on common ailments like diarrhoea. However, they had received no training in the area of disability. We prepared a one-month module on causes and identification of disability. The CHVs then went into the community and spoke to parents and began referring children to the school. In the first few years, the CHVs had to physically go to individual homes and take the children to school, as the parents all worked and could not bring them to the school on time. They were then dropped back home by the CHVs, who were our representatives in the community. Four CHVs were later employed as full-time staff on our project. Courses were also conducted for others working in the Health Department, such as Auxiliary Nurses, CHVs, Community Nurses, Multipurpose Rehabilitation Workers, *Anganwadi* workers and *Balwadi* workers. It was important that they understood how critical early education was and promoted it in the community. As they were the stakeholders they could reach out to the community and could advise mothers on issues related to their children.'

'This is how demystification of disability began in the community. The nurses were trained to do physio and speech therapy, moving the focus away from the 'specialist approach' to a 'community approach', sowing the seeds in the community to take ownership of their programs. Karuna Sadan became a kind of oasis, serving as a Resource Centre for all the children and their families in Dharavi. The community workers were very creative in designing educational aids and toys from recycled material which was cost effective and cost neutral. In fact, the success we have had in training the community workers demonstrated that disability-related needs could be addressed without specialisation.'

1. Children in the deprived areas are undernourished. We networked with existing programmes in the area. United Nations Children's Fund (UNICEF) had a nutrition programme. We immediately linked up with them.
2. The families were given fortified *atta* (wheat flour) and milk powder.
3. We also approached the Dadar Catering College to help develop some recipes of fortified *atta* and teach them to the mothers. This got the families interested in the *atta* which they started collecting regularly. A large number of students were also put on the mid-day meal programme.
4. Linking with Sion Hospital, they started their project of providing supplementary vitamins, especially Vitamin A to all children at Dharavi.
5. The backgrounds of children were very different from what we were used to in our centres. Coming from an unprivileged background, the children would use abusive language. This needed addressing. The staff learnt about the differences very quickly and adjusted.
6. Networking was essential. Many family issues like domestic violence, alcoholic and abusive fathers, polygamy and so on were addressed. We approached the Tata Institute of Social

Sciences (TISS) who sent their postgraduate trainees regularly for field placement. These trainees visited the homes of children to work on family problems.

It was found that a large number of children who had polio had actually been inoculated with the vaccine, but had still acquired polio. The cold storage chain had broken somewhere, making the vaccine ineffective. The issue was raised in the press, which brought this grave mishap in focus. Several inquiries were set up and a major anti-polio campaign was launched by Polio Plus. This helped bring down polio cases substantially (Ibid 2015).

The area of Dharavi as a whole is a hive of activity. Nine out of 10 people there have jobs, some of them within Dharavi itself, working in thousands of small workshops. Hamish McRae writes in his book *What Works* about the inclusive nurseries:

I began to understand (Dharavi) when I walked round it. My guide was Dr Mithu Alur, a long-standing friend, best known for founding one of the country's largest educational charities, SSI. The society pioneered the provision of services for people with CP and more recently has been promoting the policy of inclusion of people with handicaps into the mainstream educational system. But the particular reason for Mithu showing us around Dharavi was because of her organization's role in setting up primary schools for the poor.

After a few minutes you arrive at the school.... There is a circle of children sitting round the teacher; a few evidently handicapped in some way, bright and obviously eager to learn and all of them shining. This is the first of two shifts of children and this particular class is for infants. They are being taught the basic skills of reading, identifying objects, using their hands—the usual curriculum of any more conventional primary school.

For many of these children, this is probably the only education they will get. If you shut your eyes to the surroundings and just kneel down with the children, talk to them and play with them, as Mithu made us do, you could be anywhere in the world. Primary school kids are the same everywhere. I was told that parents want their children to be taught English, particularly if they do not speak it themselves, because they know this is a pathway towards better jobs. So the schools teach English.

Here there was a lesson. The most effective way to assist a deprived but vibrant economic region is to attend to detail and to listen to the voices on the ground. One such example, and I am sure there are many more, is the work of SSI—work which I felt privileged to catch a glimpse of. One of the key points of its operation is that it is not a 'Lady Bountiful' charity. Yes, it is a charity, but thanks in part to the fact that the educational services it provides are in part paid for, it is an economically sensitive provider. It gives people the things they really want, which among other things is education for their children. The broader message here is that anyone seeking to intervene in the hugely complex economic interactions that take place in a complicated, if informal, city must listen to the signals of the market to show what people really want, rather than impose some theoretical solution to perceived problems. If you listen to what people want, you may get it right. If you impose an external solution, even if it seems to have been successful elsewhere, you are liable to get it wrong. (McRae 2010)

A message which we found to be really true, with ground reality doing bottom-up, ground level work!

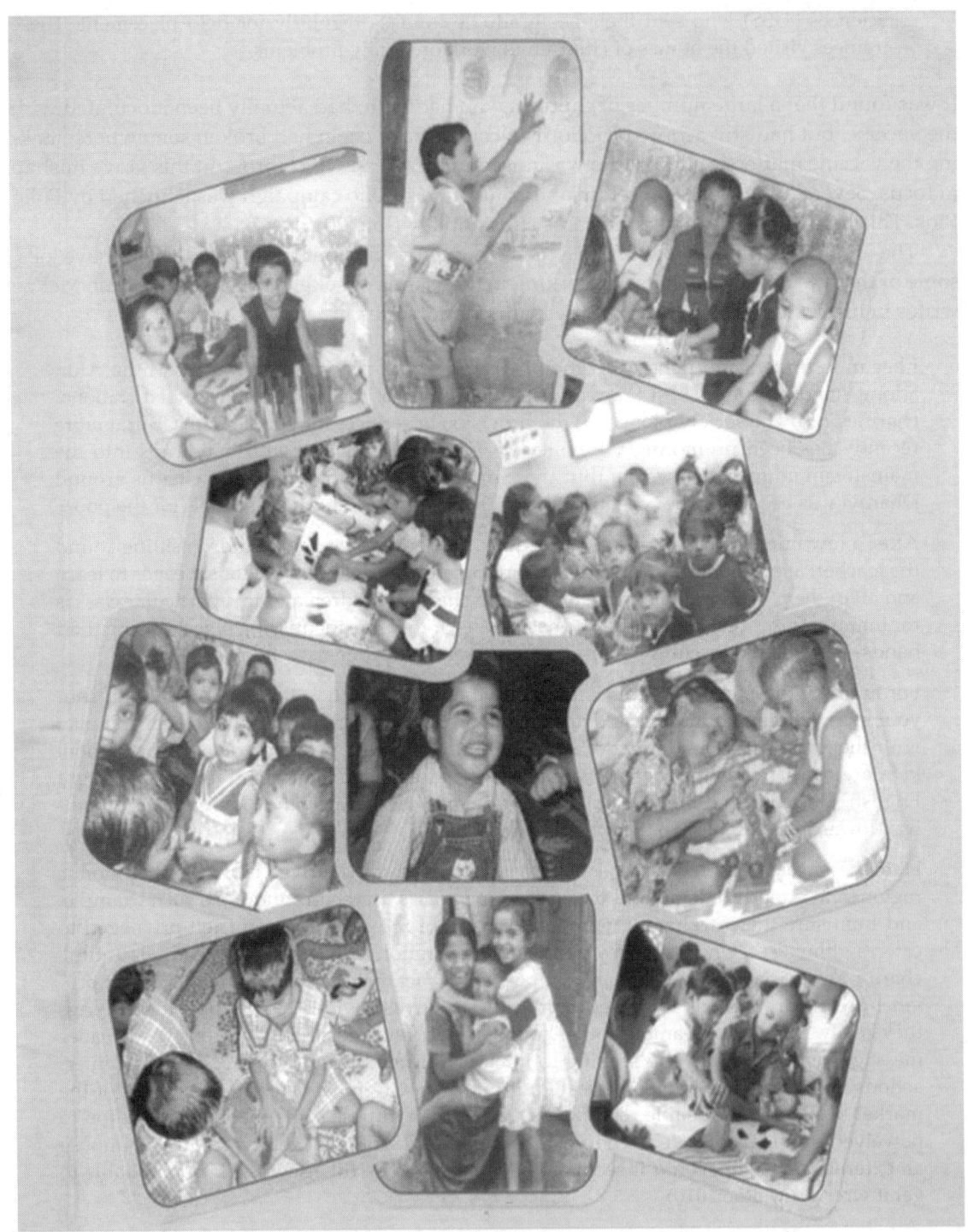

Community in Action

Photographs courtesy by Carlos Reyes Manzo, Marcia Rioux and Kunal Bhatia

Domain VI

Work Training Unit and the Skills Development Centre

Background

A research study titled 'Attitudinal Study of the Disabled Workers' showed that the most significant undercurrent running through our investigations is the intense desire of the disabled to be independent and stand on their own feet, rather than be a burden. But this is of course not possible without systematic and selective skills training in job-oriented courses. With these objectives in mind, we began the National Job Development Centre (NJDC) (Alur 1989).

A question that causes much anxiety to professionals and the family is: *what after school*?

Will the young adult leaving school have further training, will she/he be able to work, what sort of employment will she/he find? Will s/he be able to compete in open employment and if so, how can s/he be prepared.

In a small building adjacent to the centre in Colaba, the society paved the ground to set up a new unit, a work centre which would provide work facilities for young adolescents and young

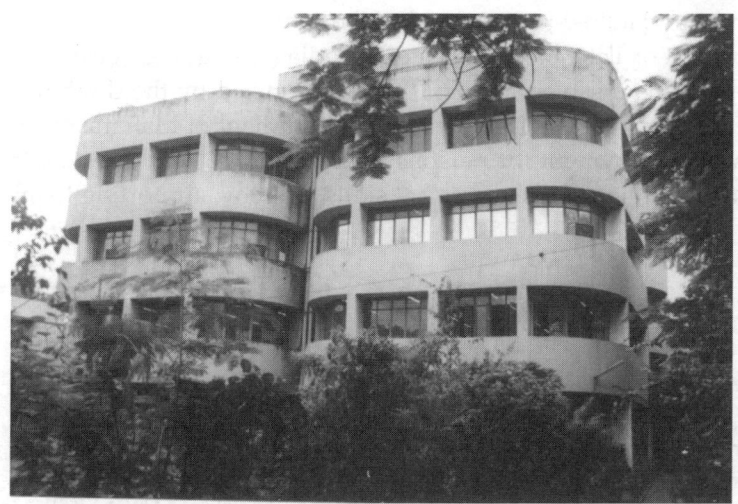

adults to deal with a variety of activities suited to their skills and aptitude. The skills introduced were carpentry, printing, office file-making, tailoring, textile printing, ceramic work, screen printing, catering and horticulture sections. They were paid a small stipend from the ministry of social welfare.

A small ray of hope for parents of severely disabled young people, who may never get employment (Annual Report 1981–82).

The hum and whirr of machines could be heard all day, as enthusiastic young trainees designed and made wooden toys, pencil holders, trays and even did special printing jobs for their clients. All this was thanks to a workshop that the Lions Club had very generously equipped with a woodworking and metalworking lathe, grinder, welding transformer, fretsaw, spray gun and a pneumatic compressor. In addition to needlework, tailoring and tie and dye, at which they were already very skilled, the girls had branched out into catering. Many office goers and students in neighbouring schools depended on our girls for their lunch every day. And they enjoyed it too, for our girls gave them a choice of 10 different menus— more than one for every day of the week. This was the first time in the city that the concept of the disabled serving the normal had been introduced.

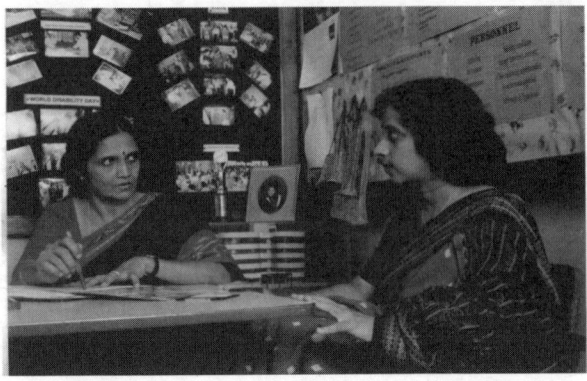

Mrs Meenakshi Balasubramanian, Director with Mrs Vandana Garware, Deputy Director, NJDC

In 1989, another beautiful area was provided to the organization by the municipal authorities. This was in Chembur and we called it the NJDC, now called the Skills Development Centre (SDC). It was set up in

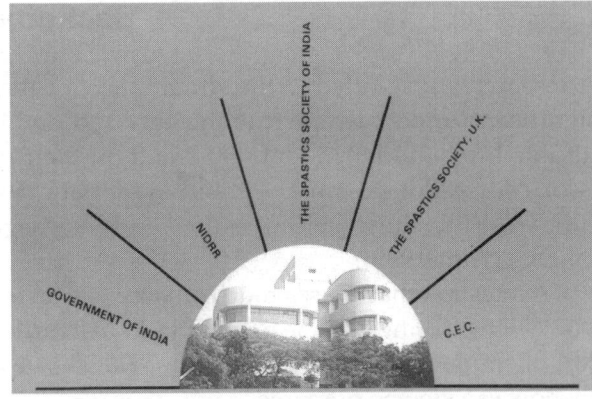

collaboration with the Spastics Society UK and the European Union. It was geared to give complete training facilities to each individual, according to his or her own ability. NJDC had been structured to create job opportunities, placement and follow-up services for all our disabled clients.

This became the vocational branch of The Spastics Society of India (SSI), as the vocational training and placement unit for multiple disabled adults. It was recognized by the disability welfare commissioner's office in the Social Justice Department (Government of Maharashtra). This was an initiative in the area of employment for persons with disability, with a vision of empowering youth with disabilities with job skills and social skills, thereby supporting them in their quest for employment.

Objectives

Following were the objectives for SDC:

- To formalize assessment strategies for employment.
- To develop context-specific models of vocational training and conducting an in-depth analysis of the person's profile, of his or her strengths and weaknesses, that can be adapted at the urban, slum and national levels.

- To research into various aspects that affect the employment process of persons with disabilities.

The fundamental goal of SDC was to provide appropriate training facilities, vocational guidance and counselling, selective employment and post-placement follow-ups. Skill training opportunities provided were through a computer applications centre. Printing, tailoring, catering and food processing, light engineering, office skills and horticulture training was also doled out. Professional training was introduced in fields such as computer skills, data entry, back office support, customer care, culinary skills, hospitality, housekeeping, accounting and library sciences. Parents, being the main stakeholders, were again included in the whole process.

Mobility Aids and the Wheelchair Division

A Mobility Aids and Wheelchair Department was set up and the first wheelchair made as a result of an Indo-Swedish collaboration. Research was led by Sathi Alur who called the first wheelchair that was rolled out 'Triumph'.

Thereafter, a development and technology centre assembled appropriate wheelchairs and other mobility aids appropriate for local conditions. The original design was obtained from Sweden, under a grant from Lutherhjalpen, together with necessary equipment and technical support.

Code of Policy and Practice

An important guide for employers was created by Dr Alur, entitled 'Code of Policy and Practice for People with Disabilities' (COPP), as a guide for the corporate sector on the experience of countries around the world in the management of disability. A reference kit by Vandana Garware was also prepared.

Reference Kit

Vandana Garware worked with Dr Mithu Alur for over a decade and served as the director of training at SDC. Dr Alur remembers she worked hard to prepare a reference kit on employment, keeping two objectives in mind: one, to empower disabled individuals and, two, to help employers to get practical information on the subject of employment. The reference kit served to provide the critical guidance needed to recruit people with disability. Besides, a short manual for potential job seekers, focusing on tips for interviews, was brought out by Malini Chib and Anita Prabhu.

Outcome

- Over 400 models of employment were developed.
- Computer training commenced as a major initiative.

- NJDC, through its training programmes, awareness campaigns, research and placement of the disabled in various models of employment, attempted to change the community's negative thinking about the disabled. A step taken in this direction was a well-researched film on employment entitled *Towards Independence*, made by Radhika Roy, which is available at SSI library.
- The most important contribution was to move employment opportunities from 'C' and 'D' category stereotyped jobs, such as basket weaving and telephone operating which disabled adults have been slotted in for decades, to high-end 'A' and 'B' category jobs.
- A review of a research study showed that although many employers felt that to employ someone with a disability is to employ a liability, the majority felt that the disabled are dependable, conscientious and productive, spending less time off work.

People Behind the Scenes

Remembering Lillian

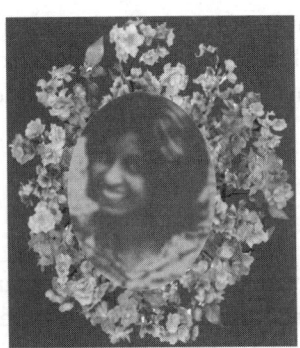

Lillian Khare was one of the 17 people present from the first day SSI came into being. She resigned from the Max Mueller Bhavan and came to offer her services in forming and establishing this society. She was elected secretary of SSI, India, for several years. The society faced a sudden and terrible shock when Lillian lost her life tragically in a car accident. With her untimely death, we lost a visionary. Her combined abilities of initiative, far-sightedness, charm and charisma made her the leader she was. A Lillian Khare Foundation was started in her name.

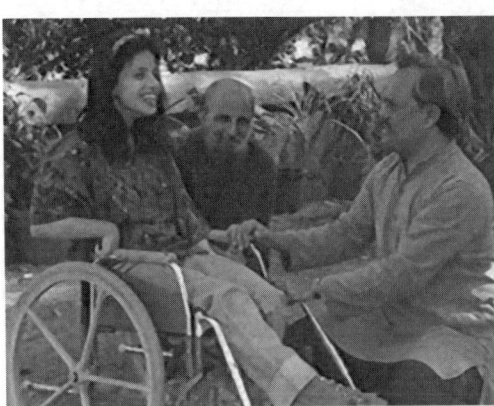

Professor Sitanshu Mehta, parent of Vipasha, with Sathi Alur examining his model of a wheelchair called 'Triumph'

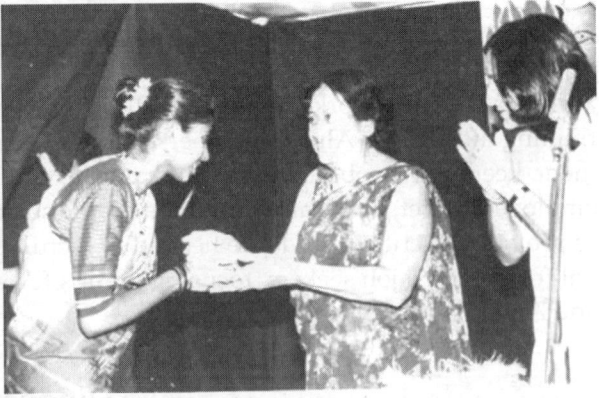

Mrs Nergesh Palkhivala, Vice Chairperson*, felicitating a student.

*Mrs Palkhivala loved the work and worked behind the scenes for over the first 10 years.

Remembering Nargis

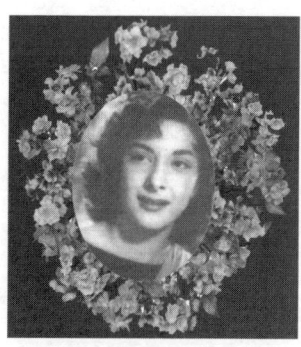

Shrimati Nargis Dutt

Nargis Dutt was one of the pioneers of SSI. She dedicated her life for the service of children with disabilities and whose dream it was to include them into mainstream life. Her association started in 1973, a year after SSI was formed. From that time Nargisji (as we knew her) was an active participant in our activities, a tireless fighter for the cause of spastics and one never to take 'no' for an answer.

She was a dedicated social worker and the first patron of SSI. Nargis was a great artiste who brought joy into the lives of millions of people through her films. She was also a compassionate soul, sensitive to human problems and sufferings of the people, a fine human being.

It was Mrs Dutt's dream to consolidate the work of the society by establishing a national institute for research into the prevention and management of CP. She worked indefatigably towards this cause and was instrumental in getting the government to grant land to the society in Bombay. She had done the spadework right up to the time she left for New York in 1980 in a critically ill condition. I remember sending a cable in 1981 to her at the Sloan Kettering Hospital, saying: 'Congratulations, you are a lady of property.' When Nargisji returned to India, she ignored her grave condition and said to me in her typical fashion, 'We must now work hard to build the national institute for CP as we had planned. I don't want to be a person in a committee. I want to work and come to office.' Although she is no more, we will never forget her valuable contribution to the fledgling organization. The First Lady of the Indian Screen brought in with her glamour, charm and charisma, compassion, focus and commitment, and in the decade that she worked with us, helped to put the children suffering from cerebral palsy on the map of the country ... and personally I lost someone who I loved like an Elder Sister.

Domain VII

(i) Expansion of Services on the National Level: From Schools to Institution Building

Background

As The Spastics Society of India (SSI) completed 10 years of pioneering services, it grew from a small single unit with just three students to a rigorously professional and ardently passionate organization with operations in four cities, providing extensive services for the cerebral palsy (CP) population of India and reaching out to help similar organizations in other countries.

One of the highlights of the second decade was that many of the students did extremely well with the education they received. Many went onto universities for higher studies. Today, some are accountants, lawyers, authors, computer analysts and librarians.

Another highlight of the second decade was that the work was appreciated by the Government of India and it came forward to assist us. Appropriate land was identified and given to the society for its expansion plans. Many policymakers, administrators and politicians visited the first model recommended by us, made suggestions and reached out to support the work.

This section also tells the story of how members of Malini's family and others supported the cause of CP in the country. It narrates how the organization expanded in Kolkata, Bangalore, Delhi, Chennai, Jaipur and Bombay (Mumbai) and most interesting accounts from our partners have come in to bring the story alive, as if it all happened yesterday! It records how a five-year plan crafted by Sathi Alur, honorary advisor, chartered accountant and developmental economist, began the decade laying out the vision for the next five years.

Training awareness and sensitization was taken on throughout the country and in international forums, broadening the expansion to the Asia-Pacific area. We also began training in 18 different countries[1] through the Community Initiative in Inclusion (CII) course run by the organization in association with the Women's Council, UK. Workshops, seminars and conferences were planned and facilitated and the outcomes recorded and disseminated.

[1]India, Bangladesh, Pakistan, Nepal, Sri Lanka, Cambodia, Vietnam, China, Mongolia, Tonga, Tajikistan, Malaysia, Indonesia, Tibet, Myanmar, Papua New Guinea, Jordan and Iraq.

Five-year Plan

Sathi Alur conceptualized a five-year plan for the society together with Pam Stretch and Mithu Alur, which helped with the expansion of services. The five-year plan's main aim was to articulate Mithu Alur's vision in financial terms. It targeted the services which needed to be developed in specific regions of the country. It gave a figure of ₹5 crore for donors, targeting various regions in the country. The organization was given a direction on how to operationalize the five-year plan; for the first time, the ideology and vision of the founder was quantified, making it easier for donors to help the expansion. Harish Mahindra, president of SSI, said that 'for the first time, we can see the vision being translated into financial terms.' Joseph Stein, a well-known US architect based in Delhi, was willing to design a centre like the India International Centre.

The document helped greatly. The government came forward to help with land and grants. So did support from international donors like the Church of Sweden Aid, the European Union, National Institute on Disability and Rehabilitation Research (NIDRR), Washington, the Overseas Development Agency (ODA), and The Spastics Society, UK, to name a few. Thus, began the movement from a small centre to institution building, reaching out to a much larger section of society.

As a consequence of the first five-year plan, the model expanded across the nation.

The Objectives of the plan were:

- To extend holistic services, combining education and treatment under a special school setting to other centres around the country, based on the first model;
- To establish a national research centre for spastic children and for others with allied physical handicaps;
- To establish a major employment centre;
- To establish context-specific centres in rural Maharashtra and in the slums of Bombay;
- To build capacity and establish teaching units for the training of teachers, paramedical staff, community workers and primary healthcare personnel, in order to reach the handicapped in the remotest corners of India.

The objective, thus, was the expansion of SSI's services in Bombay and across the nation, moving from schools to institution building, thereby ensuring services were made available to a much larger section of society, especially the underprivileged and powerless. Below is an excerpt from a document entitled 'Reach of Services of The Spastics Society of India: Its Affiliates & Branches, in 1987', penned by the late Mrs Junie Bose-Sethi, former honorary secretary of SSI, Bombay and West Bengal Spastics Society, who devoted 15 years of her life in the service of children with CP.

'Reach of Services of The Spastics Society of India: Its Affiliates & Branches, in 1987' by Mrs Junie Bose Sethi

'All the services outlined are unfortunately packed in presently in rented premises in a small bungalow in Colaba (southern Bombay). The teacher training course (TTC) and the therapists' courses have a single classroom housed in a makeshift shed; the centre for research is situated in a portable wooden cabin. Unfortunately, there is no science laboratory or library for the children. We do not also have space for a staff room! We have indeed worked under tremendous constraints for 16 years and it has now virtually become impossible to expand.

There is an urgent need to move into a purpose-built centre. This purpose-built centre will be called the National Centre for Cerebral Palsy (NCCP) which is being constructed in Bandra and for which we are urgently collecting funds.

The society gradually broadened its range of services related to education, treatment, management and training of spastic children and young adults, training of teachers, therapists and parents of handicapped children and conducting research into the prevention of disability.

Today, there are centres for special education in Mumbai, Kolkata, New Delhi, Bengaluru, Chennai, Allahabad, Dayalpur, Pune and Kochi. From a single centre in 1972, in Bombay, centres have mushroomed all over India, giving technical expertise, solace and comfort and a professionalism combined with sympathy never before available in India' (Bose-Sethi 1987).

Also quoted below are extracts from chapters and articles about the replication of the first model.

The organizations were initially named after the parent body as SSI, Delhi, Madras, Bangalore and so on; later, when they moved away, they changed their names. Central government grants-in-aid and matching funding, and applications for land were organized and released through SSI for several years until the organizations were developed to take over as independent and autonomous organizations. The organizations that emerged were largely initiated by parents, family members and close friends.[2] The result of this was the incubation and development of services in the virgin cities of Delhi, Madras, Bangalore and Jaipur through registering local branches of SSI.

> The first special school for Cerebral Palsy (C.P.) was set up in 1973. It was followed rapidly by several schools being opened in Kolkata, Bangalore, Chennai and New Delhi. Spastics Society of Northern India in 1977, Spastics Society of Karnataka in 1980, Spastics Society of Tamil Nadu in 1980 and Spastics Society of India (Chennai) now Vidya Sagar in 1985 have been formed. Spastics Society of India, Mumbai, as a catalyst, started training of teachers and therapists and skills development. Inclusive education has received a great deal of active propagation with the establishment of a National Resource Centre for Inclusive Education at Bandra, Mumbai. Similarly, the Spastics Societies located in the Eastern, Southern and Northern regions have been very active in training, in providing technical support and networking. (Bowley and Gardner 1980)

[2] To name a few in Calcutta, it was begun by Mrs Junie Bose, Mr Abhijit Bose, Mrs Sudha Kaul and Mr Om Kaul, Mrs Perin Aibara, Mrs Shanti Talukdar, Mr Ahmed and Mrs Uma Ahmed, Mr Sen and Mrs Reena Sen, Mrs Indrani Mazumdar, Jayobrotho and Mrs Subhra Chatterjee amongst others. In Delhi Mrs Mita Nundy and Dr Samiran Nundy, Mrs Anita Shourie and Mr Arun Shourie, Dr Lotika Sarkar, Mrs Minu Jalan, Mrs Manju Dubey, Mrs Radhika Roy, Miss Gloria Burrett, Ms Shyamala Gidugu, Ms Vandana Bedi amongst others. In Bombay, Mr Ranjit Chib, Mr and Mrs Vishesh Bhatia, Ms Lillian Khare, Ms Pamela Stretch, Mr Kamal Bakshi, Mrs Nergish Pakhivala, Mr Sathi Alur and Professor Sitanshu Mehta. In Madras, Mr Natarajan, Mrs Poonam Natarajan, Rajul Padmanabhan, Usha Ramakrishna and many more who were touched by the fever and thirst to serve the country. In Bangalore, Mrs Rukmini Krishnaswamy and Mr Adhip Chowdhury. In Jaipur, Mrs Deepak Kalra and Bina Kak.

A document brought out by the Ministry of Social Justice's Rehabilitation Council of India (RCI) reinforces this by stating:

'SSI was founded in 1972 at a time when very little was known about the complicated disorder of CP. SSI, Mumbai, as a catalyst, started training of teachers and therapists and skill development. Inclusive education has received a great deal of active propagation with the establishment of the NRCI at Bandra, Mumbai. Similarly, the spastics societies located in the eastern, southern and northern regions have been very active in training, providing technical support and networking.'

'It is to the credit of Dr Mithu Alur, who pioneered the establishment of the first SSI in Mumbai, exclusively for CP. Initially, it provided education and treatment services, gradually broadening its scope to teacher training, vocational training of young adults, advocacy and awareness and support for parents and other professionals' (http://www.rehabcouncil.nic.in/writereaddata/cp.pdf).

I was very fortunate as some of the pioneers of the organizations mentioned wrote for this retrospective study and given below in the following sections are their first-hand accounts.

The Spastics Society of Eastern India (SSEI), Calcutta

Beginning with the next model set-up, in 1974 the second model, replicating the first one, was launched in the country by a mother, Sudha Kaul, together with Malini's aunt, co-founder, Junie Bose. Her husband Abhijit Bose, Ranjit Chib (Mithu's husband), Perin Aibara, Uma Ahmed and Om Kaul (Sudha's husband) were the first of the early few members. Many like-minded people like Reena Sen, Ranu Bannerjee, Jayobrotho and Subhra Chatterjee, Indrani Majumdar, Sujata Parekh and a senior citizen who blazed a trail of dedicated commitment

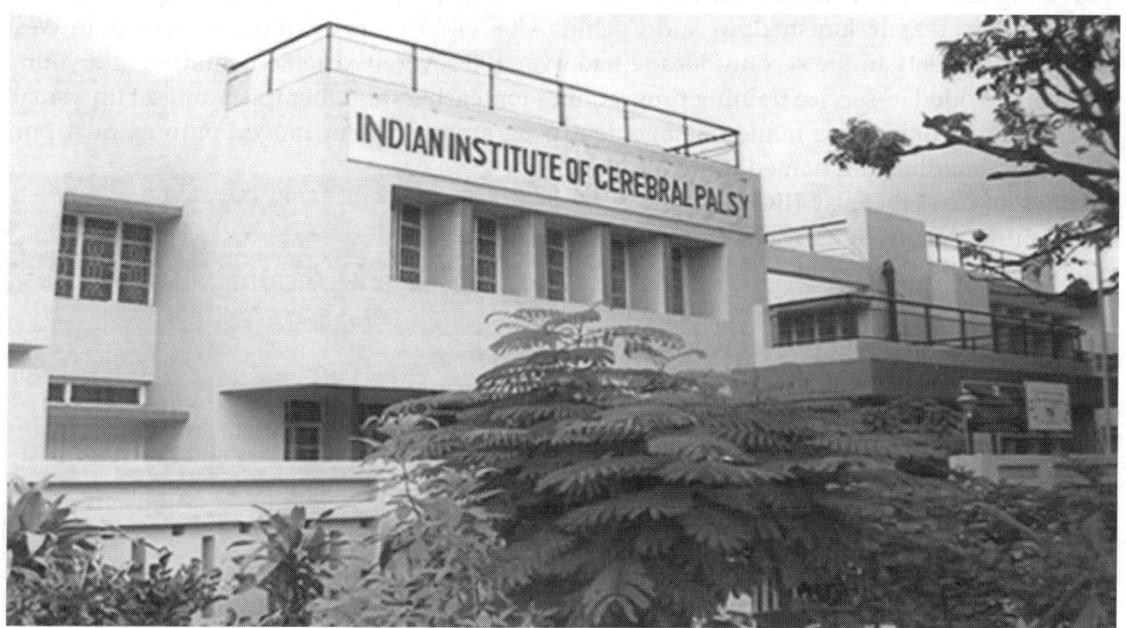

through her service, Shanti Talukdar (Dr Samiran Nundy's mother, Mani Mashi to us) joined to support this effort in West Bengal.

Sudha Kaul, co-founder, wrote in 1978:

'Like most societies for the disabled, parents of spastic children, dedicated social workers and friends brought into being the West Bengal Spastics Society in 1974 in Calcutta, two years after the pioneering work had begun in Bombay by SSI. The latter gave considerable help in inspiring and guiding us

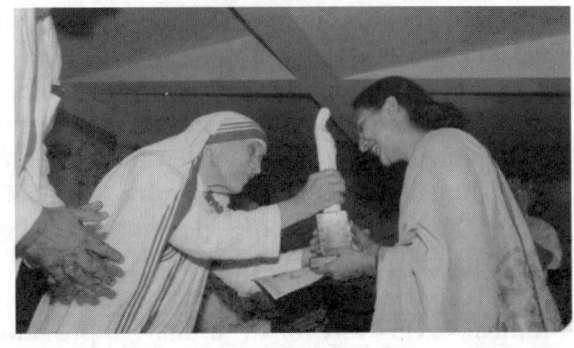

to start our organization. The main objectives of the society were (a) to provide education of spastic children in an officially recognized school of high standards, staffed by specialists well versed in the effects of CP, (b) to provide treatment and guidance to CP children and their families, (c) to create and heighten public awareness of the enormous needs of the cerebral palsied and (d) to train teachers and therapists in the special methods of overcoming the problems of CP.'

Source: It's Ability That Counts, edited and introduced by
Mithu Alur, preface by Leslie Gardner, 1978

Technical support was given by Pamela Stretch and Mithu Chib and the young fledgling society was helped to set up essential systems of intervention: screening assessment, treatment, home management, management in classrooms and how to build capacity with teachers, therapists and mothers.

Besides running a Centre for Special Education in Calcutta with an outpatient department providing services to children from all over West Bengal, it moved on to help spread services in Guwahati, Tezpur, Jamshedpur and Cochin. After eight years of valuable services in West Bengal, the society in the second decade had over 100 severely disabled children and young people, provided in-service training programmes for teachers and therapists and set up a small work training unit and a home management programme. It later moved onto its own pur-

pose-built building and named it the Indian Institute of Cerebral Palsy (IICP).

Samiran Nundy reminisces on the 40th anniversary of IICP in 2014.

A little over 40 years ago, when I was a junior doctor in Cambridge, England, we lived in a small apartment which was actually the servants' quarters of the university chaplain and had, true to Indian tradition, half our extended family staying with us. There was Malini Chib and her parents, Mithu (my wife Mita's sister) and Ranjit, as well as my mother, Santi Nundy, who had come for a holiday in the UK (probably to get away from

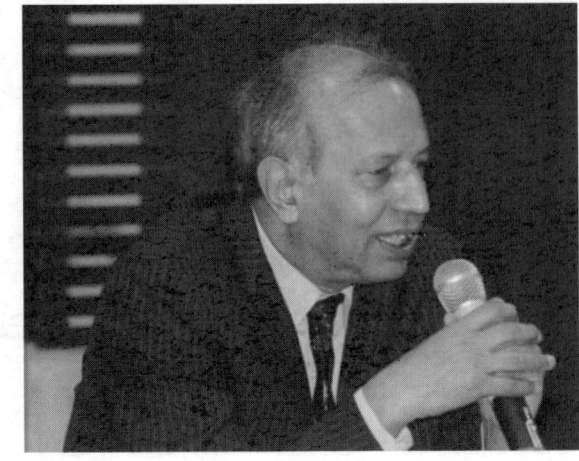

my irascible father!). Malini used to go to the Roger Ascham School in Cambridge and, when we later moved to London, to Cheyne Walk, which were top-of-the-line special schools for children with CP. I think it was there that Mithu thought of starting a similar institution in Bombay and my mother's close interaction with Malini made her think of specializing in special education.

As nothing ever deterred her, at the venerable age of 54 she enrolled herself as a full-time boarder in Brandon University in Manitoba, Canada, lived in the students' hostel and passed out with flying colours. She came home to my long-suffering and, I must say, very tolerant and liberal father, who was working elsewhere in Canada, only during the vacations to cook his favourite fish curry, *ruimaccherjhol*.

When my parents returned to India, Sudha Kaul had started SSEI and graciously and generously allowed my mother to join. In school, I think she used to play the piano, teach the mentally challenged children and look after the garden at a wage of ₹150 a month (my father said she spent more on the garden than the SSEI were paying her). I was also always a bit jealous that Sudha had supplanted my place in my mother's affections because at home she used to constantly talk about how kind Sudha was.

But how she loved the school. Even when her beloved son and his family came to Moore Avenue from Delhi, she would insist on not missing school and taking the bus to work every morning. She took piano lessons at home to become more proficient in the instrument (she didn't succeed) and would accompany us for the great Nundy family sing-song which started with Rabindra *sangeet* and ended with Christmas carols with which we would regale generally unappreciative visitors. She was an indomitable source of energy and would also cook our beloved *kyaukswe* and *balachaung* early in the morning before Mr Biswas arrived in the school bus. My daughter Karuna once asked her when and where she had been happiest and she unhesitatingly said that it was when she was working at the SSEI.

My family has been completely involved in special education for all these years with Mithu Alur in Bombay, my wife Shusmita helping to start the Spastics Society of Northern India (SSNI) (I was chairman of the governing body till she dismissed me for not being serious enough at meetings) and my mother, of course, in Calcutta.

She had a major operation in Delhi and then returned to work for four years. In the end, even when she was quite ill, she refused to stop working and came to stay with us in Delhi only two months before she died. She asked me in the end to give some of the money she had to the SSNI to help two girls with their education.

Both my mother and I are grateful to the IICP for giving her the best years of her life.

—*Samiran Nundy, 2014, Kolkata*

The Spastics Society of India, Delhi (AADI—Action for Ability Development and Inclusion)

The question 'No services in the capital!?' resulted in the first model which had been replicated in Kolkata being then developed in Delhi. It initially opened as a branch of the sister organization SSNI in 1978. It was formed under the chairmanship of Malini's aunt, Mrs Mita Nundy.

SSNI initially set up a small special school as we had done in Colaba, Mumbai, in a rented building. In the first few years, the guidance, hands-on expertise, generous sharing of knowledge and material as well as regular training by Mithu Alur and Pamela Stretch proved invaluable. Some of the earliest pioneers of SSNI were co-founders Divya Jalan and Anita Shourie and Sathi Alur, Samiran Nundy, Radhika and Prannoy Roy, Lotika Sarkar, Manjulika Dubey, Anita Shourie and Manju Dubey's mother (who was affectionately called Malti Mashi), Shyamala Gidigu, Gloria Burrett, Renu Singh, Vandana Bedi and many other like-minded people. Most of their husbands like Arun Shourie and Bimal Jalan joined the group to help support this venture.

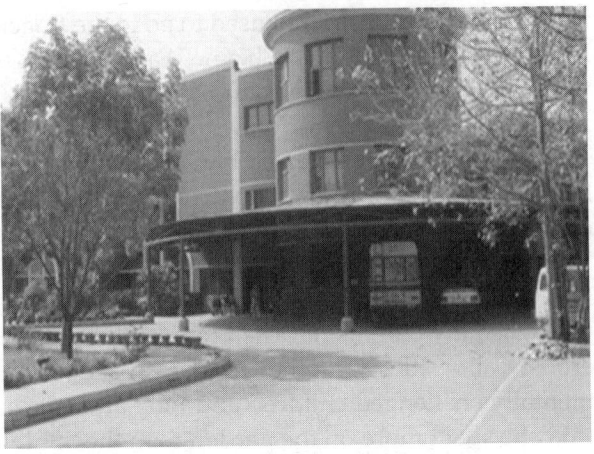

The Spastics Society of India, Delhi (now called Action for Ability Development and Inclusion (AADI))

In 1978, the late Mita Nundy spoke at the conference on 'It's Ability That Counts'. Given below is her account of the early services at international conferences held in Bombay, Delhi, Madras and Bangalore.

'The Centre for Special Education is a special school housed in the rented ground floor of a residential home. The staff consists of teachers, physio, speech and occupational therapist, social worker and principal. Thirty-five spastic children receive special education and treatment. A paediatrician, visiting the centre on a weekly basis, organizes their medical care. A social worker runs a counselling and training programme for parents. The children are admitted if they are suffering from CP and fall into the severe or moderate category of physical handicap, if their intelligence is within educable or normal range and their age between 3 and 13.'

'At present, there are an estimated two million spastics in India. After 10 years of strenuous effort, adequate facilities exist for only 300, that is less than .05 per cent spastics. There is a gap of 99.5 per cent without services. We are looking for ways to fill this huge gap. The questions that crop up are: How fast can we fill this gap? How do we make our work have maximum effect? We thought we would develop different kinds of Indian solutions and relevant intervention strategies suited to the scarcity of financial and human resources in this country.'

Three Models of Services

The Centre for Special Education, a special school in Delhi, started in 1978. A more cost-effective home management programme was started in 1979. The third project is a centre for handicapped children in the village of Dayalpur in Haryana state. The aim of the Centre for Special Education is to provide optimal conditions in an urban setting for the maximum growth and development of spastic children. The objective of the home management programme is to provide support and training for families, so as to develop the potential of the child at home, using the considerable skills and understanding that most mothers have. The objective of the

Dayalpur village project was to develop *different methods* of rehabilitation suited to the human resources and the socio-economic conditions that exist in Indian villages.

The School of Rehabilitation Sciences (SRS) was established to oversee training of urban and rural human resources in the disability area and developing skill sets for people ranging from completely non-literate to highly qualified professionals. SRS students in the early years had the privilege of learning and getting inspired by Mithu Alur.

'We are looking for ways to maximize the effect of our efforts. We feel it to be essential to work within the governmental infrastructure for healthcare in the village. This would minimize costs and, secondly, the model developed would take into account the typical limitations in the government system. Efforts could then be channelized more easily, so that advantages could outweigh the difficulties. The nature and manifestation of handicap must change with different developmental conditions. Our services have to reflect these differences. The idea of services for spastics has to be put into the correct context—an Indian context where infant mortality rates are as high as 130 per 1,000, a fact indicative of the level of absolute poverty that exists. We cannot afford to learn by trial and error as the richer countries do. We have to think and search harder for the right developmental model of providing services for the handicapped in India. This model must be sensitive to the fact that there are scarce financial and human resources in this area; to the lack of emotional and financial resources in poor families; to cultural belief systems about the nature of handicap; to the role of the family and community; and to the urban poor and a mainly rural population. We hope in the future to be able to provide some of the answers in the search for models for services for spastics in a vast subcontinent such as India.' *(Source: Late Mita Nundy in It's Ability That Counts, 1982)*

Dr Divya Jalan, one of the co-founders of the Spastics Society of Delhi, later went onto study regular schools and what kind of training regular teachers were given. This was a part of a doctoral research which earned her a PhD from the Institute of Education University of London. Very sharp intellectually and very soft emotionally, she came from an illustrious family and is married to eminent economist Bimal Jalan who helped and supported the cause too. With her sharp acumen and her vast knowledge of normal and disabled children, she partnered Mita Nundy and both of them began the centre in Delhi.

When she learnt about the retrospective study Divya Jalan reminisced:

'Mithu to me is both a long-time friend and a leader in my profession. She combines her personal and professional life seamlessly. I met her in the early 1970s, when she had just started working on setting up SSI in Bombay. I saw how, as a professional, Mithu set clear goals and put all her effort into achieving them. She pushed herself to go to endless places, meet endless people and write endless notes, till she got what people with disabilities needed.'

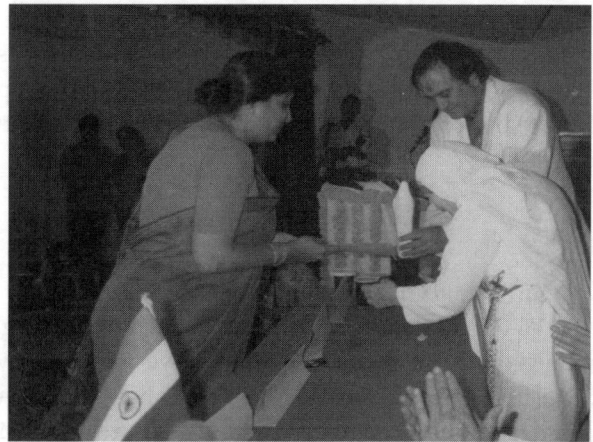

Mrs Divya Jalan, representing Mita Nundy and the Spastics Society, Delhi gets awarded by Mother Teresa for their work

'As a person, I was the recipient of Mithu's overwhelming warmth. In the early years, her ability to draw all her friends and family into her work created a community of people who were willing to go a long way with her. They saw her clarity, her effort, her professionalism and responded with time, effort, compassion and financial resources. Whole families would spend a day on the beach and many serious discussions would take place while enjoying the sea breeze and cool water.'

'Mithu sowed the first seed and continues to nurture it even today. She was the force behind starting a movement to set up services for people with CP. She, with her colleagues, set up the first institution and over time many others followed in Kolkata, Delhi, Madras, Bangalore, Lucknow, Shillong, Jaipur, Kanpur and so on. She participated in some directly and some have come up without her direct involvement. But people like me who know her and see her monumental effort draw courage to carry on working in an area which continues to be very challenging.'

'Mita (Nundy) stood tall in my doorway on our first meeting. Mithu's sister, as I saw her then, had just moved back from Boston and I had invited her for lunch with her little son. I didn't know then that this would not only be a significant friendship, but also my most important professional relationship—stormy sometimes, but always together and driven by doing what was in the best interest of the people with disability.'

'Mita had a brilliant mind and was an extremely inspiring thinker. She always had a new perspective—a way of looking at things that nobody else did. She also had great compassion and a sense of justice for the disadvantaged. Her thoughts stimulated both intellect and emotions. I was often surprised by how inspired I felt by some of her thoughts even in the twentieth year of our work together!'

'Mita was very rooted in India and always concerned about strategies being appropriate for India—services needed to be of the highest standard but also cost-effective and pro-poor. She sought to bring in Western research and academic rigour along with a more Indian and spiritual environment in our work. I did not agree with her always but never stopped marvelling at her creativity and boldness in the hundreds of things that we did agree on.'

'All of us who have spent many years in AADI together have nurtured a culture of joint ownership of work where personal achievement is always recognized but collective responsibility and achievement are celebrated. All the people who have gone through AADI under the leadership of Mita are spreading the message to strive for more compassion, wider vision and excellence.'

—*Divya Jalan, 2015*

Shyamala Gidugu, CEO, writes in 2012:
'AADI started life as a small branch of the mighty parent tree called SSI. As a testament to true growth, both organizations have matured over three decades into independent entities with distinct philosophies, programmes that have played to their strengths and differences that respect each one's uniqueness. Tagore spoke of "uniting together with differences intact", a sentiment that AADI echoes as it holds onto its dream of an equal world for all, fully aware of and truly grateful to those who challenged its being while leaving it free to evolve.'

'Persons with childhood and lifelong disabilities had no access to the outside world in India in the early 1970s. For many of us who now see people with disabilities, supported by legislations favouring their rights, fighting for equal opportunities for admission in regular schools, universities, jobs, entertainment and access to other routine services, it might be difficult to imagine how it was back then. Things *have* changed. Looking closely at the most challenging conditions within the area of disability in which multiple functions are impacted, it has been the pioneering efforts of a young mother in the early 1970s that has been the force behind the change. Mithu Alur moved beyond her challenging personal experience with her daughter to establish the first programme in India for children with neurological disabilities. Motivating, educating, inspiring, challenging, coaxing—even coercing—family, close friends, government officials, corporate executives and doctors among others, Mrs Alur succeeded in establishing the first organization in Bombay—SSI, which is now called ADAPT (Able Disabled All People Together).'

'But that was not enough…. Aware of the number of children and families still untouched by the minimal support they so needed, Mrs Alur focused on expanding services outside Bombay. Her constant question to like-minded family members and friends: 'No services in the Capital!?' resulted in the first branch being opened in Delhi in 1978: SSNI, which is now known as AADI and flourished under the chairmanship of Mrs Mita Nundy. SSNI initially set up a small special school.'

'In the first few years, the guidance, the hands-on expertise, generous sharing of knowledge and material as well as constant hand holding by Mithu Alur and Pamela Stretch proved invaluable. Some of the earliest staff of SSNI were people who had trained or worked at SSI.'

'Right from the outset, it was believed that a healthy and relevant expansion of services could only be possible when each regional centre adapted and integrated its programmes to local needs, local resources and the prevailing ethos. SSNI's additional focus on those further disadvantaged by conditions like urban poverty, rural living, and despair of wait listed parents therefore dictated the expansion of its services to include family training programmes, a vocational training unit for young adults and a rural project. The rural expansion compelled SSNI to include children with all disabilities, leading it to innovate suitable strategies to work with a more diverse group. It was during the late 1980s that SSNI used this rural experience to rethink and bring greater relevance to its programmes via the model of community-based services.'

'Following its philosophy and based on the strong foundations laid and nurtured by SSI, SSNI registered as an independent organization in 1982. It retained a strong association with SSI through a sharing of ideas around emerging issues in the disability sector, like inclusive education, rights and access. At this crucial juncture, SSI's particular contribution to every issue was its ability to involve global thinkers and evoke discussions at a macro level.' (From her close colleagues Gloria Burrett, Vandana Bedi and Shyamala Gidugu).

A Paradigm of Thinking, Knowing, Believing: Mita's Legacy for AADI

To work alongside Mita Nundy was to be immersed in a process that constantly challenged set ways of thinking, questioned a mere aping of the best of the West and focused on the real stakeholders at the heart of all our efforts: the person with disability and the caregiver. So often just by being a part of the reflective process of a case conference or the planning retreats initiated and chaired by Mita, we began to believe that complacency is a sin, that we are accountable to the people we work with, that professions need to cut across boundaries to deliver effectively in the spirit of transdisciplines and that the centre of excellence approach has to co-exist paradoxically with the responsibility to ensure the widest reach of services. The greatest impact on those of us who worked alongside Mita, however, will always be from her set of core values of justice and inclusion that stood out starkly in the prevailing context of charity and welfarism in the 1980s—values that are central to contemporary thinking, which we are still trying to do full justice to and for them to really define our organizational culture. How grateful we are to have had a prophet, visionary and teacher in our midst!

Within us even today, Mita's guiding voice provokes us to ask these questions of ourselves:

What does India really need? At a juncture when SSNI/AADI was addressing the dearth of rehabilitation professionals by exploring its own training involvement, Mita's vision challenged the existing medical model-oriented physio/occupational therapy training courses in favour of more holistic person-centred and community-oriented courses. This was too radical to be easily accepted by others and yet today forms the basis of our knowledge of relevant content in ongoing courses. At a time when AADI is changing its focus in the area of training, it is this core question that remains a beacon. Yet another example of the macro-relevance underpinning her thinking was the concept of partnerships with community-based organizations like Deepalya and Lok Jumbish which heralded a new way of working—a building of the capacities of existing professionals to address the needs of people with disabilities within the communities that they were working in. The result was a wider impact with minimum resources and ensured inclusion for people with disabilities. Today, this conceptual thinking is translated as a 'convergence' of 'disability issues' into ongoing development programmes.

Is this strategy really relevant in this context? When community-based rehabilitation (CBR) for example was making its presence felt in India, Mita was no easy convert! This stringent question was applied in full force, compelling us to read and to research for ourselves before buying into the concept. This was vintage Mita. We grumbled and how...but this was the way we learnt. A vivid image of Mita is of her in a home in rural Dayalpur, with Dr Anandlakshmi of Lady Irwin College, using sticks and mud instead of pencils and crayons to make cognitive testing more culturally relevant to and cognizant of the strengths of rural children. To see through her eyes was to realize that rural children from preschool age could recognize their own fields as different from a neighbour's rather than stay stuck with a blinkered view of narrow norms which devalued their potential.

Will the poorest gain? 'Keep an eye on the person who might not easily access your service'. It was this often asked principle that kick-started the urban CBR programme at AADI. It was a question that flowed from the deepest part of Mita. 'The poor. Think about the poor!' Years later, when she was no longer at the helm of SSNI/AADI, her informal sessions with people with leprosy, often on the street, with *bhajans* blaring from a tape recorder were high points for her. This was no duty, it was her nourishment. Mita's phone calls waking our consciences are legendary and were often met with a moan: 'Can't Mita chill? It's Sunday!' Apparently never, as long as human need was in existence. Her heart pain was never allowed to get in the way! 'Let's organize blankets, it's so cold' or 'Shuro says malaria is a real killer disease which we can prevent. Can you get 300 mosquito nets and distribute them to the poorest in the slums. I'll send Ramu with the money!' These are words that have the power to rock our consciences even today. This sense of the other seemed to emerge from a wellspring that flowed unceasingly.

Where is this service really needed? Going beyond the limits of urban-based comfort and complacency, we were compelled to proactively encourage persons from all over India to attend the training courses and return to their far-flung areas to initiate services. Stressed mothers supporting each other in Ludhiana, that young adult zooming into a pre-vocational set-up on his wheelchair, a child with CP entering school in Shillong, parents of children with CP forming an association in New Delhi to address the burning question 'Who will take care of my children when I am no more?'" or trained volunteers, teachers and trainees in Gwalior encouraged to set up independent NGOs for the most marginalized groups in urban poverty areas are a few degrees of separation from this aspect of Mita's vision.

What is the caregiver/person with disability saying? What comes to mind is a vignette of a frustrated mother who complained about her child not getting regular services at AADI. No amount of explanations or alternative support was enough. We were a weary, angry, frustrated bunch of young staff who expected Mita to support us in this stand-off. What happened was so different, as our attention was focused on the need underlying the mother's ranting and raving. We were the ones left doing a rethink of our emotions! We had to and gosh how we were reminded to 'sit on our egos that needed this appreciation for all our hard work'.

Does this programme include elements that nourish and sustain the soul for those many bleak moments of reality? Using India's theism as a valuable resource and her own spiritual practice and conviction in the power of a connect with an internal force, Mita initiated individual and group sessions with a spiritual element that helped and held many caregivers through their stress, anxiety, depression and physical exhaustion and provided persons with disabilities with a sense of meaning and sustaining spiritual strategies through their ongoing struggle. None of us at AADI can forget the day a spate of harmless questions were asked of us in Mita's soft voice: 'We focus on a child's body, mind, feelings ... what about their spirits, their souls? If they were your children wouldn't you give them a sense of their inner strength, a faith in a power they could tap into? Let's see what keeps us going when the going gets tough.... Shouldn't we share this with our students?' Mindfulness, strength-imparting mantras and spiritual discourses were regular inputs. In hindsight, this was a remarkable addition to the work, a transpersonal element that contemporary research affirms is essential for well-being.

What will build a community in the organization that will continue to share, enthuse, enjoy, challenge, develop bonds beyond professional ties, allow for unison despite differences and enable a walking of that extra mile for each other? SSNI/AADI's family-spirit legacy is the outcome where celebrating with families and sharing each other's joys and pains create a connect that goes deeper and larger than simply sharing a work vision.

Who is the next generation of workers? What do they need to develop their passion and skill? Looking way beyond the contribution of her generation and the next, Mita created an innovative supervisor's course and foresaw the value of a training component in a funding programme to complement the hands-on experiences of ADDI's workers. At least 11 staff including special educators, persons with disability, supervisors and trainers, a carpenter, basic developmental therapists and a counsellor brought back relevant information and experiences from CBR projects, vocational institutes, inclusive set-ups and academic institutions from China, Japan, USA, Africa and the UK to AADI. This was another way ahead of its time Mita-inspired plan. It is a question we need to keep asking today to ensure a continued life of the organization and its ever-widening impact. It is one way we can share and sustain Mita's dream of justice, inclusion and compassion for all (Gloria Burrett, Vandana Bedi and Syamala Gidugu in the Annual Report, 2014 of SSNI/AADI).

All three specialists and colleagues made their mark in the development of services and are outstanding human beings. Gloria is a nun now. Shyamala runs the Delhi centre. Vandana has done an amazing amount as a social activist and a professional. Mita was clearly ahead of her time and brought in some highly intellectual critiquing of our work.

In 1982, as in the first model, the third model: SSI Karnataka, in Bangalore, started with eight children in a rented building by Mithu Chib and the team from Bombay including Junie Bose, Pam Stretch, Arthur D'Mello and Sathi Alur. Rukhmani Krishnaswamy, Adhip Chaudhuri, Sheila Harlankar, Fowzia Shamim and a few others later joined to call it the Spastics Society of Karnataka. Five acres of land was allotted for this project. His Excellency the governor A.N. Bannerjee took a keen interest and inaugurated it. Well-known architects Brinda Somaya and Ranjini Kalappa of Somaya and Kalappa designed the first centre in the country and Tata Engineering Consultants came forward to assist with the structural supervision.

The centre was located in a disability friendly purpose-built school in Indiranagar.

As in the other centres, the children at the centre were roughly divided into formal academic and non-formal instruction groups depending on their intellectual abilities. The individual-based programme took into consideration not only the child's abilities, but also the child's home and community environment; with inputs from therapists, teachers, language and speech specialists, the programme formed the main basis of management and training. Special seating, word processors, calculators, adapted typewriters and computers were essential aids for these children. To this end, low-cost aids and equipment were specially designed. For non-verbal children, augmentative communicative aids were used. Perceptual dysfunctions, motor disabilities and sensory defects were a few of the difficulties the children had.

In 1982, Mithu writes:

'SSI has been in existence now for little over a decade and I am pleased to say that in this short time, we have grown and been able to extend our services to more and more spastic children all over the country. To date, we have helped nearly 5,000 children and their families in India. The Bangalore chapter was started in 1979 and the movement has grown and strengthened largely due to the generous response the society has received from government, industrialists, the people of the state of Karnataka and also because of an excellent team at work at SSI, Bangalore.'

'The government of Karnataka gave the society a prime piece of land in Indiranagar for the building of a Centre for Special Education and rehabilitation centre. We are particularly grateful to two governors who played a key role—Shri Govind Narain and Shri A.N. Bannerjee.'

—Dr Mithu Alur, SSI chairperson's message for the Bangalore centre's inauguration, 1982

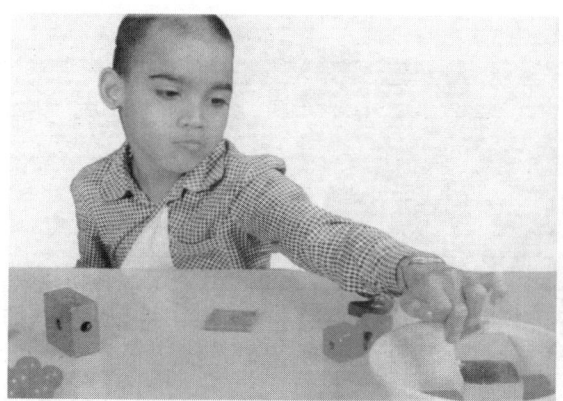 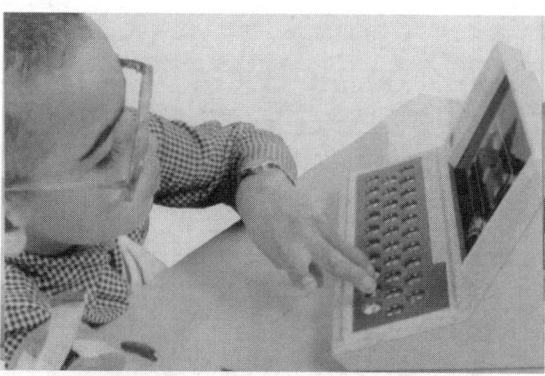

Other services provided included therapy, speech, home management, work training and community-based rehabilitation, akin to what was being delivered in Bombay and Madras. (Annual Report, 1980)

Prashanth Kamath, 15 years old, joined the Centre for Special Education in 1983. Until then, he was educated by his parents at home, who were extremely encouraging. Exposed to a lot of reading, his intelligent mind grasped things very quickly.

When he was admitted, he could hardly sit. Determination, regular exercises and encouragement of his parents have helped him to walk about with the least support today. An exceptional student, Prashanth secured 91 per cent in the Std. VII board examination. He participated in a quiz, on astronomy, organized by the Doordarshan national television network and came out with flying colours, in appreciation of which DDK Delhi awarded him a certificate.

Mrs Geetha Shankar, a teacher at the centre said, 'When we look at a child like Prashanth, we realize that a handicap cannot hinder the progress of a determined mind and brilliance will show itself; he already shows signs of being an extraordinary child.'

'Sometimes when I see a friend playing and running on the road, I feel like joining him. But when I see that I am equally intelligent, I feel consoled though I cannot run. When I come to school, I feel very happy seeing my friends and aunties. I feel like bringing all the children like me, who have not been out of their houses, to my school and play and study with them. When people pity me seeing my condition, I hope and wish that they would help me instead.'

—*Prashanth, a student at the CSE, Bangalore*

Rukmini Krishnaswamy, director of technical services, SSI, Bangalore, writes:

'Over the past three decades of my life's journey in the company of these Children of God, it has been for me a spiritual experience to learn from them as much as to teach them, to discover the true value of love, to most genuinely share feelings of joy in achievement, to give more than receive and thus discover the hidden but powerful meaning and purpose of life.'

The Spastics Society of India, Vidyasagar (Chennai)

In 1985, the fifth model of services began. Initially, again, it was a branch of SSI, Bombay and was called the Centre for Special Education, Madras. It was started by Mr and Mrs Natarajan, parents of Ishwar, together with Usha Ramakrishna and Rajul Padmanabhan. True to the

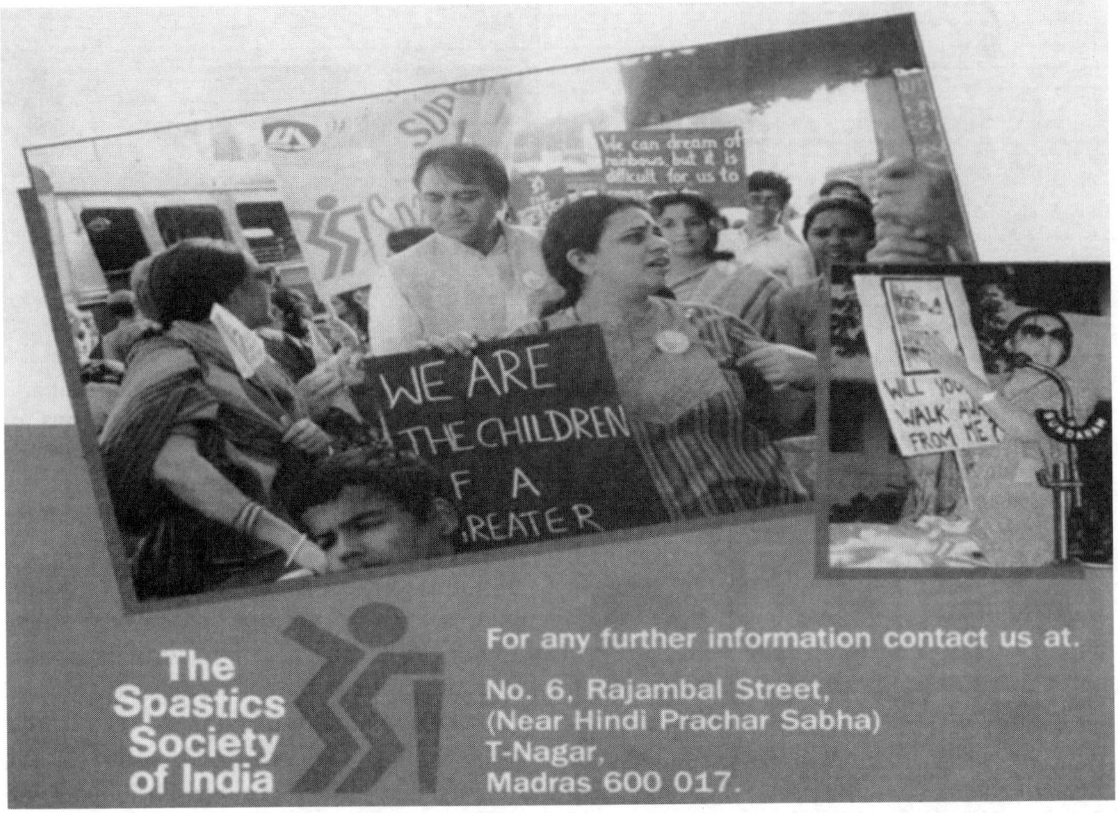

The Spastics Society of India

For any further information contact us at.

No. 6, Rajambal Street,
(Near Hindi Prachar Sabha)
T-Nagar,
Madras 600 017.

Sunil Dutt leads a rally in Chennai with Mithu Alur & Poonam Natarajan in 1984

legacy started by the parent body, services were set up in a small garage with three children—a replication of the parent organization, with the objective of providing education and treatment to this much neglected group of multiply disabled children. Later it flourished into a purpose-built centre. Land was given for this by the government, while the funds came from Denmark. The organization moved on to include a home management programme, an infant clinic, an out-patient/advisory clinic, outstation programmes and more. A key person who played a most valuable role in SSI, Madras, thus bringing Chennai and Bombay together, was Mr G. Natarajan. A visionary with an outstanding personality, hugely modest and spiritual, Nattoo (as we all lovingly called him) realized the importance of both the organizations working together. He became the first honorary secretary of the parent body, SSI, Bombay and after that the honorary treasurer. His death was deeply felt and nobody else was able to fill the gap he left

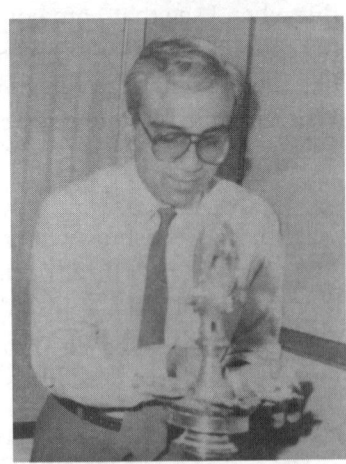

Mr G. Natarajan, Honorary Secretary and Treasurer of the Spastics Society, Mumbai, lighting the lamp at one of our functions

behind. Poonam Natarajan writes to Mithu remembering those days:

'Many memories come flooding in...of valuable
support received and Rajul, I and Team Vidyasagar are
deeply appreciative of your caring support through the
years.'

'Every parent has played a key role in making a difference and some special mentions would
include Poonam Natarajan, Eswari and Thangam from
Mayiladuthurai, Kalpana Rao, Smytha Prasad, Radha
Ramesh, Uma KS.'

Again a common thread running through the organization was the importance of parents and the family.
Aiming to involve parents closely in the management
of their children, a research unit was later introduced
and also an awareness programme to draw public
attention. Friends of the Spastics Society, or FOSS as

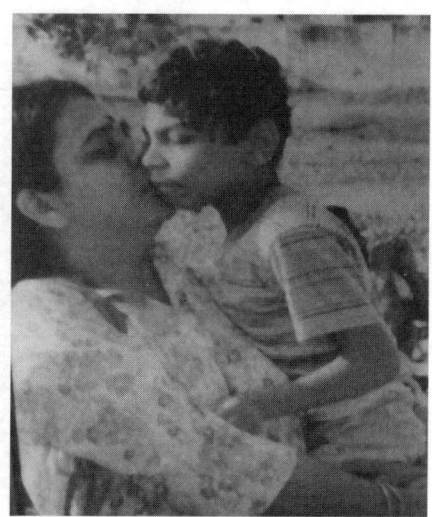

Poonam with her son Ishwar

they were called, was an active group that offered tremendous all-round help to SSI, Madras,
including fundraising, public advocacy and expansion programmes. Poonam Natarajan,
parent, founder chairperson and director of the Chennai branch of SSI joined SSI, Bombay,
Teacher Training Course (TTC) to learn how best to teach her child. Poonam then replicated modules of novel intervention such as home management, non-formal education and
extensively used community-based rehabilitation (CBR) techniques to decentralize services
around Chennai. Poonam was one of Mithu Alur's partners in the four-nation research study
on 'Developing Sustainable Educational Inclusion Policy and Practice: India, Brazil, South
Africa and England' led by international experts Tony Booth and Mel Ainscow. Later, she
became a pioneer of disability and development activities as chairperson of the Government
of India's National Trust. Poonam with her extraordinary creativity and proactivity made a
huge difference to the movement and spread awareness all over the country.

Society for Remedial Education Assessment Counselling Handicapped (REACH), Kolkata

Another organization called REACH was founded in October 1980, based on SSI model.
Purobie Bose, executive director and one of the founder members of REACH developed
extraordinary services with a relentless zeal and energy. She writes on their organization's
website:

'Our thanks to our well-wishers for their financial support and goodwill throughout these
34 years. Without this generosity, REACH could not have touched the lives of more than 10
lakh children with disabilities, their parents and society at large. We are proud of achieving
our goals and are committed to move professionally with sincerity and empathy in the years
to come.'

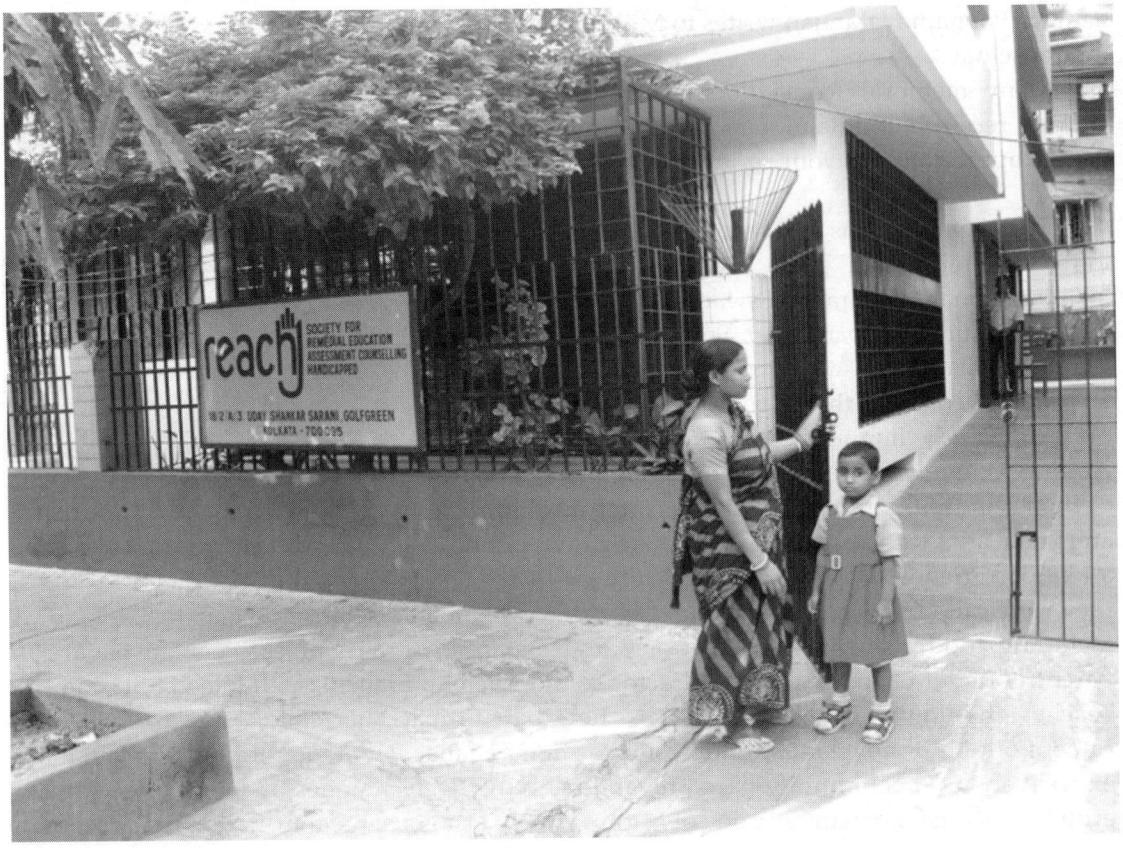

'Thanks to… Dr Mithu Alur, chairperson, SSI, Mumbai and Satyam Alur for their guidance and professional inputs in our starting up, development and growth.'

Umang—Centre for Special Education, Jaipur, Rajasthan

Another parent and pioneer of services in Rajasthan was Deepak Kalra. She came to us as a parent with her son Vickram who had CP. She had trained in child development from MS University, Baroda, and soon joined us professionally. She headed our community service Karuna Sadan at Dharavi and TTC. It was with great sadness we said goodbye to her when she left for Jaipur. Very soon, Deepak set up a string of services in Jaipur. She first began a set of services with Pearl Kavoori called Disha which the Maharani Gayatri Devi patronized. Then she moved on and set up another set of services with Bina Kak called Umang. In 2005, she was appointed the chairperson in the State Child Rights Commission. Deepak's compassion, her genuine love for disabled people and parents and her commitment to services at the grass-roots level soon made her a leader in the field and she made a deep impact to the movement.

Umang has grown from strength to strength and today:

- It reaches out to the largest number of children with brain damage in Rajasthan; over 350 families access a gamut of services at a given time.
- It has one of the most highly trained and experienced team of professionals in the state.
- Umang has been the main crusader for inclusive education in the state.

Deepak Kalra, founder trustee, Umang writes:

'My childhood friend Bina Kak (minister with the Rajasthan government) offered her house (in which she lived) to be used for starting Umang. Admiral Madhvendra Singh who had just retired as naval chief gave his support and Kumudi Singh, his wife, who is a trained special educator, became our chief resource person. The team of 11 senior staff helped me set up Disha in 1995 and offered their services free of cost till I could raise some funds.'

'The parents started putting together whatever they could, like old wheelchairs, special furniture that their children had outgrown, toys and books from their homes, friends and neighbourhood. It truly was a

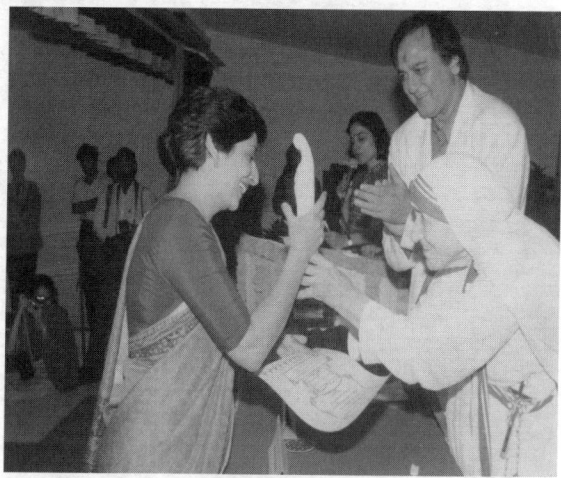

Mrs Deepak Kalra for her services to Rajasthan receives an award from Mother Teresa and Shri Sunil Dutt

cooperative/community project. The initiative and enthusiasm of staff and parents gave me the strength to make a start once again.'

'Bina and my family together gave us the capital amount to start and on 20th of December, 2005, Umang was officially registered. On the first day, when admissions were opened, over 65 children were enrolled. We started regular classes on the 2nd of January, 2006. Within three months, we had over 100 students.'

'Support also came in from friends and organizations from Delhi, Kolkata, Chennai, Bombay and Bangalore. Mithu Alur, who has been my mentor, friend, philosopher and guide, visited Umang within three months of its setting up, which gave us a lot of strength and support. The people of Jaipur, media, social organizations, corporate houses, jewellers and public enterprises came forward to lend their support.'

A Giant Step Forward: NCCP Is Born

In 1993, SSI completed 20 years in the service of people with CP and other physical disabilities and then took a giant step forward in creating NCCP for CP and other physical disabilities. This was the first purpose-built institution, addressing some of the gaps that existed consolidated under one building. It had taken around 10 years to come to fruition. It was an East-West project of international cooperation with donors mainly from Sweden and Britain. The building was a joint

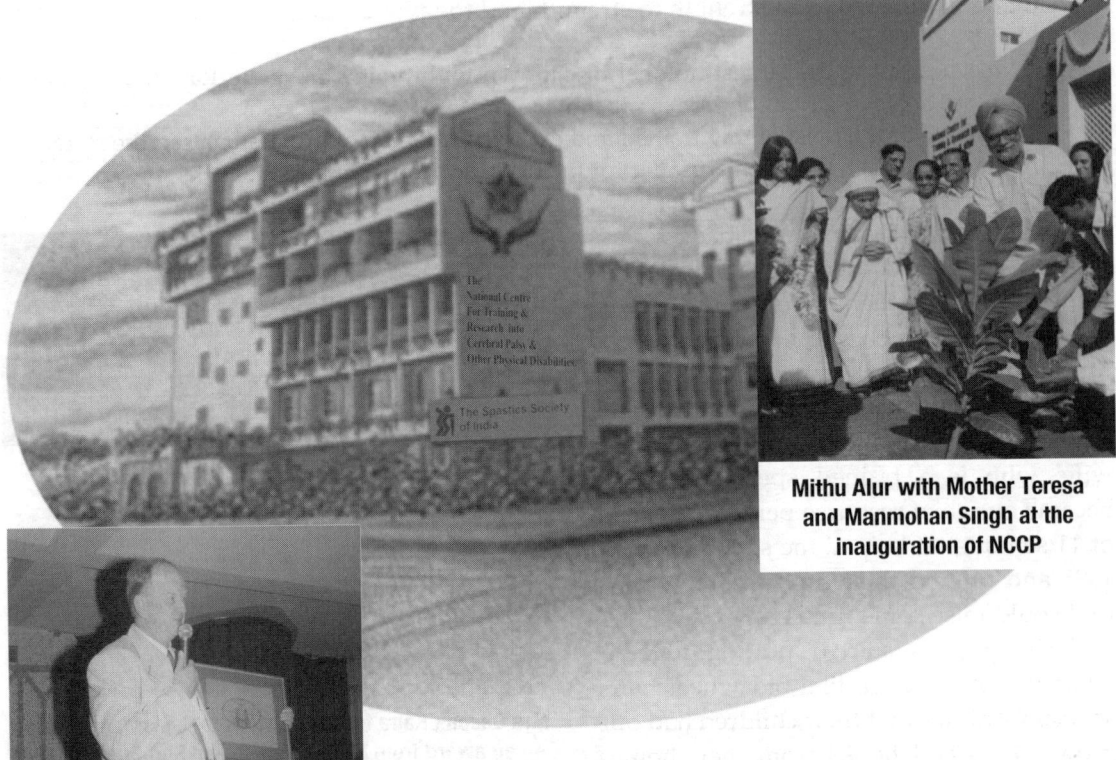

**Mithu Alur with Mother Teresa
and Manmohan Singh at the
inauguration of NCCP**

**Gerhard Egerhag, Lutherhjalpen
addressing the invitees**

effort of the Church of Sweden Aid (Lutherhjalpen), Swedish International Development Cooperation Agency (SIDA), Overseas Development Agency (ODA), Appropriate Health Resources and Technologies Action Group (AHRTAG) and SSI. The land was donated by the government of Maharashtra. It was inaugurated by Mother Theresa and Mr Manmohan Singh who was the then minister of finance. The *bhoomi puja* had taken place on the land 10 years ago, so Mother remarked: 'This is the first time I have inaugurated a building and blessed the land 10 years ago.' She also said: 'A work of love is a work of peace. Yours is a work of love.'

SSI has had a history of a close relationship with the Spastics Society, UK, since its inception. Both societies have collaborated on various projects and have provided technical support, professional backup services and information exchange through workshops and seminars over the years. NCCP is a consolidation of the last 20 years of work, nationally and internationally, with the disabled in India. The architect for the building was the renowned and eminent Charles Correa who began the designs and then involved his associate Kamu Iyer to complete it.

The national centre became the focal point of all activities related to assessment, training, education, treatment and research. Many other smaller peripheral services were set up. They included aids and appliances, computer education centre, science laboratory, library, outdoor and indoor recreational facilities, canteen, hostel and so on.

The services at the national centre presently continue to be the following:

- Early infant clinics
- Home Management
- Nursery and primary sections
- Junior and senior sections
- An education, assessment and therapy aids laboratory
- Training college for teachers, therapists and personnel
- A reference library
- Hostel for 32 outstation students
- Canteen and dining hall
- Two hundred and fifty-seater auditorium
- Clinic for adults with neurological problems
- Centre for research, publication and dissemination
- Outpatient clinics
- Resource centres for mobility, communication and other aids and appliances
- Need-based administrative, finance and management support system.

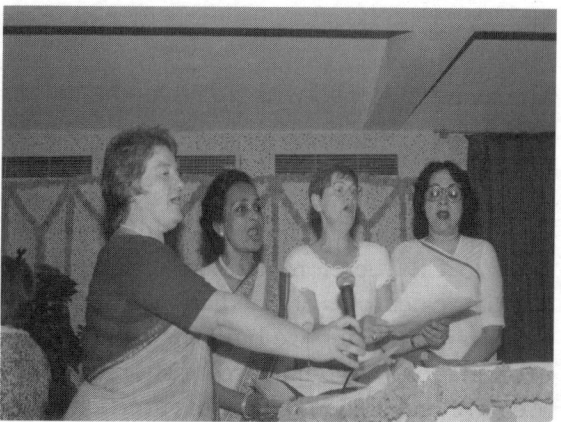

Pamela Stretch, Nirmala Mathan, Neera Benegal sing the invocation song at the inauguration of the NCCP

The national centre's new objectives focused on training which will include children, personnel, community, research and dissemination and networking with other organizations.

NCCP was to be a research-oriented demonstration model. Training and education would form the backbone of the service. Developing new assessment and evaluative techniques, remediation, teaching aids and new treatment techniques were some of the goals to be achieved. The therapeutic importance of sports, yoga, dance, recreation, music, drama, arts and crafts, work in the community and mobilization of parents' groups would be areas to be consolidated. All this would

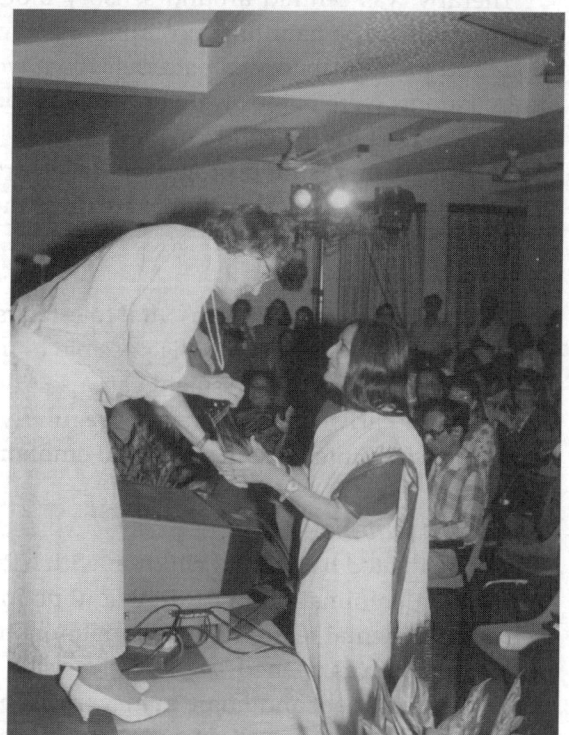

Our Swedish partners appreciating the work

be researched and recorded for dissemination purposes. Studying community attitudes, documenting information and disseminating at a macro level would be interlinked through a series of research projects. Data collection, tabulation and analysis would be carried out at every stage.

Early Infant Clinics

The sooner the child with a developmental disorder like CP receives intervention in the form of therapy and general stimulation, the better are the chances of becoming as near normal as possible.

Certain genetic, prenatal and postnatal factors place some neonates at a high risk of developing a 'central coordination disturbance' which, if not detected and managed immediately, leads to CP. Therefore, regular screening by a multidisciplinary team led by a neurologist, paediatric neurologist, paediatrician and/or neonatologist is necessary.

Over the years, we built up expertise in early infant programmes and worked in close coordination with our neurologists, neonatologists, paediatric neurologists and paediatricians. We have had a good degree of success because of this input. Therapists played a vital role in the multidisciplinary team. After a detailed assessment, an individual treatment programme was formulated for each child.

Therapy was centred around sensory-motor stimulation, interaction with the child and advising parents on handling, positioning and carrying techniques to minimize postural deviations and prevent abnormal patterns which would otherwise lead to contractures and deformities. Parents were made aware of the need for regular therapy and the importance of physical development for the child's overall growth.

Our early intervention programme was extended to hospitals, 'baby welfare clinics' and individual doctors. Research in this area was mounted.

Assessment Facilities

Before intervention starts, it was vital to establish the level at which the child is functioning so that, as treatment progresses, it is possible to monitor changes and reassess for improvement over a period of time. Assessment can also give an indication of likely problems which may develop if the early intervention is not regularly followed up. This is so for all areas of development—physical, intellectual, social and emotional.

Admission Criteria

The centre treated babies and children with CP, muscular dystrophy, spinal muscular atrophy, spina bifida, minimal brain dysfunction, polio, arthrogryposis and other bony conditions as well as mild mental retardation causing mobility difficulties. A new service for adults needing physiotherapy was opened.

In the outpatient and home management programmes, babies were admitted on an emergency basis from the age of a few weeks Those considered to be at 'high risk' of developing a disability due to known pre, peri or postnatal problems were specially focused on. Such high-risk babies were assessed and closely monitored to observe progress and for making a decision as to what kind of treatment should start.

Older children were also admitted after a thorough assessment by the various therapists and the medical social worker. All children were assessed by the clinical psychologist and/or a senior, experienced special educationist.

Nursery and Primary Sections

As early intervention greatly helps the all-round development of the child, children were then admitted as early as one and a half years into the nursery class.

In the pre-primary section, children 'learnt through play'. This form of educational input enabled children to learn the required skills to the optimum level, according to each child's capacity. The educational aids were modified and adapted to suit each handicapped child's profile of needs. Here, they acquired all the concepts essential to learn the 3 R's and learning through much-needed movement experience was introduced.

In the primary section, the educational input became more formal so that the children could come under the purview of Secondary School Certificate (SSC) and appear for officially recognized board examinations. Special attention was given to their communication difficulties.

Junior and Senior Sections

The secondary section follows the same SSC board curriculum as is followed in normal schools.

The emphasis on the secondary stream is for preparing the students educationally and emotionally to appear for the public examination, while encouraging their creative talents and preparing them for integration. Treatment is interwoven with their curriculum.

Assessment, Education and Therapy Aids Laboratory

This is another service closely linked with our research facilities. There is a battery of aids which are in regular use and we record the type of aid which is appropriate for a particular child as well as the benefit that the patient receives from its use. In this way, we are able to build up a database which can be shared with other organizations in our network.

Training College

Realizing the paucity of trained professionals in the much neglected field of disability, the following postgraduate courses are offered:

- TTC
- Management in Cerebral Palsy (MCP)

The diploma in education of the physically handicapped for teachers was of one year duration and was recognized by the Bombay University. Professional interactions, hands-on experience, wide exposure to state-of-the-art teaching techniques were the salient features of this course.

MCP was an intensive course for physio, speech and occupational therapists. The duration of the course was six weeks. It includes extensive practical experience in various treatment methods. Alumni from these courses are instrumental in spreading the reach of services, not only nationally, but internationally in countries such as Mauritius, Kenya, Uganda and Malaysia. Thus, the society was able to decentralize services on a macro level. Admissions were restricted to qualified therapists.

Library

A specialized library, containing books on various subjects like psychology, therapy, education, counselling and related topics was set up. Professional journals, magazines and other reference material were bought and subscribed to.

Hostel

Hostel facilities were available to outstation staff and students attending TTC. Facilities are also extended to outstation parents, seeking an evaluation of their child at the centre. The hostel is located on the third floor with a total of 19 rooms, some with attached baths. Other amenities include a large kitchen with basic cooking facilities, a dining hall, a recreation room equipped with TV and a visitors' lounge.

Auditorium

The 250-seater auditorium catered primarily for the society's programmes. With excellent acoustics and air conditioning, it was also to be used for concerts, cultural functions as well as an arena for the society's exhibition sales and as an art gallery.

Outpatients and Home Management Departments

The therapists at NCCP saw a large number of outpatients. Special clinics were held throughout the week for those children who could not regularly avail of the school facilities. The infant stimulation clinics received babies only a few weeks old. Residential facilities were available for outstation families attending these clinics. Families found this to be of great help because majority of our clientele came from low socio-economic backgrounds and could not afford the long-term care and treatment of the handicapped person.

Administration and Finance

The national centre is administered by a small team of finance and administrative personnel. These two areas are of critical importance for providing the infrastructure for the effective delivery of services to our patients.

Research

The primary objective of research will be to network with professionals by augmenting the database and through interaction and information exchange with other organizations. The projects undertaken have been classified in the following categories: education, training, treatment, CBR and attitudes.

A research advisory council is to be formed, comprising different organizations working in the field of rehabilitation with national and international collaboration. The best publications submitted will be published in international journals.

Research in specific disability areas is a new, unexplored field in the country. Therefore it is essential to disseminate information, not only through technical papers but also through lecture series, seminars, workshops, symposia, group discussions and publications. Medical and psychological problems, electromyogram (EMG) studies, yoga and treatment of CP, remediation or correction of learning disabilities, discipline problems, behaviour modification, integration and mainstreaming disabled children into ordinary schools … are some of the areas in which research was to be mounted.

There was a phenomenal response and requests came flooding in from all over India. By the end of the decade, the map of India looked like that given below:

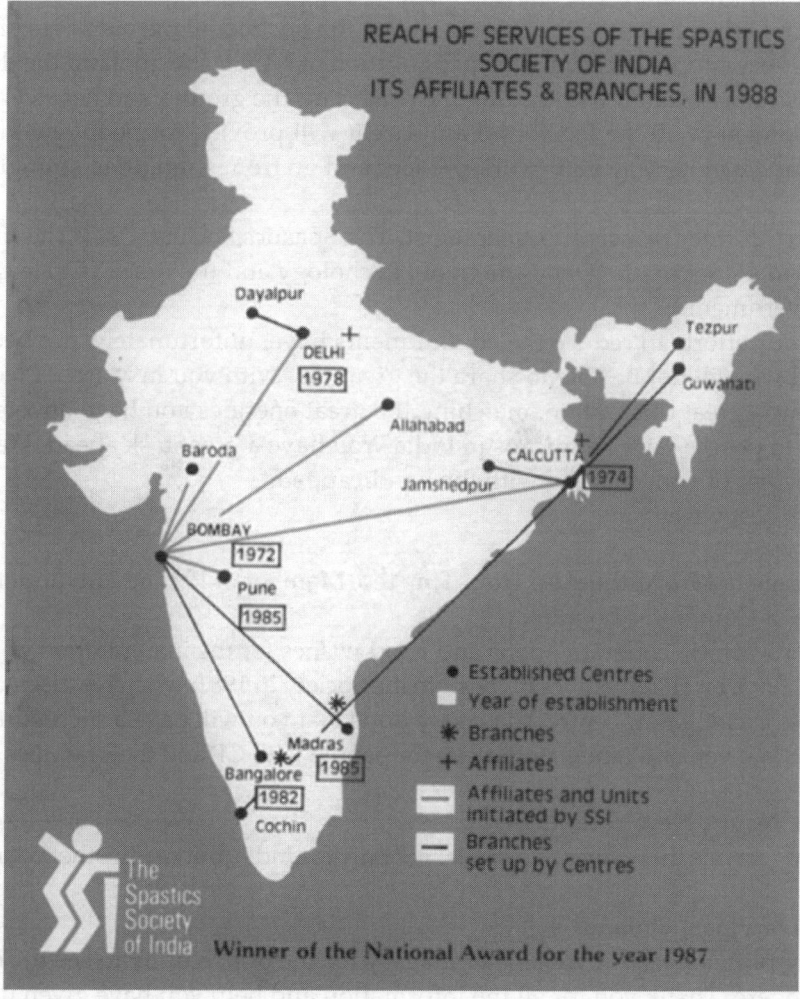

This figure is not to scale. It does not represent any authentic national or international boundaries and is used for illustrative purposes only.

Albert Schweitzer once said, 'All work that is worth anything is done in faith that the seed will sprout.' The seed sown in 1972 by SSI, Bombay sprouted, bore fruit and continues to serve hundreds.

What They Said

Margaretha Ringstrom, executive director (On behalf of the Church of Sweden Aid/Lutherhjalpen):
'Dear friends in The Spastics Society of India, Bombay!'
'Lutherhjalpen rejoices with you today. All of us would have wanted to be there. We are happy and proud to be your partners in caring for God's children. May our symbol "The Equals" always be the symbol of our relationship.'

Anthony Hewson, chairman, The Spastics Society, UK:
'Dear Mrs Alur, I am delighted to be able to convey to you, and all the members of SSI, my best wishes on this very special occasion, the inauguration of NCCP. We applaud the dedicated and selfless endeavour associated with getting the project off the ground and have very high hopes for the development of all the facilities. I am sure it will provide for people with CP in India, their families and carers. May your work prosper and go from strength to strength.'

Leslie Gardner*, former principal psychologist, The Spastics Society, UK (*The first psychologist who trained us, set up the Department of Psychology and the first TTC. He came through the British government.):
'Dear Mithu, our efforts to reduce the commitments have, unfortunately, not been successful and I'm afraid we will not be able to share the great day with you in March. I feel sure it will be a happy day, a great celebration, matching the great energies you have devoted to furthering the rights of people with handicaps in India. You have a great task ahead. We pray for the continuing success of your mission with the handicapped.'
'With our very best wishes.'

Personal message to Mrs Mithu Alur from Tim Yeo, Member of Parliament, undersecretary for health, House of Commons, London:
'I send you my warmest congratulations and good wishes for the inauguration of NCCP on the 21st of March, 1993. I well remember my visit to the Society in 1981, when we discussed the establishment of this exciting new centre. I sincerely hope that you will have a successful day and the excellent work that you and others undertake for people with CP and their families will flourish.'

Ken and Lind Reston, New York, USA:
'A splendid programme that serves as a model not only for India, but many other countries as well.'

Sepp and Eila Jarvinan, Finland:
'An interesting place to visit … we are very happy for the opportunity to see the centre and its happy atmosphere. Thank you for all the information and help you have given us.'

Margaret Yekutiel, Israel:
'I suppose I count as a "visitor", but I feel as though I'm coming home when I come here. So much change and progress and colour since I was here in 1993. Congratulations!'

Church of Sweden Aid, Lutherhjalpen:
'We are very thankful for our visit here in your centre and happy of all the people we met here.'

Sanjeev Chowdhury, Vice Consul, Canadian Consulate:
'Excellent facility! What a lovely place!'

Beppie Spee, social worker, Holland:
'I am very happy to see that things can be organized, so good as in this centre. The library is very well kept and even in The Netherlands, we can learn from this. About the school, I think you all are doing a great job here.'

The American Academy for CP and Developmental Medicine:
'What a Model program! Extremely impressive and inspirational to us. I look forward to some collaborative efforts between your centre and the American Academy for Cerebral Palsy and Developmental Medicine. We feel as if we've come around the world and yet we are at home!'

Patricia Hayden:
'Thank you for showing us your excellent programme, more importantly, thank you for having the courage to be advocate for the social and political reforms needed for all our children.'

Ekkehard Henschke, Ex-Chief Librarian of City Library of Cologne, Germany:
'I was very much impressed about teaching and training disabled children and their mothers for a better future. Many thanks to all of the teachers, therapists and volunteers. Good luck and much success.'

Christer Akesson, International Project Coordinator, Church of Sweden Aid:
'Thank you for sharing this beautiful resource centre—"The house of happiness and hope".'

Gunilla and Olof Milton, SIDA, Stockholm:
'I will be thinking of you, especially on that day to wish you ... every success in your continued work to spread information on methods to avoid complications for babies at the time of birth and to assist those children who have been born with defects so as to alleviate possible handicaps. For you ..., this day will mark a well-earned reward for your untiring and—as it seemed in the early stages of the planning period—endless effort to create something you believed so strongly in and which meets a great demand. With our best wishes and warmest regards.'

Tord Larsen and Ingvar Javer, Eracare (Triumph Wheelchair Collaborators), Sweden:
'Dear Sathi, Ingvar and I are thinking about you and all the activities at SSI and the inauguration which you have just ahead of you. Even if we will not be there in person, our thoughts will
be with you. We do admire all the work you have done, the great things that you, together with
your staff, have been able to accomplish. The one who deserves the most on your great day of
celebration is Mithu who has been carrying a heavy workload and your daughter, Malini, who
has been your inspiration. You should be feeling good to see what you together have been able
to accomplish. Ingvar and I wish you and your project all the best for the future and we are at
your side whenever you need us.'

Doug Patterson, Canadian Consul:
'Thank you for the tour of your outstanding school... Best wishes.'

Commissioner for Disabilities, Rajasthan:
'It is really inclusive education. The philosophy of inclusion is learnt here.'

Brian Dickson, Deputy High Commissioner, Canadian High Commission, New Delhi:
'Congratulations on your pioneering work, on your enthusiasm and on the difference you are
making in people's lives.'

Gerhard Egerhag, Finance Director, Church of Sweden Aid, Lutherhjalpen:
'Dear friends, it was a great joy to come back to SSI about 10 years after the memorial inauguration when I and my wife could take part. I am very happy to see the progress work and that
the building has been well maintained and been of service for this many years. Thank you and
best wishes.'

Lindo Libront, Programme Coordinator, Canadian International Development Agency (CIDA),
Canada:
'Dear friends, thank you very much for giving me your time to explain your programming. I
learnt a great deal. All the staff are professional and energetic. I hope that you and Canada can
maintain a partnership into the future.'

Martin Thummelm, Deputy Consul General of Germany in Mumbai:
'Dear friends, I thank you most warmly for the wonderful reception and introduction to your
work. You are a true model not just to India.'

Dr Felicity Armstrong, University of London:
'The work here is inspirational and a real learning experience.'

Fleur Bothwich, Ernst & Young, London:
'Thank you so much for opening your doors to us and sharing such a wealth of background
to your work. You are truly doing the change you want to see and as the mother of a disabled

child, I am deeply moved to see what quality of life you are giving these young people. I do hope we can find ways for Ernst & Young to support you.'

Pankaj Joshi, Joint Secretary (DD), Ministry of Social Justice and Empowerment:
'Very inspiring and thought-provoking visit. I got first hand lessons on inclusive education and multi-level teaching. I wish if government could collaborate/partner with this organization in its present and future endeavour. Best wishes to all!'

Namrata Thapa, Deputy Secretary, Government of Sikkim:
'It is wonderful and amazing to see such dedicated teachers who are putting everything to do this wonderful service. Best of luck.'

Shweta, lawyer, Justice and Peace Commission, Mumbai:
'It is a learning experience being here and seeing ADAPT's activities. Thanks for having me here.'

Dr I.C. Verma, Delhi:
'The institute is doing wonderful work, and importantly spreading this around India. Keep it up.'

Late president of India, Dr A.P.J. Abdul Kalam:
'If a country is to be corruption free and become a nation of beautiful minds, I strongly feel there are three key societal members who can make a difference. They are the father, the mother and the teacher. If we work and sweat for the great vision with ignited minds, the transformation leading to the birth of a vibrant developed India will happen. You have begun it here.'

(ii) Expansion of Services on the International Level

a. International Collaborations

We have had many international collaborations and each has enriched our knowledge base. Technical support came in a big way from the UK which has been our partner for the longest period of time and also where Malini and I were educated. Some important players, mentioned earlier, who helped in setting up the technical services were Leslie Gardner, Pamela Stretch, Edwina Baher, Klaus Wedell, Seamus Hegarty, Tim Yeo, Lord Alfred Morris, Mark Vaughan, Richard Rieser, Tony Booth, Jennifer Evans, Alex Crawford, Sheila Wirz, Prue Chalker, Frances Moore, Antonia Derry, Pat Yaxley, Ruth Whitehouse, Baroness Flather and other venerable members of the Women's Council. Felicity Armstrong and Len Barton from the Institute of Education, Joyce Smith and Joy Weeks and many, many others from the British Council, Institute of Education and the DFID (Department For International Development) helped to promote the development of our services. From Sweden, Lutherhjalpen and SIDA helped in setting up NCCP as a national focal point for research and intervention. Mr Olof Milon, Einar Helander Margaretta and Bjorn Ringstrom, Horsten Mansonth, Pastor Thorsten Ramonth, Gerhard Egerhag, Malene Campbell, Carin Gardbring, director Christer Akesson were all instrumental in making this happen. Our engagement with the Government of India was most useful, too. In the case of Sweden, our Indian ambassador Kamal Bakshi stepped in to help us. With regard to Canada, the Roeher Institute, Toronto and CIDA promoted research and demonstration through the establishment of NRCI. Our partners have been Marcia Rioux, Melanie Boyd, Cam Crawford, Michael Bach, Gary Bunch, Jack Pearpoint and Doris Rajan. Here, again, personal contacts of Sathi Alur helped in joining hands with organizations and collaborating to design NRCI, which was to tackle legislation and policy with engagement on a macro level.

When we began the National Job Development Centre (NJDC), our engagement with government helped and the USA was drawn in. The building of infrastructure for skills development for youth and adults with disabilities began with a tripartite partnership, an Indo-American collaboration with the Government of India and NIDRR and the National Institute of Health, Washington DC, provided technical assistance for skills development of youth and adults with disabilities. This programme was implemented by the Government of India under an Indo-US Intergovernmental Protocol. Paul Ackerman and others provided valuable assistance in this. Daniel Mont and Sathi Alur, consultants to the World Bank, trained the team on mapping and screening, and Mitchell Loeb and Kristen Miller, experts from the National Centre for Health Statistics, National Institute of Health Washington, DC and the Q Bank, contributed to the Statistical Methodology. Robust data about the numbers of disabled people and the concentration of disabled people in areas are not available and mapping is an exercise that trains enumerators to identify, screen and plan the intervention needed through a process of need analysis.

This kind of training helped the organization to engage with Germany. A visit from the German chancellor Angela Merkel led to an Indo-German collaboration between ADAPT, BMZ (the German development agency) and CBM (Christian Blind Mission) in mapping all out of school children through a very huge project. People from BMZ were Hanni Walters, Sian Tesni and our CBM partners were Bridgetta Mary Prema, Sara Verghese, Anthony Joseph and Sheila S. who worked closely with our own team.

b. International Course: Community Initiatives in Inclusion (CII)

Another international project was a six-month, Asia-Pacific CII course for master trainers which began in 2001. The course aimed at training the trainers and planners of community disability services. The course has been supported by the Centre for International Health and

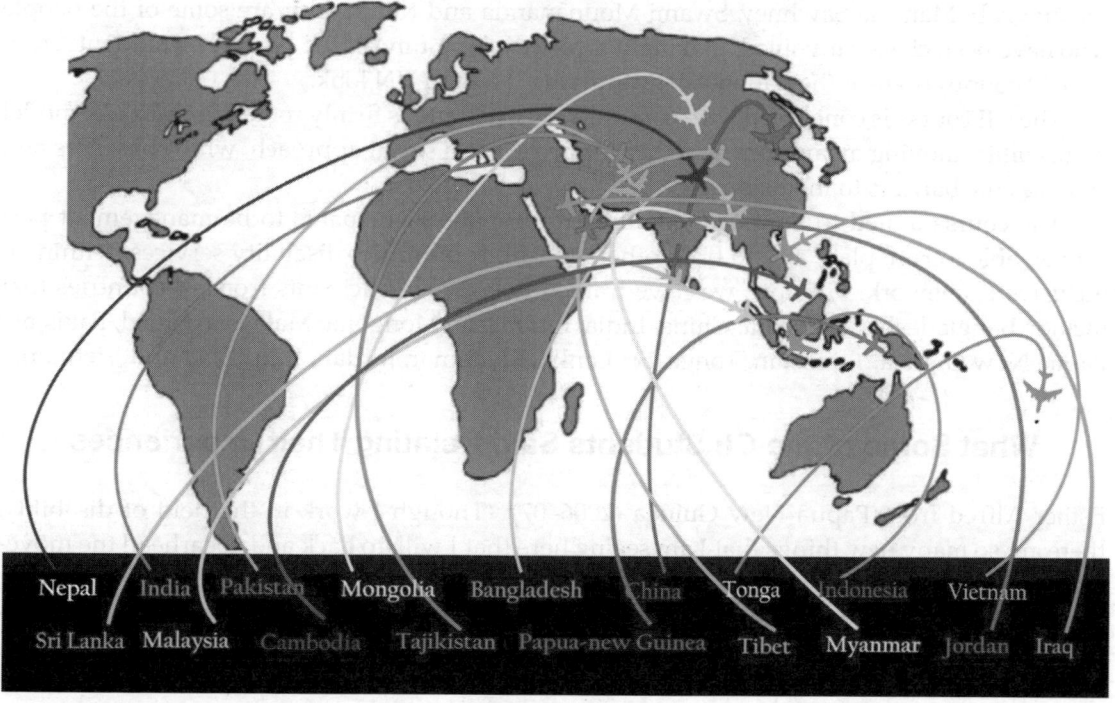

Nepal   India   Pakistan   Mongolia   Bangladesh   China   Tonga   Indonesia   Vietnam

Sri Lanka   Malaysia   Cambodia   Tajikistan   Papua-new Guinea   Tibet   Myanmar   Jordan   Iraq

Asia-Pacific Reach

Development (CIHD), London and is sponsored by the Women's Council and ADAPT (formerly SSI), Mumbai. Dr Sheila Wirz and Dr Prue Chalker, from the Institute of Child Health of Great Ormonde Street, together with Mithu Alur conceptualized the first course while Dr Frances Moore and Antonia Derry of the Women's Council crystallized the ideas with the council's support. Dr Wirz was a very respected academic, researcher, author in her field and had vast experience in CBR with numerous publications to her name. She had been associated with disability issues in England, India, Sri Lanka and Africa for over two decades and with our work at SSI for a very long time. Dr Moore is the honorary technical advisor to the Women's Council. It has been a great pleasure to work with Frances who has been involved at the ground level activities of providing services to the community all over the world during her stint with Save the Children. We are fortunate to have a person with her meticulousness in her professional work, her feeling for the underprivileged and above all a very humane and unpretentious person. Antonia Derry has been the backbone of the CII course. Hugely modest about her contribution, she has been responsible for the smooth movement of finance and administration. A very senior person with her experiences with Save the Children and various other organizations across the world, she has worked with marginalized groups in many developing countries. It has been a pleasure to work with the present chairperson, Pat Yaxley, a skilled writer and communicator. Many of the members of the Women's Council have visited us over the last 14 years. One of them has been Baroness Shreela Flather who has graced CII inauguration ceremonies and hosts the annual meeting of the council at the House of Lords. Alex Crawford has been supporting our inclusive nurseries and now has begun sponsoring students from Nepal. From the Indian side, Ami Gumashta, Sharmila Dhonde, Deepshikha Mathur, Varsha Hooja, Sujatha Verma, Malini Chib, Maneeta Sawhney, Swami Mounananda and Mithu Alur are some of the people who have been closely involved, making it a very exciting time of the year when students from over 12 countries are at the national centre, giving it a mini UN look.

The CII course is concerned with community issues and is firmly rooted in the social model of disability, moving away from a medical approach to a social approach, which observes and analyzes the barriers to inclusion.

The course aimed to and shall continue to prepare participants to be management personnel, able to run, plan, and to train others to run, community disability services, within an inclusive framework. Till now, we have trained over 200 participants from 18 countries that include Bangladesh, Cambodia, China, India, Indonesia, Mongolia, Malaysia, Nepal, Pakistan, Papua New Guinea, Tajikistan, Tonga, Sri Lanka, Myanmar, Jordan, Iraq, Tibet and Vietnam.

What Some of the CII Students Said Relating Their Experiences

Esther Alfred from Papua New Guinea (2006–07): 'Though I work in the field of disability, there are so many new things that I am seeing here that I will go back and spearhead the movement of inclusion in my country.'

Manju Regumi from Nepal (2003–04): 'NRCI has started the CII course. For the twenty-first century, it is the most important thing because only "inclusion" can end war or terrorism. World globalization is only possible through inclusion.'

Sadia Afrose from Bangladesh (2003–04): 'The CII course is a guideline for me. In the practice of inclusion, there were many questions in my mind. I got the answers here. The knowledge and experience that I gained from this course will be my strength in the journey of inclusion.'

Otgonbileg Yura, Mongolia (2003–04): 'In Mongolia, we don't have inclusion. This is a new concept for Mongolia. There is a need to change attitudes in Mongolia because how you think leads to how you react and behave. During the three months, I learnt a lot about inclusion. I want to start inclusive education in Mongolia.'

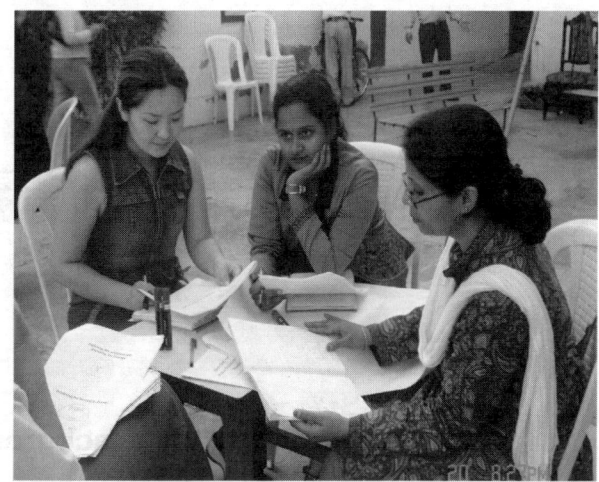
CII students

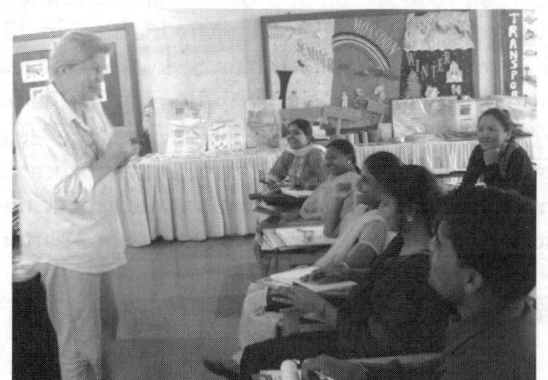
Mrs Frances Moore interacting with the CII students

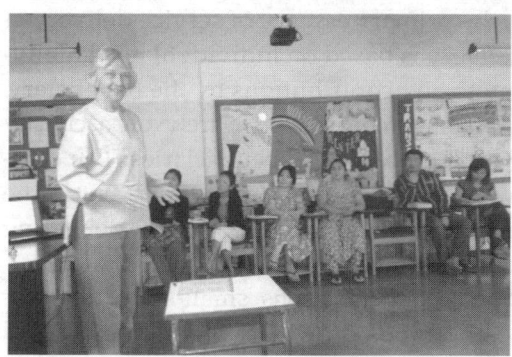
Dr Sheila Wirz taking a session on policy

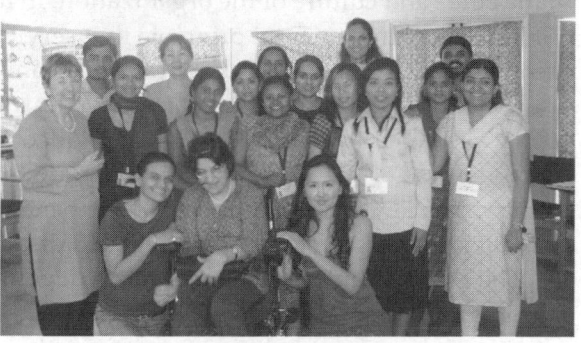
Mrs Prue Chalker and Dr Sharmila Donde, Ms Malini Chib with the CII students

(iii) Economics and Sustainability

Background

In the early years, I realized it was crucial to get the Government of India involved in order to pioneer the very first service for the disabled in India. I began at the top, meeting the then prime minister Mrs Indira Gandhi to locate an appropriate space. In the beginning, I was sent to the most bizarre places by people. Eventually, when Mrs Indira Gandhi intervened, we were able to get an idyllic bungalow overlooking the Arabian Sea within the leafy and safe precincts of the army cantonment territory to begin the service in Bombay, Maharashtra. There has been no looking back after this. The recognition of our work was clearly reflected in the government again helping to locate lands to expand services at Bandra, create a vocational training centre in Chembur and help locate similar land in Chennai, Bangalore and other cities where services were replicated and led by a dedicated, committed team who became our partners in this journey.

The Original Charity Model Framework

The organization was founded on the core principle of service delivery domain and not for profit ideology—offering services at a time when nothing was known in the country about CP and spastics. It had its roots deeply embedded in these values which form the very basis of the ethos and culture of the organization. In fact, the primary essence of service delivery at SSI lies in the fundamental principle that service delivery is based on individual need, delivered in a holistic manner and not related in any way to any contributions by the beneficiary.

Four decades ago, the organization's financial management rested purely on a charity framework. Clearly all services were provided free or at no cost to all beneficiaries. The charity model was of prime importance in laying the foundations of a service non-existent in the country. The key was to reach out to the beneficiaries and convey the methods of delivering education for persons with CP and related disabilities and to empower them.

The charity framework of operations depended on ad hoc donations, small-scale fundraising programmes and government grants. With the enormous growth of services and allied activities, it became a challenge to continue the charity model of operations.

In the early 1990s, the organization eventually was faced with a key question: To shut down operations under the charity model framework or to move towards a sustainable framework of operations?

Innovative Financial Management Towards Sustainability

We existed with the help of government grant-in-aid for 16 years. The bureaucracy and paperwork involved in operating with government grants was very time consuming and tough for a handful of staff. It only added to the challenges and financial sustainability became critical. It was vital to shift from a grant-in-aid organization set-up to an independent, non-government organization (NGO). This was a crucial move introduced by Mr Sathi Alur. The organization evolved its service delivery domain dynamically. On a parallel level, it had to evolve from a complete charity model towards a sustainable one, under the umbrella of a non-profit organization.

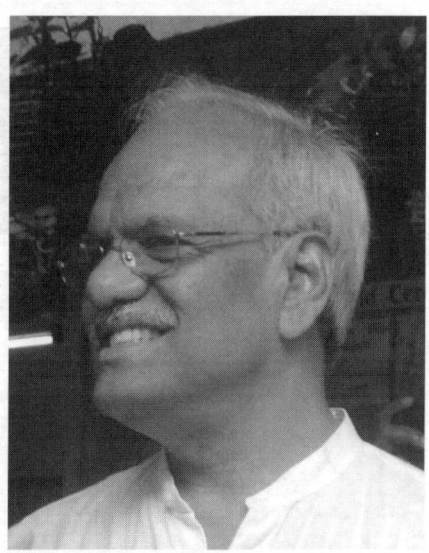

Mr Sathi Alur, Honorary Finance Advisor

The critical issue for NGOs in this sector was to ensure a continuum of services and to make the service sustainable. It was of key importance to move from a charity framework to an entitlement-based one. This required a careful consideration of the various participants in the programme: such as the services providers, primary beneficiaries, families, the wider community and the government. In order to ensure sustainability, it was necessary that each of the stakeholders understood the process and contributed. This way they would take ownership. Ami Gumashta (who assisted Sathi Alur) writes in 2005: 'Moving on the path of sustainability, we tried to highlight some of the achievements that we have made from following the principles of this model. We have also tried to establish an economic relationship between the beneficiaries as well as the cost of the services. We have tried to empower the beneficiary, so that he or she can evaluate the quality of service as well as the cost of the service which was attached to the beneficiary. Once they start paying the cost, they start questioning the quality. We have tried to instil in them the idea of entitlement.'

'We have been engaged in this process for the last 10 years and are amongst few NGOs in the country who have created a model of sustainable services through a comprehensive organization of stakeholder responsibility.' The processes introduced have been indicated in Figure 7.1.

Eventually, it paved the way for international partnerships and collaborations with like-minded partners like Danida (Denmark), SIDA (Sweden), European Union (Britain), NIDRR (USA) and so on. It also provided the organization an opportunity to innovate and venture into otherwise untreaded territories of developmental work. We were grateful that our own contacts (my husband Sathi's and mine) helped in forging these alliances.

How Did We Do This?

Over the years, fundraising has evolved in a creative manner, from film premieres to art and craft exhibitions, 'I Can' bazaars and *melas*, greeting cards, charity balls, carnivals and annual concerts. These are fundraising traditions which have carried on remarkably for four decades.

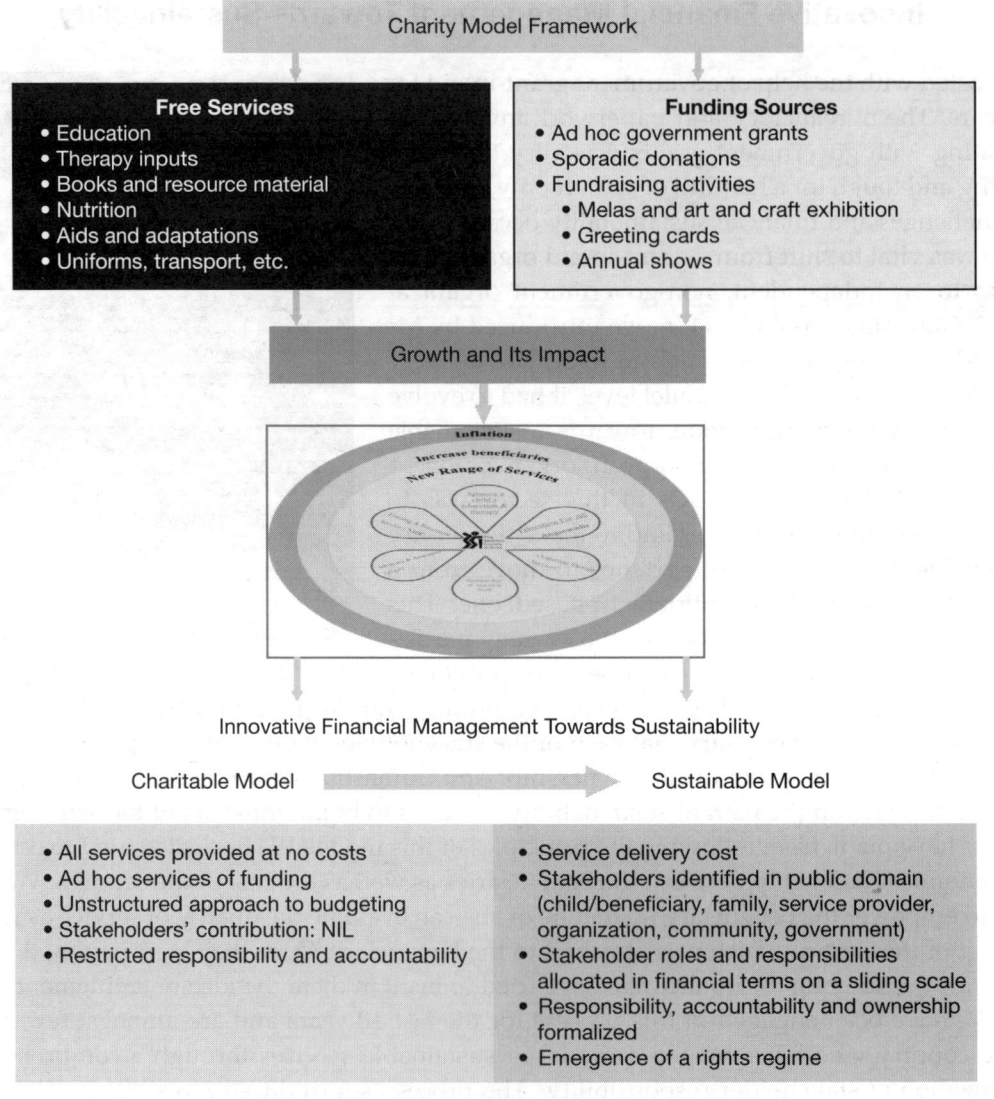

Figure 7.1. An Economic Evolution: Moving from a Charity Model to Sustainable Model

Source: S. Alur and A. Gumashta, extract from paper presented at an internal Board Meeting in Bombay.

A study of the annual reports reflects unique new initiatives each year and the seriousness and importance of fundraising as the organization grew. We enjoyed the fundraising activities, immensely. I remember Junie and all of us sitting on the floor in the verandah, sticking envelopes for invitations and for greeting cards…These memories reveal a unique joy in the activity of fundraising. Today, the spirit continues to be the same as the organization embraces new paths of fundraising involving schools. Individual-level fundraising for scholarship corpus and annual sponsorships continue to grow.

I remember a story when the British high commissioner donated the organization three Land Rovers. When I met His Royal Highness Prince Charles at Raj Bhavan, he said in his usual humorous manner, 'Has it happened? I would believe it when I see it!'

The annual report of 1981–82 reports: 'On behalf of His Royal Highness Prince Charles, Mr Colin Imray, the deputy high commissioner of the UK, graciously handed over the keys of three sturdy British Land Rovers the prince had gifted to the Society.'

On home ground, the Tata Engineering and Locomotive Company Ltd donated a 40-seater bus. This was the first bus for the organization and was used to bring the children to school. Thereafter, Tatas continued to provide buses through the years. Mahindra, too, donated vehicles to the organization. In fact, Mr Harish Mahindra came forward to become the first president of the organization.

To name a few other Indian organizations who came forward to help: IDBI Bank, Hongkong Bank, Larsen & Toubro, State Bank of India, Industrial Credit and Investment Corporation of India, Volkart Foundation, Indian Oil Corporation and so on.

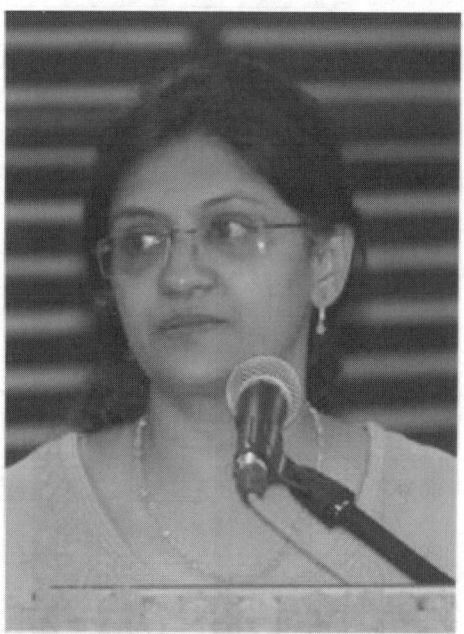

Mrs Ami Gumashta*, Honorary Director, Finance

*Ami Gumashta has been in the organization around 18 years. A Chartered Accountant by profession, she together with Sathi Alur made a valuable contribution in setting up the Department of Finance and Revenue Generation making all systems transparent and setting up strong financial systems.

This reflects the deep involvement of the corporate sector in India even before corporate social responsibility (CSR) was formalized in the country. Relationship building with corporate and public sector undertakings continues and has grown with time, along with the involvement of foundations, service organizations and other trusts who continually support the cause. The gradual evolution has been represented in Figure 7.2.

International Initiatives for Fundraising Were Also Undertaken

NCCP was built with funds from SIDA and the Church of Sweden Aid, Lutherhjalpen. NJDC was built with funds from NIDRR and The Spastics Society, UK. International fundraising contributed to creating the first ever corpus of the organization in the early 1990s. Contributions by the Church of Sweden, Lutherjhalpen have made it possible for the organization's core central service to function.

Following the visit of His Highnesses Romeo and Diana Leblanc Governor General of Canada and his wife in the early 2000s two International projects began. They were the National Resource Centre for Inclusion and the UNICEF Research projects, both supported by the Canadian International Development Agency. These projects are key milestones in developmental work in inclusion of disabled people in India and for influencing policy change. ADAPT recently completed another key international project funded by the BMZ, following the visit of Chancellor Angela Merkel, which has been yet another key milestone in developmental work in the community.

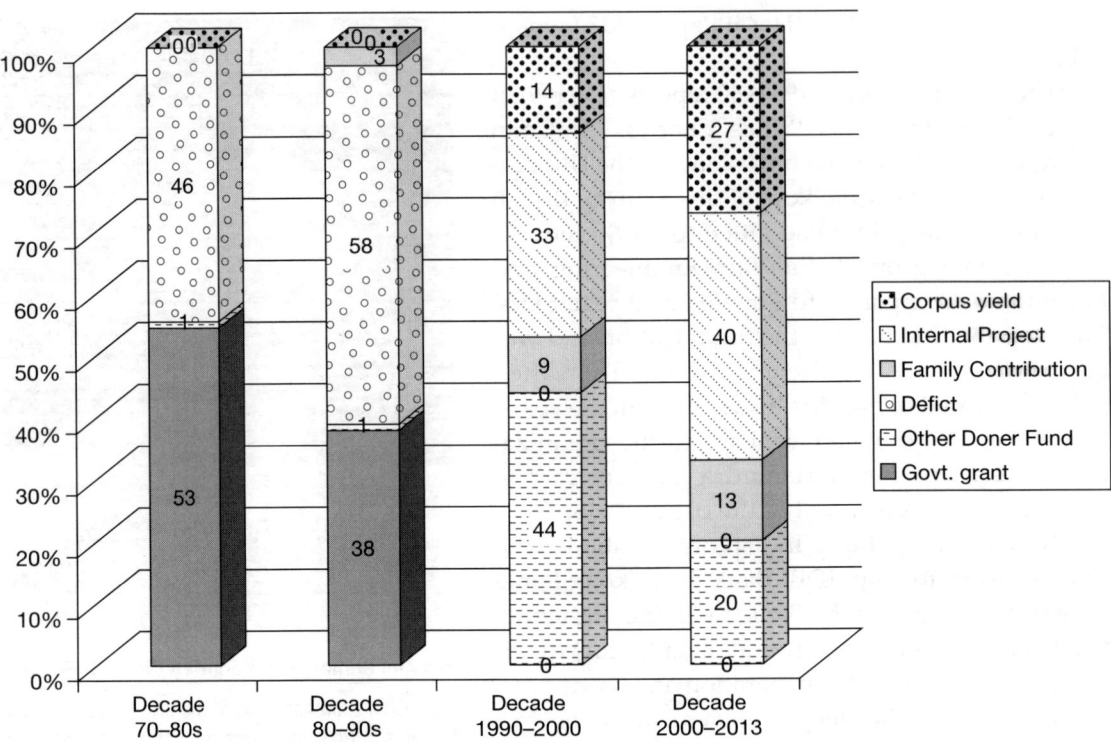

Figure 7.2. Graphical Representation Reflecting the Economic Evolution over Four Decades (in Percentage)

Source: S. Alur and A. Gumashta, extract from paper presented at an internal Board Meeting in Bombay.

The constant endeavour to promote international partnerships has been a key input in fundraising for new collaborations and initiatives from early days and these have served as platforms for exchange of ideas, sharing best practices and developing demonstration models and action research projects.

Fundraising is an ideology which has percolated through all stakeholders at all levels at ADAPT through this journey of four decades. We continue to raise funds at the service levels by way of sponsorships, scholarships and earmarked donations. Corpus donations through individuals and foundations are an ongoing part of the revenue generation programme for future sustainability. Project grants with like-minded partners like corporate houses, public sector companies and foundations has been a key outcome of the CSR initiative which has strengthened over the years. Work has transcended to a different plane due to the efforts of international donor agencies and associations over the years.

Lessons Learnt

The main principle has been family and community involvement. This is based on the broad philosophy of inclusion to draw in all participants in the community and using the resources of the various stakeholders in a unique way through *melas*, exhibitions and concerts. It has been a crucial stepping stone for this ever-growing organization to venture into new initiatives and has resulted in invaluable family participation and community participation.

- Community participation through individual sponsorships and scholarship provisioning support has evolved over the years as a part of the service level fundraising along with family participation within the sustainability framework.
- The service providers generate and attach value to the services delivered, bridging accountability and responsibility. The balance is underwritten by SSI.
- Raising revenue through various imaginative ways has supported the organization.

Outcome: The Sustainable Model

- Every stakeholder is an active participant in the financial viability and sustainability of our inclusive ideology. This remains the core of our continuity of services and sustainability for more than four decades now.
- Revenue generation and appropriate financial management emerged as a core activity to support financial sustainability.
- A planned programme of revenue generation for both corpus (restricted funds) and operations was set up and continuous financial management of budget and cost control was done.
- Whilst the beneficiary families contribute on a sliding scale, based on their socio-economic status, they also become empowered within a rights regime framework, questioning and assuring quality of service.
- Stakeholder involvement through family and service providers' participation contribute to service delivery fundraising. Community participation involving individual and corporates contribute to providing the safety net by the parent organization.
- Fundraising initiatives, portfolio management, corporate partnerships and international collaborations have resulted in assigning financial responsibility on a macro level.
- This strong foundation has been a key decisive element in newer initiatives of the organization in the field of developmental work.

As SSI completes 40 years of dedicated services to the nation, many lessons have been learnt along this remarkable journey in trying to achieve economic sustainability. Among the lessons learnt is that change can be initiated, attitudes can be changed and reformative action can happen without being a part of a political party.

Conclusion

It is a recognition of the quality of work done when the Government of India included the Spastics Society amongst the first batch of 47 NGOs eligible for receiving CSR funds.

The chapter of pioneering in a virgin territory was now over. The work would now move much more towards advocacy and awareness campaigns about the needs of disabled people, changing community attitudes and legislation and government policies to benefit the disabled at a broad-based, macro level throughout the country.

People Behind the Scenes

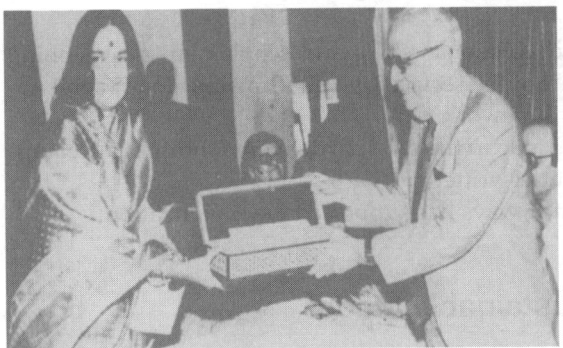

Dr Alur receives the N.D. Diwan Memorial Award from the former Vice President of India, Shri Hidayatullah

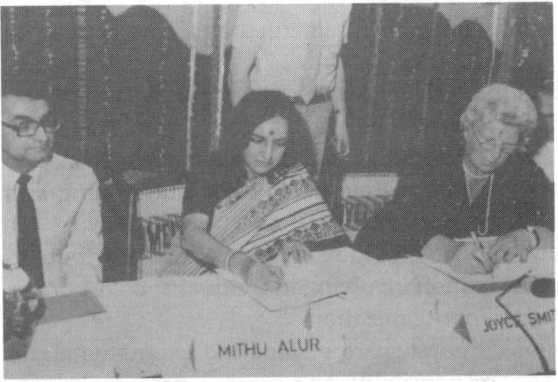

Mr Y. Malegam, Dr Alur and Mrs Smith sign a historic agreement for the Institute for Research, Assessment, Training and Employment (IRATE)

The society has been very fortunate in having the support of great visionaries who have helped to nurture and guide the movement in its efforts to serve the interests of the people afflicted with CP. It was, in the truest sense, a family movement.

Late Mita Nundy, Pamela Stretch, Poonam Natarajan, Usha Ramakrishnan, Mr Natarajan, Rajul Padmanabhan, Perin Aibara, the late Lilian Khare, Divya Jalan, Sheila Christie, Anita Shourie, Sudha Kaul and Varsha Hooja from Bombay are but a few names. One can write a book on just the people who have given themselves so completely, who have fought so many battles and who have stood steadfast in their single-minded purpose of putting spastics on the map of India.

In this context, one must mention the many government officials all over the country (especially, the ministry of social welfare) who recognized the need for services for spastics and came forward to help establish these services—Kamal Bakshi, Pranab Dasgupta, Moni Malhotra, Salman Haider, Bhaskar Ghosh, Yogesh Chandra, Mrs Joan Dias, a former governor of Maharashtra and

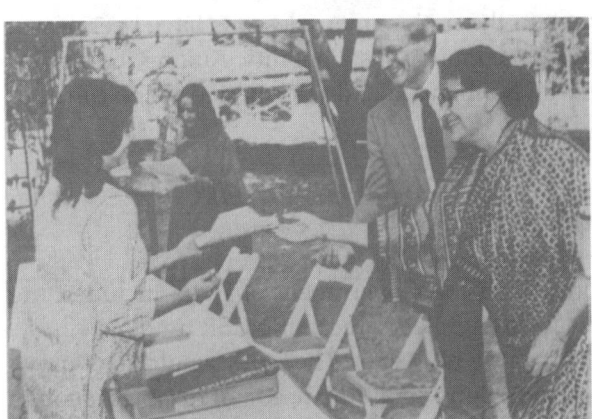

Ms Lobo receives her certificate from Mrs Uma Banerjee and Professor Klaus Wedell

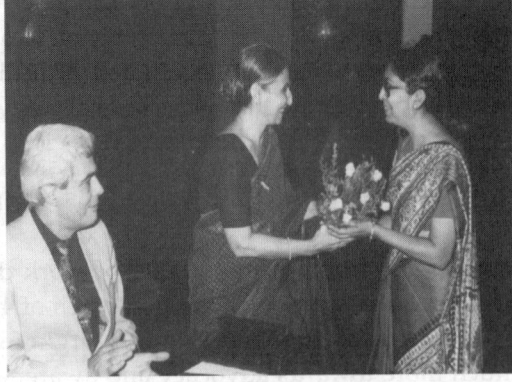

Sheriff of Bombay, Shrimati Mehboob Nasrulla, and Joachim Buehler, Director, Max Mueller Bhavan, being greeted by Sheila Christie

our chief patron Air Chief Marshal I.H. Latif and Begum Bilkees Latif. The trustees of the SSIs all over the country are giving help and support steadfastly behind the scenes. Above all one must always remember the encouragement and support extended to the society by our late prime minister, Smt Indira Gandhi, who by reaching out to a distressed parent, helped to start the movement for spastics in India.

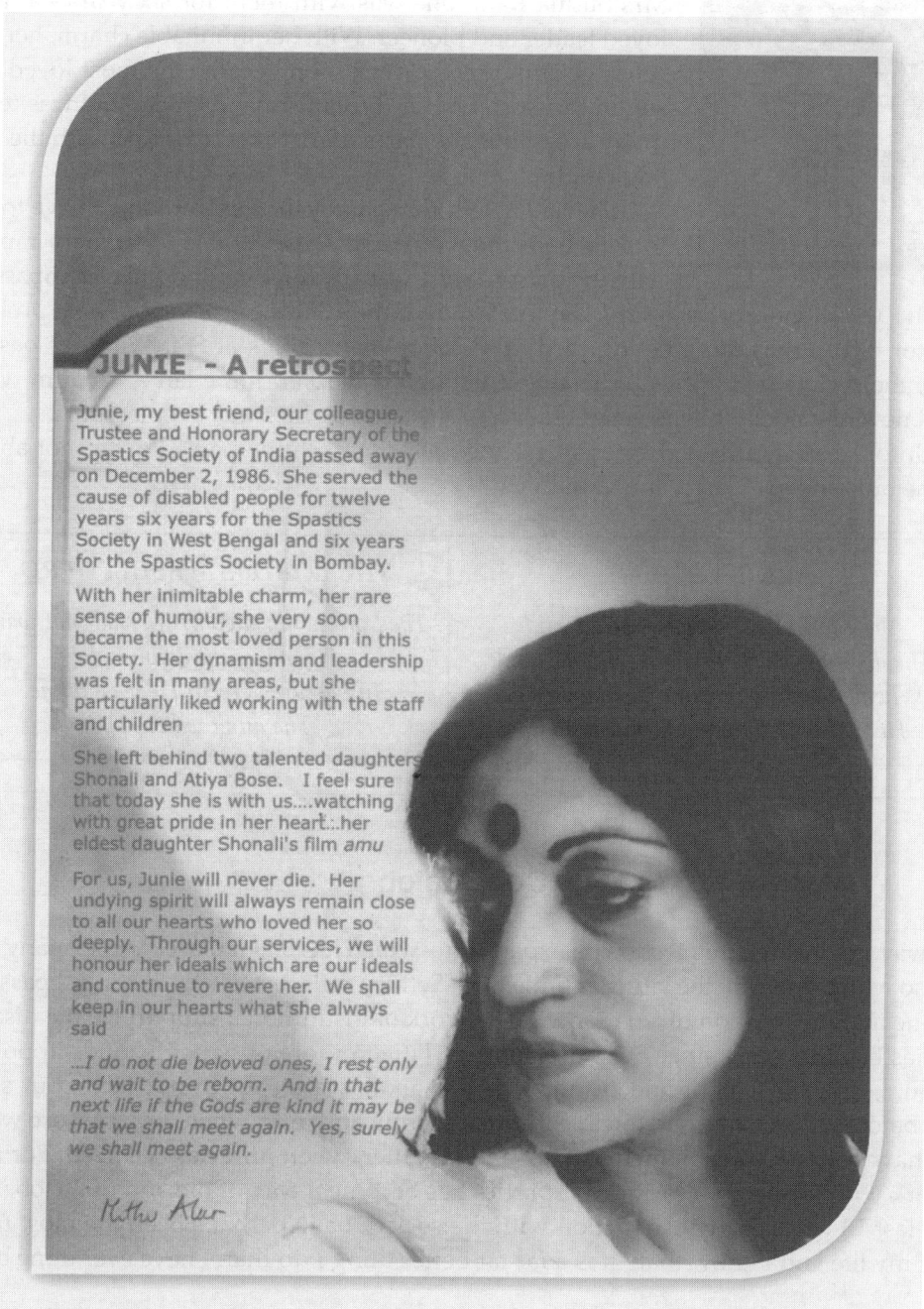

JUNIE - A retrospect

Junie, my best friend, our colleague, Trustee and Honorary Secretary of the Spastics Society of India passed away on December 2, 1986. She served the cause of disabled people for twelve years six years for the Spastics Society in West Bengal and six years for the Spastics Society in Bombay.

With her inimitable charm, her rare sense of humour, she very soon became the most loved person in this Society. Her dynamism and leadership was felt in many areas, but she particularly liked working with the staff and children

She left behind two talented daughters Shonali and Atiya Bose. I feel sure that today she is with us....watching with great pride in her heart...her eldest daughter Shonali's film *amu*

For us, Junie will never die. Her undying spirit will always remain close to all our hearts who loved her so deeply. Through our services, we will honour her ideals which are our ideals and continue to revere her. We shall keep in our hearts what she always said

...I do not die beloved ones, I rest only and wait to be reborn. And in that next life if the Gods are kind it may be that we shall meet again. Yes, surely we shall meet again.

Kutku Alur

Remembering Junie

Junie Passes Away...

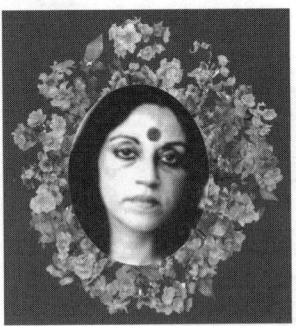

In 1974, Junie started the West Bengal Spastics Society with Mrs Sudha Kaul. She was with them for six years—a much loved leader and pioneer. With her inimitable charm, her rare sense of humour, she very soon became the most loved person in this society. Her dynamism and leadership was felt in many areas, but she particularly liked working with the staff and children.

She had a very rare charisma. She would just have to talk to somebody, anybody and she was able to set up a rapport with the person. She was truly humane and full of compassion.

She was honorary secretary, deputy head of the centre, director of slum projects, director of fundraising, greeting cards and school campaigns at SSI. With her passing away, the society lost a most crucial and dedicated worker. Junie left a vacuum which could never be filled; it is no exaggeration to say that her loss was irreplaceable.

Unfortunately, although present for the *bhoomi puja*, Junie passed away, not able to see the building she had planned with us.

ABIDE WITH ME	THE LORD IS MY SHEPHERD
Abide with me, fast falls the eventide, *The darkness deepens, Lord with me abide,* *When other helpers fail and comforts flee* *Help of the helpless, O abide with me.*	*The Lord is my shepherd, I shall not want* *He makes me down to lie* *In pastures green! He leadeth me* *The quiet waters by.*

Conclusion

An apt way to conclude this section on expansion—which has taken place over so many years—is to do so with a quote by the late Mrs Junie Bose-Sethi; it reflects the love, tears and passion that have gone into the creation of a nationwide network of institutional support for the disabled:

'It has been 15 years since SSI was founded. Fifteen years of struggle, of disappointment and failure, of achievement and triumph. Many doors were shut in our faces, but so many opened before us. We have had terrible times of sorrow and tears when we lost those we loved, but we have also had our moments of joy and laughter, when miracles occurred. For all of us who work with the society, caring for spastics has become a way of life and not a job. And for me, the last 13 years of my association with the society have perhaps been the most fulfilling years of my life and I know that "it is a far far better thing I do than I have ever done before".'

Remembering Sunil Bhai

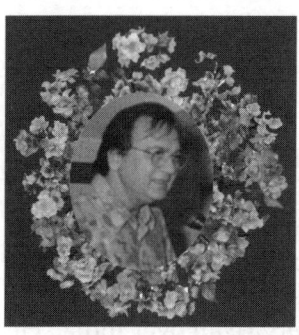

'In 2005, as we soared high and imbibed new knowledge, we came crashing down with the death of our beloved patron Shri Sunil Dutt who had played a key role in developing NRCI. His death left a void.'

'I have been a close friend of the Dutt family for 35 years and know them to be extremely genuine and warm people. The relationship began with my friendship with Nargis Dutt who became a close friend and the first patron of SSI. It is the personal side of my relationship with them that makes the passing away of Sunil Dutt a painful one.'

'In 1970, when I was keen to begin a movement for the education of disabled people in our country, I was given the names of 10 eminent people by Mrs Indira Gandhi, people in the city of Bombay who were helpful and supportive of the kind of work that I was about to venture into. Amongst the names were Nargis and Sunil Dutt. My husband and I set out for the stately home of the Dutt family in Pali Hill. Nargis was utterly affectionate and charming and agreed to be the first patron of SSI. She said she had always wanted to be a doctor and would like to begin reading about CP, the medical term for the jargon 'spastic'. My husband and I were thrilled and began planning the structure and organization of the society. For a decade, while she helped build the organization, she became a friend, elder sister, confidante and, of course as she said, a worker. For all these 10 years, Sunil did not visit us as he said that he could not bear the suffering of our disabled children.'

'But soon after Nargis' death, Sunil Bhai, as I called him, rang up and said he would like to carry on his wife's work but did not need a title. I persuaded him to accept a title. He took up the mantle then and became the next patron. My relationship with him again went far beyond a professional one. I was fortunate to connect with the humane side of him. I was fortunate in seeing his warmth, affection, care and sincerity. He was one of the few people in this city who was always aware of my pain as a mother of a disabled person, doubly compounded by the fact that we live in a disability-unfriendly country, ignorant about how to include people who are different into the mainstream and into our lives. He reached out to my disabled daughter, Malini, encouraging her. He proudly called her up to light the lamp with him and said, 'Our Malini has got a double Masters and has done not only her mother proud but all of us and our country proud.' He loved the restaurant Busaba that Nikhil, my son, had opened and just a week before his death, when he met my husband Sathi, he had promised that he would be there with the family. Not having my extended family here in Bombay (as they live in Delhi and Kolkata), Sunil Bhai was our family supporting us through all our ups and downs and joining in all our joys and sorrows.'

'I had longer innings with him than Nargis as we worked together for the betterment of people's lives for over 23 years. In all this period of development of the movement, I also found him to be hugely professional. I found that he liked to read everything on any subject he was speaking on. He never got tired of this. I had innumerable functions with him but he was hardly ever unprepared. He was also hugely humorous and a skilled communicator and would say, 'I am not a professor, I don't know big words and I can't give scholarly or learned lectures like Mithu!' With a simple sentence like that he would get the audience laughing and give a simple down to earth talk, reaching out with much more ease than I had with all my preparation on the subject. He was also not a typical politician who only talks but never really walks the talk. He had a sharp memory for anything we discussed and would always ask if we had followed up a job. It was a great learning situation for me to observe the meticulous manner in which he could micromanage events, yet have a bigger vision as a goal.'

'I always thought he was too ambitious for me. He was one of the few people who was passionate in his appreciation of my work and would keep asking me, 'Why is the media not covering it more? Why is the work invisible? We must see that your ideas are scaled out on a macro level… we must have the same kind of service all over India.' He was happy to keep it an apolitical body and respected my decision on this. He would not want the organization to be thought of as his own party's monopoly and would not use our premises for any of his meetings or election work. Never would he send patients just to please someone from his constituency; if he did send a family, he respected my technical judgement, assessment of the situation and recommendations. This showed again his inherent respect for our work combined with his desire for being ethical in his practices.'

'However, what was strange was the slight disconnect that existed in our development work, where he was proud of the work on one level but did not really push it out too much in the public domain. Although very proud and always encouraging of the work, he seemed to have been very protective of his role, as he was about his family, so the work was more personal not public.'

'Alas, Sunil Bhai, although the work has spread to over 16 states out of 31, we could not fulfil some of your desires because of the maladies that exist in the delivery of services in this country where implementation is given short shrift.'

'Sunil Dutt's demise is the passing away of that one public figure who was staunchly behind the cause and behind what I have been doing for 35 years in this country. He was the only national figure, the only minister who has been closely involved over decades in serving the disabled, the needy, the poor, the helpless, regardless of the fact that they are powerless and depoliticized. He is the only public figure who had the courage of his convictions, the tenacity to keep going on, the spirit to reach out to people without working out what he would get out of his help and support. He was a true Gandhian and the country has lost a true patriot.'

'And I … I have lost a friend, a fighter for the cause … a spiritual and emotional relationship which resulted in so much work over the years is over. The splendour will remain, the wonderful moments are unquenchable, the essence of his spirit, his atman, will not die, but the outside looks bleak, the journey long, Himalayan and tiring…'

'Maybe in another life, Sunil Bhai, we shall meet again, surely we will meet again… meanwhile we shall never forget you.'

—Mithu Alur, 2015

Domain VIII

Research and Transformation of Ideology: A Shift from Special Education to Inclusive Education

Background

Twenty years passed by and fast. We were in a mad hurry to establish basic services for the country. The main aim was to technically, financially and administratively help as much as possible. The idea was to let a hundred flowers bloom; let as many children receive services as possible. We realized that this could be best achieved by decentralizing services. Most of the resulting partner organizations were hugely creative. Often a stakeholder's own child or a child related to them was involved; this was an additional reason to make it a grass-roots service. We worked with families and disabled people and when the service had consolidated and our partners had learnt the ropes, we would move away, encouraging them to be independent. We were all foot soldiers and derived happiness from working with children and parents. They were our central focus. We emphasized activities like art and crafts, painting competitions, drama, sports and holidays which not only brought a great deal of variety and fun into the work, but focused on the abilities of children rather than disabilities, basically what they could do instead of what they couldn't.

However, 'mainstreaming' or 'integrating' children with special needs is not easy. While some may blend into ordinary class and thrive, others cannot fit in with the pace of normal education. Some may have problems of behaviour which may disrupt the class. Much has been written on this subject and space does not permit me to go into detail. Each child with special needs presents its own individual problem which needs to be carefully worked out, before placing the child into a normal school.

What of Malini? What was she doing and what was her thinking? Here is an excerpt from her book *One Little Finger*.

'I am a special school survivor. When I went to special schools the medical model prevailed.'

It was the age of labelling
It was the age of medical attention
It was the age where working for the disabled was considered charitable work.

It was the age where there were no rights for disabled people.
It was the age where disabled people were voiceless and devalued from society
In special schools we were ghettoized
In special schools our rights were hidden and never to be revealed
In special schools our voices went unheard
In special schools we remained helpless and children of charity (Chib 2010)

'I challenged special education and special schools. Being a product of special schools, I realize that in a special school a disabled person is caged. The disabled student is violently overprotected with every need of his/her met. He/she is not allowed to think or fend for themselves. I consider myself a special school survivor and have given lectures how harmful special school can be and can disempower the disabled child's growth, instead of empowering them.'

'Anyway, ... just to reflect back for those of you who don't know my educational background, I began life at Cheyne Centre in England which had the unfortunate name of Cheyne Centre Hospital for Sick Children.... Because it was a teaching hospital, it had to do a lot of demonstrating about whatever they were teaching.... I was ... I believe a very good guinea pig and would perform for all the doctors and workshops how well I read.... How well I communicated ... and so on. This was in the late 1960s ... here again everything was compartmentalized ... speech therapy for my poor speech, occupational therapy (OT) for my poor hand function ... physical therapy (PT) for my mobility ... we had to be fixed ... cured, made normal.... My special educator, a dear lady, Mrs Pritchard, did not get on with the therapist and often they were not communicating with each other and my mother had to be the intermediary ... so much for interdisciplinary rapport.'

'In the early 1970s, I returned home to India thinking how wonderful ... getting back home.... A shock awaited us. There were no schools.... My mother opened a special school instead of putting me into a mainstream school like my brother ... she started the first school for people like me called the Centre for Special Education. I spent eight years here ... lovely school, great fun ... but my education got seriously hampered by the fact that there were no trained teachers ... there was no syllabus to follow ... as they were very liberated educationists! And developed the curriculum in a broad style so to say ... we were really their guinea pigs in what they saw to be a very innovative experiment ... to me—everything we did was special— we were a new breed of people who were praised for whatever we did ... excellent very good girl ... how well you have done that were expressions I grew up with.'

'I had serious problems with academics ... in my writing and communication ... I went to another special school, this time it was the UK ... the Spastics Society Higher Secondary school, Thomas Delarue in Kent for two years to do my GCSES. In Delarue, disabled people were ghettoized. We were kept away from our peers.'

'There were specialized buses, specialized people to help us. To be let loose in society was unthinkable.'

'My idea of special schools is that they imprisoned disabled people. Disabled people are secluded from the hub and buzz of life. Whatever we did was triumphant, disabled people were cosseted and kept in cotton wool by special educators!'

'In the end, it resulted in living in an environment where disabled people were not seen or heard. I wrote articles which made the intelligentsia think and sit up. I first wrote on disabled people themselves and how the "World Does Not Owe Us a Living" and how we as disabled people have to be equally contributing and giving. I found most often disabled people would sit back and demand things to be done for them.'

'I also touched upon sex and disability, which made people sit up and look aghast and think to themselves: "What, you want sex too. There's never an end to what you disabled people want! Sex too. In your deformed body. Your needs are really unrealistic". But once they read what I had to say, I think they agreed sex is a basic need and everyone is entitled to it.'

'The most important reason for the low self-image of disabled people, however, is this: the lack of opportunity to handle their own affairs. History bears witness to the fact that people who can handle their own affairs, or are strong enough to snatch this right from others, are always looked upon with respect and enjoy greater self-esteem than those who sit back and allow things to be done to or for them.'

'My two Masters', the first in women's studies and the other in information technology, and my time in London has helped me reflect on what I missed. In London as an adult I began to reflect … after being in an inclusive setting for more than 15 years, I realized that my whole thought process changed.'

I agree with my friend Jack Pearpoint,

Inclusion isn't a new program or something one 'does' to or for someone else. It is a deeply rooted spiritual concept that one lives. It is not a trendy product or fad to be discarded. It is not a new label—'the inclusion kids'—not a bandwagon.

People are either included or excluded. One cannot be a little bit pregnant or a little bit included (like the myth of 'inclusive' recess or lunch). One is either 'in' or 'out'. One either belongs or doesn't belong. If we exclude people, we are programming them for the fight of their lives—to get in and to belong.

Inclusion means the need to belong to something and as a child this is essential (Ibid 2010).

The Spastics Society of India (SSI) was now in the third decade of service. I had been invited to the London School of Economics as a visiting academic and spent much of my time during those two years studying the latest developments in the field of special education. I returned from London end of June 1995 after a two-year period of study, which I draw on, in this section, to investigate research perspectives, what had been happening in the international scene, our own transformation in ideology from a special schooling to inclusive education and how we spread awareness through various workshops conferences.

a. Special Schools Versus Inclusive Schools

The world had moved on. A new approach had taken over. No longer was it right to look at disabled people as if they were diseased or incapacitated. Earlier, the focus was on the disabled person as a 'dysfunctioning individual'—focusing on his or her deficits and diseases. Current thinking concentrated on a 'dysfunctioning environment' and societal conditions, which aggravate individual limitations. This is called the social model and it focused on an 'enabling environment', putting the problem of persons with disabilities back into the collective responsibility of society as a whole. The argument favoured globally today is that it is *society* that should adapt to a disabled person, rather than the disabled person having to be 'normalized' to fit into society.

There was a move away from segregating disabled children into special schools, to integrating them into mainstream schools and this seemed to have taken place over the last two decades.

I learnt that it had become a question of human rights and changes in social policy backed by legislation to protect the rights of disabled children, asserting that they should not be removed from their community and must be educated with their peers in ordinary schools.

Acts of Parliament, International Declarations such as the Convention on the Rights of the Child, the Jomtien, Dakar, Salamanca declarations and more recently the UN Convention on the Rights of Persons with Disabilities (UNCRPD) reiterated that education must be accessible to 'all' children and 'all' must include children with disabilities as well.

There was a new approach to disability: a shift away from the *medical* model, which had earlier focused on factors wrong within the child, to a *social* model of factors wrong within the environment (Wedell 1985). The trend was to modify the environment and the curriculum and to differentiate the need of each child with special needs. Researchers and professionals were now of the opinion that there are enabling factors in the environment which various paradigms could help to normalize the life of a child with special needs. Special schools kept children in special schools; regular schools introduced children with special needs into inclusive classes. The practicality of normalizing a child's life and enabling the child to be a part of the school population included ramps, adjusted toilets, computers in the classroom curriculum, examination modification, attitudinal and pedagogical changes and, basically, an open disability-friendly environment which included the child's peer group, the teachers and the community. Children could belong to a special unit attached to a regular school and do certain activities together with their peer group, or special classes in ordinary schools could be used for remedial or extra teaching, allowing all children to mix freely to do certain subjects together.

Well-known writers and philosophers like Michel Foucault have argued extensively questioning the concepts of normality and abnormality and that it is *society that creates these walls and labels and it is society that needs to change.*

Why Inclusion?

There is a strong research base to support the education of children with disabilities alongside their non-disabled peers. Special schools, separate classes, lower student to teacher ratios, controlled environments and specially trained staff do not demonstrate the effectiveness of these programmes (Lipsky and Gardner1997). Some researchers have even felt that other than a smaller class size, 'there is little that is special about the special education system'. On the other hand, students with disabilities in inclusive classrooms show academic gains in a number of areas, including improved performance on standardized tests, mastery of individualized education programme (IEP) goals, grades, on task behaviour and motivation to learn (Alur 2000). Inclusive classrooms do not interfere with the academic performance of students without disabilities either with respect to the amount of allocated time or the instructional time. In addition, strategies used in inclusive classrooms—peer tutoring, cooperative learning and differentiated instruction—are beneficial to all learners (Duflow 2003).

Inclusion is...

A philosophy. It is a belief in every person's inherent right to participate fully in society. Inclusion implies acceptance of differences. It means making room for a person who would otherwise be excluded. Translating this philosophy into reality is a process that requires collaboration, teamwork, flexibility, a willingness to take risks and support from a whole array of individuals, services and institutions.

A practice. It is the educational process by which all students, even those with disabilities, are educated together, with sufficient support, in age-appropriate, regular education programmes in their neighbourhood schools. The goal of inclusive education is to prepare all students for productive lives as full, participating members of their communities.

Evolving. As people learn more about inclusion, they understand that 'full inclusion' means that all students can be a part of the regular education system—even if their curricular goals and needs differ from those of their classmates.

Rewarding for all people involved. When inclusion is carried out appropriately, research has demonstrated benefits to all students. Friendships develop, students without disabilities learn to appreciate differences and students with disabilities are more motivated. All of this is carried home and into the community.

Ten reasons for inclusion:

Centre for Studies on Inclusive Education (CSIE)

Human Rights

1. All children have a right to learn together.
2. Children should not be devalued or discriminated against by being excluded or sent away because of their disability.
3. Disabled adults, describing themselves as special school survivors, are demanding an end to segregation.
4. There are no legitimate reasons to separate children for their education. Children belong together—with advantages and benefits for everyone. They do not need to be protected from each other.

Good Education

5. Research shows children do better, academically and socially, in integrated settings.
6. There is no teaching or care in a segregated setting that cannot be provided in a general education setting.
7. Given commitment and support, inclusive education is a more efficient use of education resources.

Good Social Sense

8. Segregation teaches children to be fearful, ignorant and breeds prejudice.
9. All children need an education that will help them develop relationships and prepare them for life in the mainstream.
10. Only inclusion has the potential to reduce fear and to build friendships, respect and understanding.

Source: Vaughan, M., Centre for Studies of Inclusive Education, CSIE, Bristol, UK

Inclusion has been referred to as:

- Valuing all students and staff equally
- Increasing the participation of students in, and reducing their exclusion from, the cultures, curricula and communities of local schools
- Restructuring the cultures, policies and practices in schools so that they respond to the diversity of students in their locality
- Reducing barriers to learning and ensuring participation of all students, not only those with impairments or those who are categorized as having 'special educational needs'.
- Learning from attempts to overcome barriers to access and participation of particular students to make changes for the benefit of students more widely
- Viewing the difference between students as resources to support learning rather than problems to be overcome
- Acknowledging the right of students to education in their locality
- Improving schools for staff as well as students
- Emphasizing the role of schools in building community and developing values as well as increasing achievement
- Fostering mutually sustaining relationships between schools and communities
- Recognizing that inclusion in education is one aspect of inclusion in society

(Source: Booth and Ainscow 2000. Index For Inclusion,
CSIE—Centre for Studies of Inclusive Education.)

Inclusive education within a human rights framework had taken centre stage.

The other noteworthy point is that inclusive education is not special education. It does not refer only to children with special needs; it refers to all children facing some sort of barrier to learning and participation in the classroom. Inclusion is improved access to education. It is a high-quality education individualized to each child's needs. Children are not seen as one homogeneous mass, but individuals, with their own levels of functioning, who work at their own pace. It is an exciting concept, a new approach to teaching children. Here the belief is that no child is a failure and each learner's challenge is special. Inclusive education is really education for all (EFA). In the Indian context, this denotes children from poor socio-economic backgrounds, the girl child facing cultural barriers, children from impoverished disadvantaged backgrounds and children with special needs facing systemic institutional barriers.

It has been written that the introduction of one system does not mean that the old system has to be suppressed, instead it means widening the scope and action of such a system. The inclusive education and special school concepts are not competitive but complementary to each other. This spirit would go a long way in establishing a base for the harmonious growth of services for persons with disabilities in India. I thought, therefore, that special schools can change their role and play a vital role for the betterment of inclusive education in the following ways:

1. Serve as resource centres for a cluster of general education schools which are involved in inclusive education.
2. Organize in-service courses for the teachers of general schools in methods of handling children with disabilities.

3. Share special equipment with general schools for enriching learning experience of children with disabilities.
4. Undertake action research studies on disability-related issues and disseminate information to general schools.
5. Initiate community-based rehabilitation (CBR) services to provide alternative education and rehabilitation to persons with disabilities in their own localities.

Strategies for including all students:

1. Foster students' involvement in extracurricular activities.
2. A group meets to develop an integration plan and work to implement the plan.
3. Training teachers and administrators on how to successfully integrate students.
4. Giving all students strategies for effectively interacting with each other.
5. Cooperative learning strategies and opportunities for all students.
6. Environmental accommodations and accessibility.
7. Integrate therapy/related support services—speech, OT/PT and so on—delivered in general education settings.
8. Anticipating difficult behaviour and intervening before they happen.
9. Students learning at their own pace together
10. Allow and encourage parents to have dreams, hopes and goals for their children.
11. Eliminate 'plateau'. Believe that all children can learn and succeed.

Source: (Australia) Sarah's Special Needs Resource Page on the net:
www.2000888.com/www/tizx/seri/general.htm

Inclusive education is one of the viable approaches to make this dream come true. Inclusive education is not a threat to special schools. Setting up a special school with all the necessary resources like infrastructure, equipment and manpower warrants a huge capital outlay. In a developing country like India, which cannot afford huge investments, an alternative system becomes imperative so as to bring all disabled children under the umbrella of education.

Although we have been pioneers in the field of special schools, I felt the need of the day was now to move away from it wherever possible and look for alternative paradigms for educating our children. I decided to research further the kind of culture-specific paradigm most suitable for India for integrating our children into ordinary schools.

b. Research: Invisible Children: A Study of Policy Exclusion (1993–99)

Background

During my work of over 16 years in the slums of Dharavi in Mumbai, I noticed that children with disabilities were not included in the government's Integrated Child Development Scheme (ICDS), one of the world's largest preschool services providing basic welfare and psycho-social services through their nurseries or *anganwadis* for women and children.

The ICDS operates amongst the poorest sections of the population, amongst people living in the peri-urban slums of inner cities, in peripheral tribal forested and hilly areas, in the remote rural villages of India and is considered to be the world's largest package of services for women and children. It functioned on a mammoth scale, requiring multisectoral operations (Siraj-Blatchford 1994; Sood 1987; Swaminathan 1996; Verma 1994). The objectives of the ICDS had been drawn up by several ministries (health, agriculture and community development, rural and tribal development, education and welfare) together with international agencies such as United Nations Children's Fund (UNICEF), World Food Programme (WFP), CARE (US) and the World Bank. From our own work in the slums of Mumbai, we knew the ICDS was leaving children with disabilities entirely outside of its nutritional supplement and other programmes. They were simply not enrolled. Even in ICDS health and nutrition programmes reaching into the tribal, rural and slum areas of India, children with disabilities were not getting nutrition, or any of the other components of the programme, even though they were at least as equally impoverished as other children in the community. While health, nutrition and psycho-social services were given to the poorest who were called scheduled caste and schedule tribe,[1] disabled children within these groups were not enrolled. They were not entitled to even basic healthcare and nutrition, such as immunization or vitamins.

This was a violation of human rights and unacceptable.

Why then has this comprehensive service delivery package excluded disabled children? How is India going to be able to achieve education for all if children with special needs are not brought into existing services? While non-governmental organizations (NGOs) are doing yeoman service, there were still 98 per cent of those in need who remain outside the scope of services. Should only these few children that we can handle be the privileged ones to receive the best possible service?

Policy is not made in a vacuum. Barton and Tomlinson (1984) write that policy issues are embedded in a broader and complex socio-economic and political context, which generally cater to the needs of the wider society. It involves the whole educational system, as well as professionals working within the system, rather than simply looking at it as the needs of individual children (Ibid 1984).There is a need to acquire wider social, historical and political perspectives on the policies, practices and processes which make up special education (Tomlinson 1982). It was important to examine the broader framework in which policy gets embedded and to question this, so I undertook my doctoral research which could further inform work in this area (Alur 2010a). In 1994, I began examining the ICDS and the larger policy for the disabled in the country under the supervision of the well-known writer and researcher Jennifer Evans at the Institute of Education (IOE), University of London. My examiners were the well-known academics and authors Professor Sally Tomlinson and Professor Tony Booth (Alur 2000). I examined why and

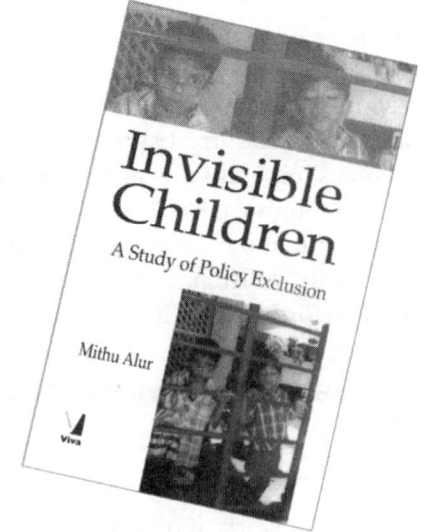

how such a major social policy in the country had omitted the disabled child from its agenda, the socio-cultural attitudes towards disability in the Indian subcontinent and explored the wider historical, political and ideological framework in which Indian social policy for the disabled exists and within which the ICDS policy and practice may have become embedded.

Findings

The investigation concluded (as already discussed in the earlier section on contextual analyses) with the finding that various factors have led to disabled children being left out of the ICDS programmes. The research found that exclusion was rooted in the very formulation of the ICDS policy and programme framework. Disability was simply not identified or defined in any policy. This failed to happen in part because just at the time the ICDS was being formulated the ministry of education was bifurcated and the ministry of welfare created. When responsibility for disability was being transferred from the ministry of education (now human resources and development) to that of welfare, the issue of education of children with disabilities lost focus. The objectives of the ministry of welfare were to 'rehabilitate' rather than to 'educate'. The ministry was meant to act 'as a nodal agency in coordinating services for the disabled'. In the specific context of the ICDS, although it may have been the intention to include disabled children in the term 'all' children, there was a *gap between policy stated and policy enacted as the ICDS did not include them in practice.*

There was an over-reliance on voluntary action or NGOs to deliver services. The NGOs themselves were part of the problem. They were focused on service delivery, their specialist role and fundraising, while disabled people and their advocates were left politically weak and unable to mobilize more systemic policy change. This had taken the matter out of the public domain and placed it within a charity framework. Negative attitudes, ignorance and a lack of awareness that prevailed towards disability had also contributed to this exclusion out of the programmes of the ICDS (Alur 2003).

International donor agencies had also been ambivalent. Partner international agencies had failed to set clear parameters in policy formulation at the outset and had not insisted that national policy-makers target their child-centred health/education programmes to include children with disabilities.

The findings indicated that, due to ill-defined policy objectives during the policy formulation stage, policy remained silent on the issue, not clarifying that 'all' meant disabled children as well. Implementation strategies for the inclusion of disabled children, therefore, were not worked out, which led to the non-inclusion of disabled children from the programmes.

The ICDS policy of non-inclusion of children with disabilities was symptomatic of a wider malaise in India, preventing children with disabilities from getting access to existing provisions and services available to others: without a clear-cut policy directive from the top, a massive exclusion was perpetuated at the ground level. The absence of a clear policy directive had left this segment of the population at a critical 0–5 years. A radical change in approach to the problem had to take place. It was critical to change, but change also had to come from within. Gandhiji said, 'We must be the change we seek.' And so began the transformation of SSI in Mumbai, moving towards inclusion.

c. Developing Sustainable Educational Inclusive Policy and Practice: UK, South Africa, Brazil and India—An International Research Study—UNESCO Project (2000)

We began doing another research broadening project ourselves. This was called the United Nations Educational, Scientific and Cultural Organization (UNESCO) Four Nation (UK, South Africa, Brazil and India) Research Project.

The UNESCO project was initiated by well-known authors and academics Professors Tony Booth and Mel Ainscow from the UK to conduct a research and development project on inclusive education, policy and practice.

It planned to draw on the knowledge and experience of researchers and practitioners from the above-mentioned countries. They were selected with the aim of making a major contribution to each other's development and broadening the scope of understanding inclusion.

The term inclusion was being used in a broader perspective, as it should be. Inclusion referred to all children facing some sort of barriers to learning. It was not restricted to only children with special educational needs but drew in children who were socially disadvantaged. Inclusion

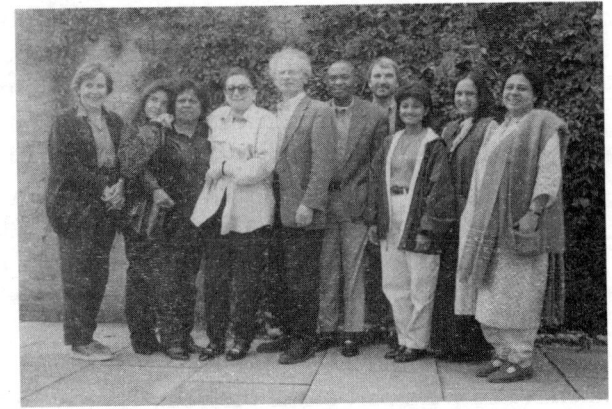

The UNESCO team at the Cambridge University

has been defined by various writers as a process of increasing the participation of all students, reducing their exclusion from cultures, curricula and communities. It is a never-ending process, dependent on continuous pedagogical and organizational development with the mainstream.

Two or three researchers were identified in each country. Heading the team from UK were Professor Tony Booth and Professor Mel Ainscow; from India was Dr Mithu Alur, research associate Poonam Natarajan, director, SSI Vidyasagar, Chennai, and team.[2] Brazil was represented by Rosita Edler Carvalho and Monica Pereira de Santos. South Africa was represented by Marie Schoemann, Nithi Muthukrishna and Sulochani Jairaj.

The objectives of the project were:

- To identify the factors causing exclusion and maximize the participation of all students within the development area under an education for all paradigm.
- To build context-based, culture-specific models of inclusion which will be sustainable.
- To coordinate with the state and local authority and draw them into the project to ensure sustainability.
- To develop inclusion policy and practice within that pilot area and evaluate progress over a three-year period.

[2] Mrs Varsha Hooja, Dr Madhuri Pai, Mrs Usha Ramakrishnan, Mrs Rajul Padmanabhan and Mrs Anuradha Naidu.

In each country, researchers identified an administrative district or sub-district within the organization of services. The district contained a number of schools and other educational facilities and reflected a range of issues, including maybe some of the more intractable barriers to learning within that country. In India, Maharashtra and Tamil Nadu were selected as research sites, where development work was both at the national and state level.

Findings

Some of the findings that emerged from the study were that various factors have excluded children from education.

- Failure to adopt the right strategy, more specifically, the large birth rate, consequent rapid growth of population which continually increased the size of the problem, the high dropout rates due to low motivation and ineffective teaching, the socio-cultural traditions against the girl child and the disabled child, and the general low allocation provided to education, remained the main barriers to learning in a national analysis.
- The inability of the government to raise the financial resources needed to support this massive programme of Universalization of Primary Education (UPE) had led to large numbers of children being left out of education.
- The disabled child remained out of programmes. The government's conceptualization of the problem remained ingrained in the belief that the education and management of disabled children needed voluntary action. This had become the norm.
- The pedagogic issues had not addressed this problem and the teachers were not aware of the needs of the disabled child.

Lessons Learnt

- Demonstration of inclusive education was critical as was the training of teachers.
- Each region had different context- and culture-specific needs and appropriate solutions needed to be worked out for each of these. One needed to develop an idea of a code of practice that was separate for the rural, urban, tribal and peri-urban areas (Alur and Natarajan 2000).

d. The National Resource Centre for Inclusion (NRCI), an Indo-Canadian Project (1999–2004)

Background

Following the findings of the research on policy for the disabled in India and the UNESCO project, we began to look for opportunities and resources to transform SSI to demonstrate inclusive education and reposition our own objectives to advance policy change.

It was around the same time that the governor general of Canada, Their Excellencies Romeo Le Blanc, and his wife Diana Fowler Le Blanc, visited SSI. They were keen to see worthwhile social projects and the government arranged that they see ours. They were very pleased with what they saw and hearing about a need for a macro level policy inclusion of children, they

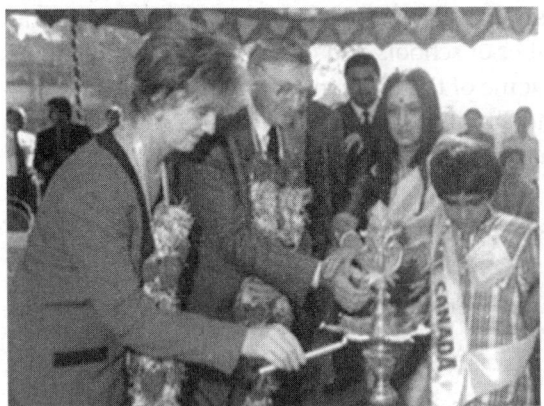

Governor General of Canada Romeo Le Blanc and Mrs Diana Le Blanc with Mithu Alur and a student lighting the lamp

The Spastics Society of India & The Roeher Institute launch The National Resource Centre for Inclusion—India an Indo-Canadian Project supported by Canadian International Development Agency (CIDA)

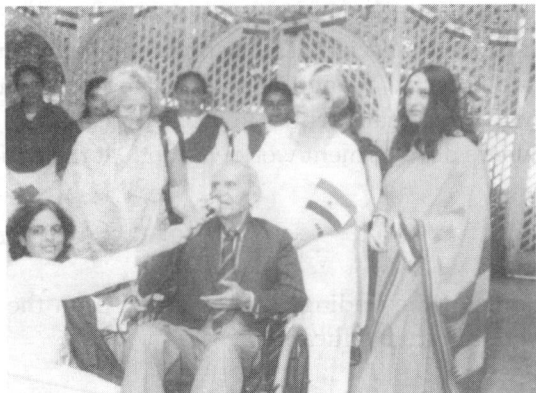

Left to Right: Mrs Varsha Hooja, Mrs Bose and Mr Bose, Dr Marcia Rioux and Dr Mithu Alur at the inaugural ceremony of NRCI

evinced an interest in future collaboration. Later in the year, we put in an application to the Canadian International Development Agency (CIDA) for funds for starting NRCI.

CIDA approved our five-year proposal; with our shift in ideology, we transformed the National Centre for Cerebral Palsy (NCCP) to the NRCI with an agenda for initiating change.

NRCI was born in 1999 in partnership with the Roeher Institute, Canada, and supported by CIDA. The mission statement was to develop, promote and sustain education policy, as also delivery systems and practices in the target region of India, with the intent to confirm and promote the realization of universal EFA, irrespective of disability, social disadvantage or gender.

From its early days as a special school in Colaba, and its broader reach through a network of special education services in Mumbai and India, we planned to make NRCI a driving force for inclusive education in India. The plan of action was conceptualized and headed by the principal investigators, Dr Marcia Rioux,

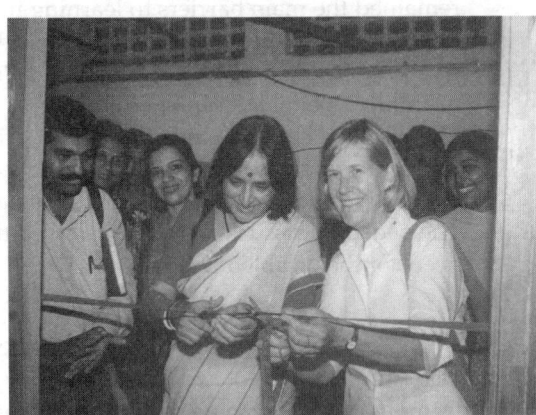

Dr Marcia Rioux and Dr Mithu Alur in the community opening the first inclusive nursery

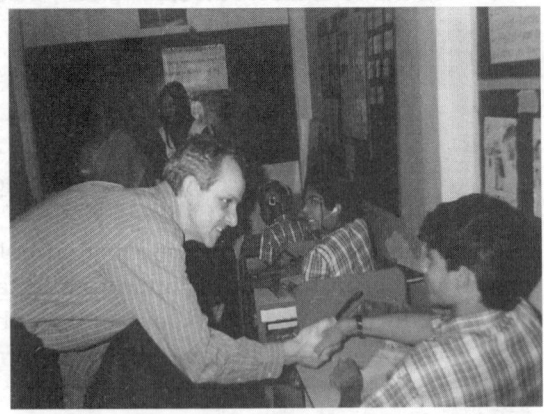

Dr Michael Bach at the Colaba Centre congratulating a student

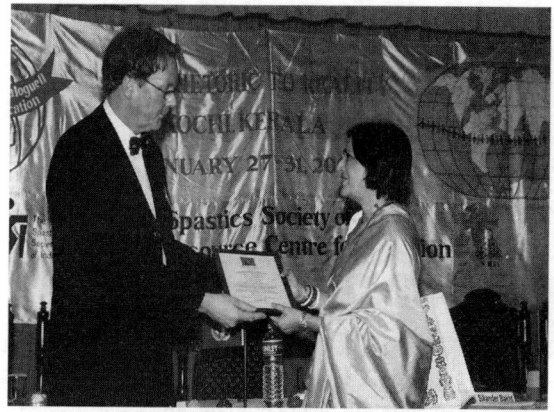

Mr Mark Vaughan, Co-founder of the Centre for Studies in Inclusive Education, giving The Marsha Forest Award to Mithu Alur from Jack Pearpoint

Canada and Dr Mithu Alur, India (advisors attached to the project were Mr Kamal Bakshi, Mr Sathi Alur, Mr Vasant Karmarkar, Professor Sitanshu Mehta. Playing a leading role was patron Shri Sunil Dutt).

A Project Implementation Plan (PIP) was created to set out a project management, implementation and accountability framework to guide the initiative.[3] We followed a Result Based Management (RBM) approach, which stated the key deliverables and performance indicators within an accountability framework. A detailed plan for implementation within a short- and long-term timeframe was drawn up for each year within the five-year work plan. This became the backbone of the project.

A charter for NRCI was created within the human rights framework with operational principles which would take policy into action.[4]

Implementation was carried out by a large team of practitioners and researchers, dealing with policy, from the Roeher Institute (Canada's leading organization dealing with reformative action and on policy change) and ourselves from India.[5]

Goals and Objectives

The project's broader goal was to support social and economic policy reforms in India within a human rights context. Additionally, the project aimed to:

- Demonstrate the access of children to educational opportunities irrespective of disability, gender and social disadvantage
- Promote the exchange of information and ideas on sustainable inclusion policy and practice

---

[3] NRCI-I was headed and administered by the Principal Coordinator, India, Dr Mithu Alur and Principal Coordinator, Canada, Dr Marcia Rioux. The project administration was done by Mr Cameron Crawford, president, Roeher Institute, Canada. The technical resource team at NRCI-I from Canada consisted of Dr Michael Bach, vice president, Roeher Institute, Dr Vianne Timmons, Dean of Education, University of Prince Edward Island and Dr Gary Bunch, Professor and researcher at York University in Toronto.

[4] Kamal Bakshi, Mark Vaughan, Gary Bunch, Cameron Crawford, Michael Bach, Vianne Timmons, Sathi Alur and Professor Sitanshu Mehta contributed to its creation. Several research studies contributed to a code of practice, described in the last section of this chapter.

[5] From Canada they were Dr Marcia Rioux, Dr Michael Bach, Dr Vianne Timmons, Dr Cameron Crawford and Professor Gary Bunch. From SSI there were Mrs Varsha Hooja, Dr Madhuri Pai, Mrs Ami Gumashta, Mrs Diane Saldanha, Mrs Priya Dutt Roncon, Ms Malini Chib, Dr Anita Prabhu, Dr Shabnam Rangwalla, Ms Sangita Jagtiani, Mrs Deepshika Mathur, Dr Sharmila Donde, Dr Urvashi Shah and Dr Anuradha Sovani guided the researchers. Our advisors were Mr Sunil Dutt, Dr Vasant Karmarkar, Mr Kamal Bakshi, Mr Sathi Alur, Professor Sitanshu Mehta and many others.

- Develop a cadre of resources (human and technological) to support a sustainable model for universal primary education
- Foster community attitudes, professional practices and legislative measures supportive of inclusive education and a social model of disability

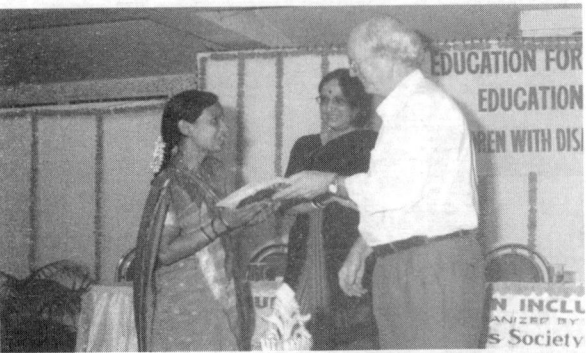

Professor Gary Bunch one of our Canadian partners facilitating one of our students

We broadened our perspective and used the term inclusion within the context and culture specificity of India. In our case, inclusion addressed children facing barriers of some kind and excluded from existing educational programmes owing to the following:

- The socially disadvantaged child caught in the grip of poverty
- The girl child who faced formidable cultural barriers
- The child with disability facing systemic bias

NRCI focused on change at three levels:

1. The *micro level* was the level of classroom and school values and culture. It examined two key areas: *School Development and Training*. This has been called *The Whole School Approach*
2. The *mezzo level* was the level of the community. Based on an action research, we developed inclusive services within the community which we called *The Whole Community Approach*.
3. The *macro* level looked at policy, legislation at the local, state, national and international level, which we called *The Whole Policy Approach*. It examined existing policies, their impact on practice and the changes needed. The whole policy approach describes the rights group that focused on moving away from service delivery to the matter of rights and entitlements.

This multidimensional approach helped us to change policy in India (Alur and Bach 2010).

A Four Unit Model

Four major units under four team coordinators were created. The four units were:

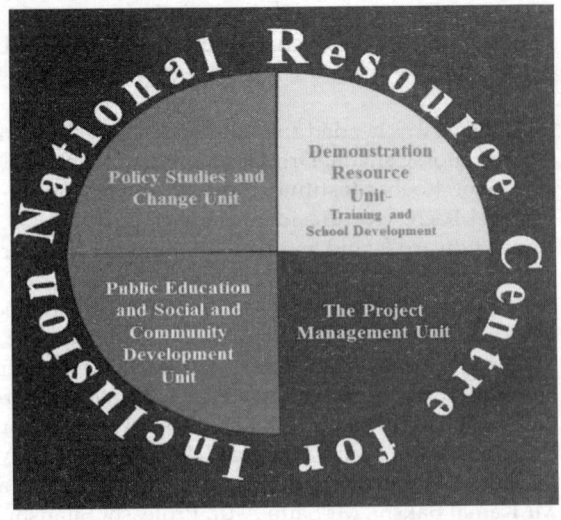

- Policy studies and change unit was directed towards the development of an Indian national policy of inclusive education.

- Demonstration resource unit to examine and develop pedagogical practices for inclusion within the specific context of India.
- Public education and social and community development unit to ensure that information on policy and practice concerning effective inclusive education was made broadly available to policy-makers, educators, parents and other stakeholders in education throughout the subcontinent.
- Project management unit to monitor the progress.

The aim was to desegregate special schools and introduce inclusive forms of education to demonstrate how all children can learn side by side regardless of disability, gender, class, religion or caste; to create a model that could be moved into the context of education for all, including the child with disability; to change policy on a larger level to address the massive exclusion happening in the country; and to demonstrate practice on how to include children with disability into classrooms and the programmes of the government. We opened up our own centres to children without disabilities from socially disadvantaged backgrounds, demonstrating how special schools can desegregate and also to demonstrate how EFA can take place.

The objective went onto lead the movement towards reconstructing a more inclusive community where not only disabled children are included but also other children, who have barriers to learning, moving towards the wider goal of achieving EFA.

Across the world, descriptive labels that create barriers to inclusion in society are being cast aside in an attempt to eliminate discrimination towards a defined group. The word 'spastics', originally used to define persons with cerebral palsy (CP), is not an appropriate form of address today.

In 2007, SSI changed its name to Able Disabled All People Together (ADAPT). The change was initiated with the aim to eliminate forms of address that create labels and barriers. ADAPT also reflects the growing aims and larger vision of the organization to create an inclusive and disability-friendly society.

A Whole School Approach to Inclusive Education: Dismantling the Specialist School

Problems Encountered

We encountered four major sets of barriers:

- Attitudes
- Access
- Curriculum and class size
- Training and support systems

Staff and parents were unsure of 'how' this would work and their apprehensions and fear contributed to a non-acceptance of the concept of inclusion. Parents of children with disability were unhappy with the introduction of inclusive classes within SSI set-up and worried their children would not get the same individual attention. Later they had fears about their children 'coping' in a regular classroom with so many children. Parents of children without disability felt they would pick up 'bad speech' or 'involuntary movements'.

Principals in regular schools initially rejected the idea and felt their staff would leave. Their attitudes were based primarily on a charity model of disability and believed that inclusive education was more a parental choice and responsibility, rather than *a child's right and a school responsibility*.

We first had to address the philosophical

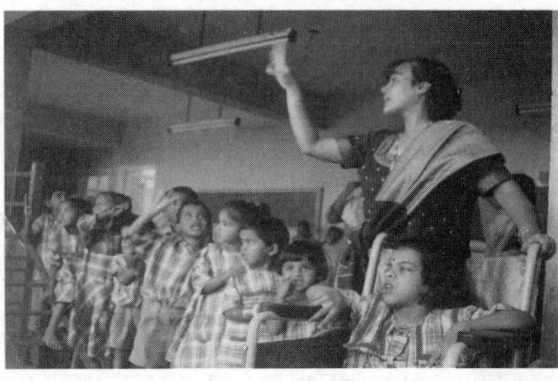

The first Inclusive Nursery

and ideological aspects of our own organization and then move towards restructuring it within a human rights and policy framework. The main aim was how to operationalize inclusive education. All of our earlier activities had to be reoriented towards a *new social model* and an approach that moved towards inclusive education.

One of our earliest steps was to create an *inclusive admissions policy* and open our schools in Colaba and Bandra to socially disadvantaged, out of school children with a special focus on the girl child. We admitted disadvantaged children from the neighbouring slum settlements in the preschool age range of 3–6 years. With the new policy, we also began admitting, in addition to children with CP (who had been our focus for so many years), children with Down's syndrome, Attention Deficit Hyperactive Disorder (ADHD), autism, dyslexia, sensory impairment and children who were intellectually challenged.

The existing special school was converted into a demonstration resource centre contributing to two major areas of inclusion: school development and training. Alternative paradigms were developed whereby children from SSI special schools moved out into ordinary schools that have developed inclusive practices (NRCI-I 1999).

Outcome

- Inclusion was hugely successful, much more than envisaged.
- Over the years, 110 students with disability have been included in mainstream schools.[6]
- Different paradigms of inclusion were developed:

   Paradigm 1: Socially disadvantaged children with and without disability with a focus on the girl child were included in district resource centre (DRC) schools.

   Paradigm 2: Students with and without disability were included in partner mainstream schools from DRC.

   Paradigm 3: Inclusive activities for art and crafts, painting, dramatics and sports were carried out with partner mainstream schools.

[6] List of names available in the NRCI library.

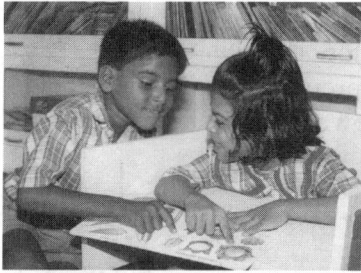 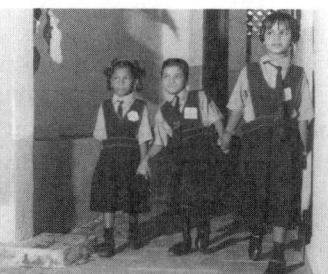 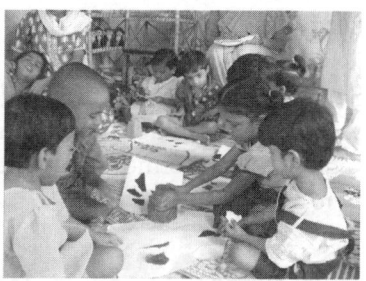

- The inclusive education coordination committee began to provide need-based support in the areas of education, therapy, counselling and adaptation to the schools.[7]
- Partnerships were developed with 91 mainstream schools which admitted students with disability.[8]
- All training programmes and courses focused on the philosophy of inclusion. In-service training, workshops, regular group parent meetings led to a shift in the attitudes of staff and parents. Orientation programmes were also held for regular, mainstream schools on disability and inclusion.
- Regular teachers and students in these schools were sensitized to disability.
- Modules on training for all stakeholders (teachers, parents, heads of schools, bureaucrats and policy-makers) emerged, based on the experience of inclusion and the research studies conducted.
- Six action research studies were set up to get an overall view of attitude change and outcomes among key stakeholders in mainstream schools—students with disabilities who had transitioned from SSI schools, teachers and principals in mainstream schools and parents of the students with disabilities.
- Special schools moved to becoming resource centres.[9]
- The resource support required from NRCI lessened over the years. If there were no hired helpers, family members—uncles, aunts and even neighbours—came forward to help. This then was a community effort, very cost-effective.
- Instructional resource material entitled 'Culturally Appropriate Policy Practice (CAPP III): The Whole School Approach' was created by us as a resource kit targeting children of 6–14 years. It focused on the micro level of classroom and school values and culture/policies/practice.

Inclusion Stories from Teachers

Ayush Srinivasan

Ayush, who was included in Swami Vivekanand School, was initially hesitant about the transition to a mainstream school. His uncle later stated, 'The family is happy with the school; Ayush is doing well, thanks to your staff who guided the school on matters of curricular modification.' Ayush went on to receive a First Class in his M.Com course, making everyone very proud.

[7] Progress reports of NRCI
[8] List of names available in the NRCI library
[9] Photographs courtesy: Carlos Reyes Manzo.

Urvi Pithodia

Urvi, at age 10, was included in Guru Harkishan School. She topped her Senior Secondary Certificate (SSC) exams, making everyone proud. She would say, 'I can do as well as anyone else and will not let you down.' Sadly, today Urvi is no more, but she will always be remembered with fondness here at ADAPT.

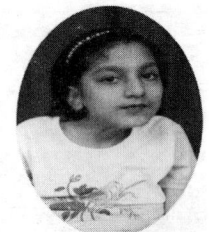

Vimla Christi

Vimla Christi was at SSI (now ADAPT) till her fifth standard, after which she went to Gandhi Memorial, a mainstream school. Vimla did well in school and college, securing work with Eureka Forbes. To this day, Vimla remains grateful to ADAPT for introducing her to inclusive education which changed her life!

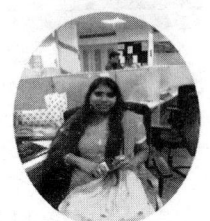

Royce Fred

Royce, included in St. Stanislaus High School in his third standard, blended very well with his peers academically and socially. Some years later, he visited ADAPT with some of his classmates as a part of his school's social service programme and proudly took his classmates around to show them the services at the centre.

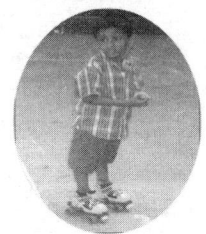

Ansh Walmiki

Ansh, who has speech impairment, was included in St Joseph's School in his second standard. Later, his mother returned to ADAPT and said to the teachers, 'Ansh is confident, determined and even competitive thanks to all of you who never doubted Ansh's potential, keeping your faith in him constant.'

Lessons Learnt About Transforming Schools, Pedagogy and Community

- A vast majority of teachers remain unaware of the needs of students with disabilities and this continues to be a major barrier to inclusion. Almost universally, the curriculum in schools is inflexible and rigid, expecting all students to measure up to certain norms. Flexibility in the curriculum was a hugely positive tool, being cost-effective.
- Inclusion is a process of change that must begin from within oneself. This is essential if one is to face the challenge of addressing diversity and understanding concepts of equality, human rights and social justice. It is a process, a journey, not a fixed outcome.
- Inclusion needs to be demonstrated. The stakeholders—parents, families, teachers, principals, the community, the policy-makers, and the administrators—would join the journey once they see that the experiment works.
- Developing teachers' capacities for an inclusive curriculum and pedagogical approach, such as differentiation of the curriculum, mixed ability teaching, supporting different learning styles and so on requires ongoing, regular and intensive training.

- Limited physical access was a significant barrier and financial constraints were identified as the key reason. In some instances, the aids and devices developed for students at SSI could not be used as effectively in the mainstream schools.
- Lack of accessibility was one of the main concerns. There were no lifts or accessible toilets. Classrooms were congested and would not accommodate wheelchairs. There was no provision for modified furniture for children with disability in regular classrooms and transportation to the school was also a huge barrier.
- Coordination between schools and therapy centres to deliver services needed requires much more development to fill this gap. This is where a few human resource and capacity issues emerged.
- There was a lack of training to deal with children with disability. Management and teachers felt that children with disability needed special teachers (Alur and Bach 2010).
- Parents can be trained to be the resource support that inclusive schools needed.

Gender Strategy

We were very keen on working out our gender strategies as well … Gandhi had written:

'To call women a weaker sex is a libel; it is man's injustice to women. If by strength is meant brute strength, then indeed a woman is less brute than man. If by strength is meant moral power, woman is immensely man's superior. Without her, man could not be. If non-violence is the law of our being, the future is with women.' Unfortunately, gender discrimination continues to be a problem in Indian society. Traditional patriarchal norms have relegated women to secondary status. In the lower socio-economic strata, gender inequality is very stark.

In Dharavi, at times the girls are pulled out of school to look after younger siblings or assist mothers in income-generating activities at home. We developed our own gender policy. The first imperative was to start with school attendance.

i.   For School Attendance: Inclusive Preschools

- Encouraged all children to attend school. There are government facilities like attendance allowance and free mid-day meals, which can be availed of only if the school attendance is more than 70 per cent.
- Conducted poster campaigns and meetings with parents to make them aware that education is the right of every child. Moreover, education of the girl child is free till the 12th grade.
- Provided assistance for school enrolment. Many parents did not have birth certificates of children. Assistance to get duplicate copies or affidavits was given.
- Informed the community that a preschool facility was available close to their residence, therefore the safety of girls is not compromised since they do not have to travel far. Once a girl attends preschool, primary school enrolment is almost automatic.
- A valuable manual of inexpensive aids, called 'Upkaran', was worked out by Ranjana Das.

ii. For Addressing the Issue of Equality and Gender Subordination
- An easy to understand resource kit was developed in local languages. Photographs and illustrations were liberally used to increase readability. The kit addressed health, nutrition, hygiene, gender and literacy issues.

- Capacity-building programmes were arranged in multiple languages. The programmes were conducted by women whom locals knew and respected.
- Increased women's access and control over private resources, especially food for pregnant women and family income. This was achieved through *mahila mandal* programmes.
- Women were made aware of their right to access public resources such as ICDS, formal education, water, sanitation and subsidized food (fair price or ration grains). What was also brought to their attention was that action should be taken if the rights are violated.
- Encouraged women to become leaders in the community. For example, occupy decision-making positions; obtain membership of political bodies (such as panchayats).
- Made women aware of their rights and imparted information about the laws and actions that should be taken in case of domestic violence, child abuse or sexual abuse. Women police officers were invited to address the *mahila mandals* and talk about filing an First Information Report (FIR).
- Special programmes were organized for women to understand financial management, opening bank accounts and starting small saving groups.
- Home-bound employment to supplement income was arranged. Women were given job work in making costume jewellery and embroidery.
- A research project into the difficulties of the girl child was launched, keeping in mind girls with disabilities.
- *Mahila mandals* and a service called *nari ka shakti* was opened for women with disabilities and mothers, providing them with a small stipend.

e. Developing Inclusive Education Practice in Early Childhood in Mumbai: The Whole Community Approach—UNICEF/SSI Project (2001)

Community or the Mezzo Level

Another Research Study Began

Research shows that the first five years of a child's development constitutes the most critical period of his or her life. It has also been shown that there are certain critical periods in the child's life, when he or she learns at an optimal level. Research also reinforces the theory that the most formative years are before the child comes to school. This argument holds true for *all* children, including disabled children. The consequences of inadequate stimulation at an early age have been found to be far greater for disabled children, as it is during this period that the child with a disability is best able to improve abilities and develop efficient 'compensatory' patterns (Alur 1999). In addition, poverty and disability have a strong reinforcing correlation. People with disabilities are poorer, as a group, than the general population and are the 'poorest of the poor'. On an average, disabled people receive less education and are likely to leave school with fewer qualifications than others. These findings hold for both developing and developed countries.

At the mezzo level, we began a two-year action research project based in the slums of Dharavi entitled 'Inclusive Education Practice in Early Childhood in Mumbai, India' in collaboration with UNICEF supported by CIDA. This was all a result of the visit of the governor general of Canada, Romeo Le Blanc and Mrs Diana Le Blanc.

This action research project was conceived to demonstrate how disabled children under the age of six could be included in an existing preschool programme in the slum areas in Mumbai. The main idea was to address the exclusion taking place from government nurseries or *anganwadis*.

The principal investigators of the project were Dr Marcia Rioux, Ph.D. human rights, Canada, who has worked in the fields of human rights, social policy and disability since 1973 and has a PhD in social policy and jurisprudence from Boalt Hall Law School at the University of California, Berkeley, and myself with my own doctorate on policy in India combined with practical experience of 30 years in the field. My doctorate was entitled 'Invisible Children: A Study of Policy Exclusion'.

From CIDA, Canada, the team included Ms Tracie Hewitt, development officer, Ms Melanie Boyd, development officer, Ms Sumeeta Bannerjee, programme officer, New Delhi and Mr David Spring, senior advisor, CIDA, Canada.

The research consultants who did the micro qualitative tracking and evaluation of the children and parents were Dr Urvashi Shah and Dr Anuradha Sovani[10] and the research agency for the macro quantitative research was Mr Partha Rakshit of AC Nielsen. The researchers were practitioners from SSI and the project coordinator was Dr Maria Baretto. UNICEF was represented by Dr Prakash Gurnani, Chetana Kohli and Deepika Shrivastava.[11]

The project's focus on early childhood education was based on the recognition that the first five years of a child's development are formative years. The project had two key components, the intervention modules and the research studies. The former aimed to demonstrate the 'how' of inclusion and the latter to track the changes in the children and the community over two years.

To indicate the 'how' of inclusive practice, we studied and worked out

- How children with disabilities can be put into existing services
- What kind of tools are needed to identify children with disabilities
- What modifications are needed within the classroom which will ensure the children's participation within the class

  - How can training be conducted
  - How is the community empowered

- What kinds of awareness spreading and sensitization programmes are to be conducted to facilitate the community's acceptance of children and families with disabled children
- How to demonstrate this within the existing preschool programmes, so that it has systemic implications.

[10] Dr Urvashi Shah, who has a doctorate in neuropsychology from the University of Bombay, has been involved in research studies. Anuradha Sovani, a clinical psychologist and psychotherapist, was a reader at the Mumbai University and had written extensively on child mental health.

[11] The action research team consisted of Ms Ami Gumashta, Ms Mary Bunch, Ms Deepshika Mathur, Ms Anuradha Dutt, Dr Shabnam Rangwalla, Dr Anita Prabhu, Ms Sangeeta Jagtiani, Ms Ritika Sahni, Ms Susan Barla, Dr Sharmila Donde, Mr Ishwar Tayade, Ms Gulab Sayed, Ms Shraddha More, Ms Malini Chib, Ms Varsha Hooja and Ms Taruna Kumari.

The Objectives of the Project

- Identify effective and appropriate practices for the promotion of inclusive education.
- Track changes if any and move towards developing a code of practice for the community

Project Design

- The study encompassed six impoverished slums of Mumbai, with a 1,000 households from each site. The total population of children was 600, with a 100 children from each site. Multilingual and multireligious communities were characteristic of these slums.

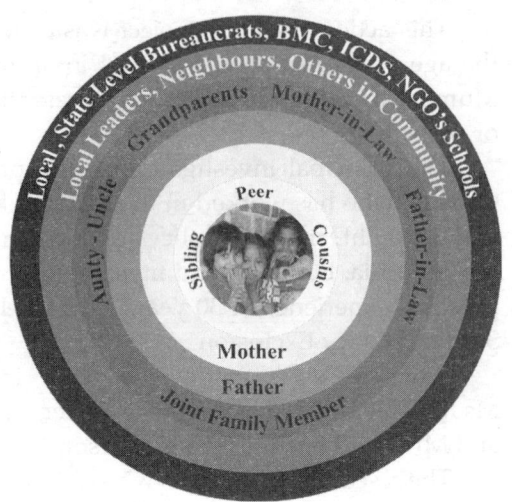

Process of Change: An Ethnographic Participatory Approach to Empower and Build them

- The identification of disability: a new diagnostic tool was developed
- An ecological inventory was developed creating a knowledge base of children's backgrounds through an observation guide.
- The enrichment programme—a collaborative, participatory approach in developing a curriculum context-specific to the community was introduced
- Siblings, cousins, mother, father, grandparents, mothers-in-law, fathers-in-law, joint family members, aunts and uncles, local leaders, neighbours and others in the community were all a part of the training and capacity building.
- Local and state level bureaucrats, Brihanmumbai Municipal Corporation (BMC), ICDS, NGOs and schools were also trained.
- The three D's and the three R's were used.

The Three D's

Deinstitutionalization

Rather than providing primary interventions in specialized settings, inclusion entails moving away from specialized settings to the community setting and involving parents. Moving from an institutional base to a community base was not easy. Many trained specialists have a biomedical approach and are used to well-resourced rooms, beds for examinations and technical aids and find it difficult to shed their

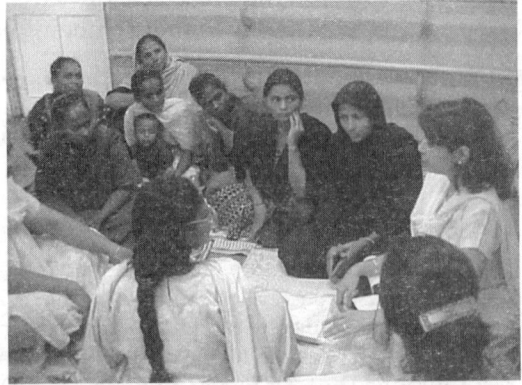

Sangeeta Jagtiani, Deputy Head Education, holding a parent workshop

aura of professionalism. Professionals moving from an institutional base to a community base needed training and understanding to appreciate that the usual well-resourced, institution-based equipment was never going to be available in places where there were no services for anyone. All professionals were taught to take up multifaceted roles. They did not limit themselves to only their area of expertise but also provided broad-based inputs to all fields of intervention that the child may need.

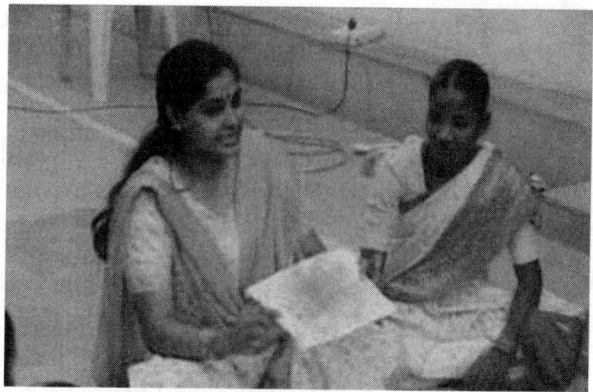

Deepshika Mathur, Deputy Director Training sharing the work done by students with their parents

Demystification of 'Disability'

It was necessary to demystify the processes framed by the 'specialist approach'. Simple methods of handling their children at home and at inclusive schools were introduced. Workshops for regular teachers continued. We took a number of steps to build support and engage parents and community leaders. We trained the siblings of the children attending our preschool.

Deprofessionalization

- Technical jargon makes the parents feel alienated when they are needed to work together with the specialists in partnership.
- More regular education preschool teachers believe they are able to meet the needs of children with disabilities in their classes, when intervention is supportive of their expertise and respects their contribution.

The Three New 'R's for Deprofessionalization

Inclusion of children need not only be done by professionals. But it usually is. It is dominated by a highly professional attitude that has its roots in a specialist approach cloaked in the medical model. This creates a barrier. In a context where there were few professionals, the aim became to introduce a more cooperative and collaborative partnership instead of an authoritarian and hierarchical one. Professionals have to be retrained in approaching the new context and culture in which they were operating. A system and process of deprofessionalization, which I have called the Three R's, is necessary:

- Retraining into a new context and culture of the community.
- Relocation away from the institute to the community, which meant developing more community-based initiatives.
- Redeployment of time: in the institute, several jobs were chalked out; these had to be worked out and another set of priorities introduced into their agenda.

Findings Across Sites

The overall results were very positive. Improvements were noted in development and learning for both, children with and without disabilities. The spirit of the project can be summed up as 'by the community, for the community, with the community', which emerged as a powerful intervention strategy. Here, implementation of inclusive education may simply involve the positive reinforcement of a well-established community, based on inclusive attitudes and practices.

A critical learning lesson is to initiate and focus on a holistic programme involving parents and community as major stakeholders and transferring the ownership to them.

The 'Dharavi Ugam' programme is the most exciting programme in inclusive education I have seen anywhere. I have been privileged to visit the programme frequently as a consultant.

While many believe that inclusion of all learners with disabilities is impossible due to lack of funding, teacher education, negative impacts and other dynamics, Ugam programme in Dharavi proves that nothing is impossible when there is vision, sound leadership and the belief that no child should be segregated from her or his typical peers.

Source: Professor Gary Bunch (Alur and Bach 2005a)

Education is deeply valued in these communities but the struggle for daily survival, the challenge of fulfilling the basic needs of *roti* (food), *kapda* (clothing) and *makaan* (housing) was so difficult that unless education is offered within the community, close to the homes and at minimum cost, it will not be pursued.

Across all communities and across all groups of people, we found support for inclusion—'that is how it should be'—but most were unsure how it could be put into place. If shown the way the seed of inclusion could easily bloom into a healthy way of life.

Listening to the voices of the community and understanding their needs and their reality is critical if inclusion is to succeed. The challenge before us is to ensure that these voices do not fade away and we all join hands to fulfil a universal aspiration for a more inclusive world.

Source: Dr Urvashi Shah and Dr Anuradha Sovani (Ibid 2005a)

When this is scaled out, inclusion will become a reality for four to five million children in India (Alur and Rioux 2003) caught in heartbreaking and terrible circumstances and for millions in similar circumstances in other areas of the world both rich and poor. Universal education has to be the rallying cry for this millennium.

Source: Dr Urvashi Shah and Dr Anuradha Sovani (Alur and Timmons 2009)

Inclusion is possible with limited resources if there is a commitment and a continuum of support in the right spirit. Yet the larger goal of achieving full inclusion through changing state programmes to include children with disabilities has to be pursued systematically. The removal of systemic barriers requires a commitment from the top levels of government and such a commitment is beginning to emerge. The next step will be to produce a blueprint for replicability for implementation on a macro level (Alur and Rioux 2003).

Inclusive education is about organizational transformation. When working with teachers, we need to present inclusive practice as good pedagogy. We cannot just say this, we have to demonstrate it and produce research that presents evidence to teachers.

Source: Vianne Timmons (Alur and Bach 2005a)

I see inclusive values as concerned with equity, compassion and respect for diversity, human rights, participation, community, joy, honesty and sustainability.

Source: Alur and Timmons 2009; Booth 2008

Inclusive education is achievable when leadership and capacity are developed at the classroom and school level; when positive and supportive relationships are developed with parents and the broader school community and when enabling public policies are put into effect.

Source: Alur and Timmons 2009

Outcome

- All children were put into local regular schools.
- Professionals learnt to listen to the voices of children and parents and developed a new approach suited to the poor in the community. Professionals or the resource support team became the community support team. Change in the balance of influence took place.
- Tapping existing resources such as the efforts of civil society and working with the community are valuable resources for advancing one's beliefs. It is critical to ensure that some basic services are available and for this it is necessary to identify *key resources* to achieve this. The one way this is possible is through *community and family participation*. The cornerstone of my inclusive policy is *cost-neutral*. The cost-neutral philosophy requires key elements to be resourced such as: empowering disabled people and their parents to lobby for their rights in the area of practice ... inclusive practices within the child's community and neighbourhood.
- By demonstrating the implementation of inclusion in six impoverished slums

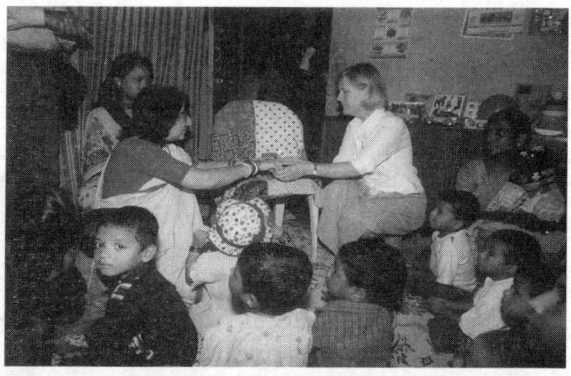

Dr Marcia Rioux with Dr Mithu Alur in the Community

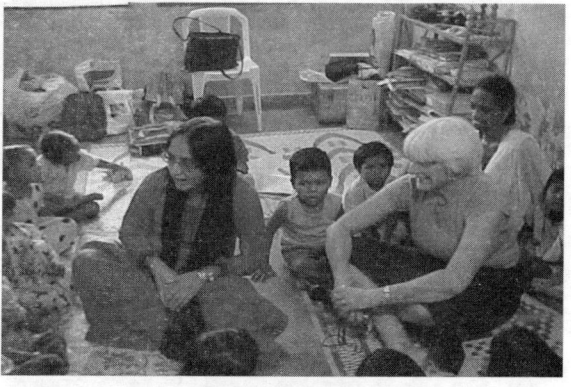

Mithu Alur and Jennifer Evans in an inclusive nursery in the Community

of Mumbai, this project joins a growing body of research that shows that inclusion is not only possible in rich countries, it is also possible in countries facing significant poverty and disadvantage.

- A code of practice, consisting of a very valuable instructional material emerged, supported by UNICEF (2005). CAPP II is in the form of manuals and flip charts and emphasizes the whole community approach to inclusive education consisting of 16 manuals written by Jennifer Evans, well-known lecturer, writer, and researcher from IOE and myself. Flip charts to be used to conduct interactive workshop training sessions for teachers of preschool inclusive nurseries were designed. (They are in both text and pictures. The content is provided in a question and answer format.)
- It is targeted at training for teaching at the preschool level age group of 3–5 years. The manuals have been written on four levels. Level 1: policy-makers, academics, administrators, non-governmental agencies; Level 2: professionals; Level 3: master trainers; Level 4: *anganwadi* multipurpose workers. They have been grouped in six basic themes of policy, community, education, training, meeting individual needs and managing inclusive classrooms.
- The flip charts are in four modules:
  Module 1: ideology and philosophy; Module 2: early childhood care and development; Module 3: inclusive educational inputs; Module 4: community.

f. Developing Rural Services—Mithu Alur Foundation (MAF) 2009

The Mithu Alur Foundation, Rural and District Work

In the words of Gandhiji, 'the real India is not in its few cities, but in the villages.'

MAF was conceptualized under the aegis of ADAPT and set up to fill this gap. The vision was to create and demonstrate an inclusive village model in a district in Maharashtra which would combine education, healthcare, employment, empowerment and services, an extension of ADAPT's work.

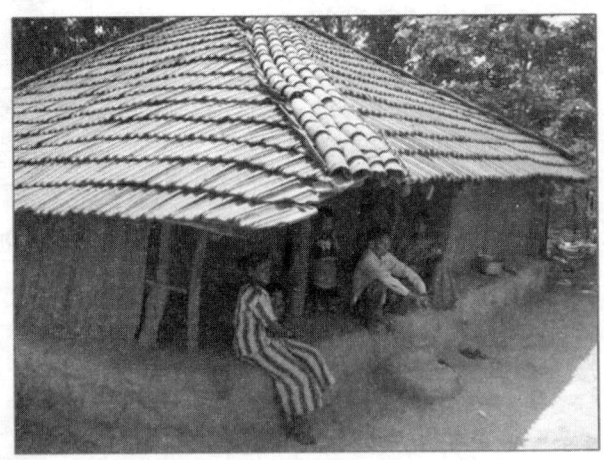

During our data collection in the rural areas it became obvious that caste barriers, negative attitudes, stereotypes based on misinformation and lack of awareness about disability issues were the main problems facing the rural disabled. Studies on the reach of services showed that the rural disabled were almost totally deprived of rehabilitation services.

The gap between the rural poor and the urban affluent (30 per cent) is getting wider and a small section of urban India reaps the benefits of economic progress, leaving out of the safety net, the 70 per cent disadvantaged social sector and those in need of dire assistance. The time had come to understand rural needs better and help to make villages more self-sufficient.

The idea was not to set up new services but to work in collaboration with the gram panchayats (village governing body) in the area and engage with the existing government services to ensure and support sustainable development and ownership of the programmes introduced as well as partner with the corporate sector through their corporate social responsibility (CSR) programmes.

Our first project was in Pelhar, a cluster of 22 villages in Vasai taluka, Thane district, near Mumbai. With a population of 20,000, Pelhar has a functioning gram panchayat and a primary health centre as well as *anganwadis* and primary schools. The main occupations of the people are agriculture, manual and migrant labour, woodcutting and shopkeeping.

Recognizing the importance of using local resources, materials and workforce and learning from our research with UNICEF in Dharavi, we mobilized the community and partnered with the villagers for all activities and developmental programmes. Four multipurpose workers, among them a woman with disability, from the villages of Pelhar were employed by the foundation. They are the key link to the local communities and receive ongoing training in community mobilization skills.

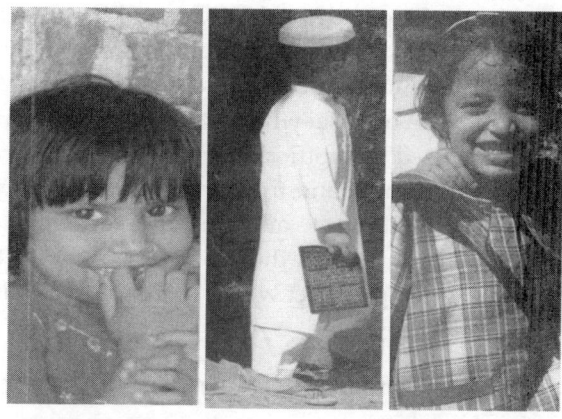

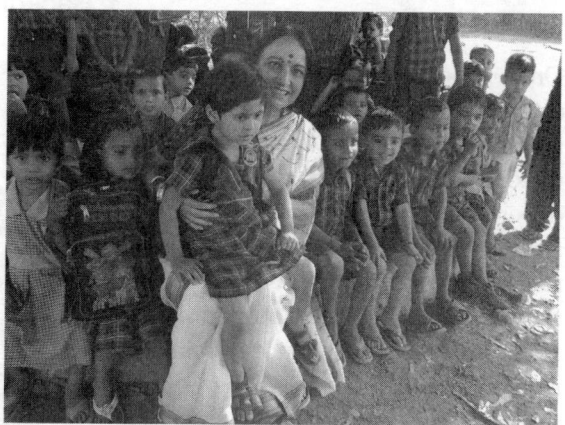

Dr Mithu Alur with the children, Pelhar, Vasai block

We first held camps to identify the health and therapy needs of the children. Students identified with disabilities were provided therapy and remedial services either at the MAF centre or at their villages through a mobile van. Parents were encouraged to admit their children into mainstream schools and a continuum of support was and continues to be provided to the schools and the students to sustain their inclusion.

At the community level, street plays were used to increase awareness on inclusive education. The villagers were helped to get 'Aadhar' cards.[12] A self-help group was begun of mothers of disabled children who now have monthly savings accounts.

A Disabled Persons Organisation (DPO) has developed with 22 members. Collaboration with the Primary Health Centre (PHC) enabled us to refer our beneficiaries to them for health services. A tie-up with the rural outreach centre of the King Edward Memorial (KEM) Hospital and the Rama Krishna Mission facilitated treatment for the people of Pelhar.

---

[12] Aadhar card is a basic, universal identity over which registrars and agencies across the country build their identity-based applications including subsidies.

Networking with local NGOs working for tribal upliftment such as Samarthan in Vasai and Sramjivi Sramjivi Vikas in Usgaon has ensured a wider coverage. All these activities increased our visibility and trust within the community. At the district level, linkages were established with the MLA of Vasai who also runs an NGO and with the local health and education authorities. We liaised with officials of the National Rural Health Mission (NRHM), social welfare and justice department and the Sarva Shiksha Abhiyan (SSA). In the Vasai taluka, networks were established with block- and cluster-level school officials.

Our learning from the work of MAF facilitated our move onto the next research called Shiksha Sankalp project which focused on making *districts inclusive*.

g. Developing a Sustainable District Model: Shiksha Sankalp (2010–13)

Background

One of the greatest problems faced while estimating anything in relation to disability in India is the fact that figures are hard to come by and when available they vary depending on the definitions, the source, the methodology and the scientific instruments used in identifying and measuring the degree of disability. Coupled with this is the lack of the convergence of ministries in providing synergic services, thereby leading to the malfunctioning of the block resource centres (BRCs) and district resource centres (DRCs). To address the need for robust data that will help bridge existing gaps in services for the disabled, SSI embarked upon a project that has demonstrated a service delivery model at the district level.

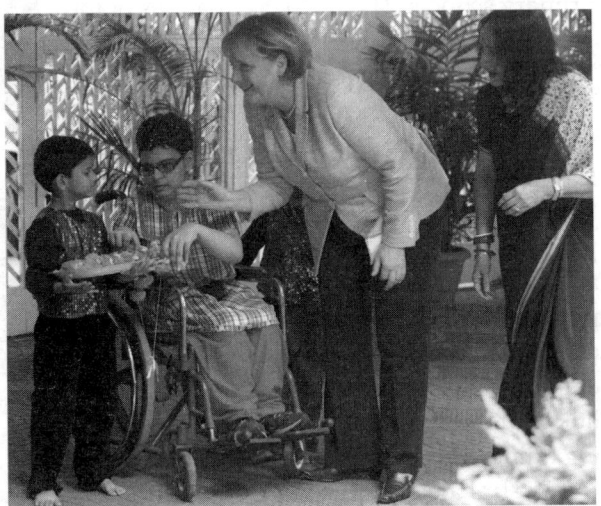

Dr Angela Merkel at NRCI

It all began with the visit of the German chancellor. She was keen to see an effective social project and the government arranged her visit to SSI.

Her Excellency, Dr Angela Merkel visited the NRCI in 2007. Following her visit, Dr Alur and the ADAPT team explored the possibility of seeking support from Germany to develop model community-based resource support centres in two hubs—the urban 'A' Ward at Colaba and the rural Pelhar region in Vasai taluka, Thane—that could possibly be replicated across the nation. The project, entitled Shiksha Sankalp, was co-funded by BMZ (Federal Ministry of Economic Cooperation and Development), CBM (Christian Blind Mission) and ADAPT.

Shiksha Sankalp seeks to develop a sustainable model for inclusion of children with disabilities within mainstream (public) educational institutions in the two urban and rural catchment areas. The project demonstrates a service delivery model at the macro level in a three-tiered manner (scaled, sustainable and replicable) whereby all children with disabilities identified within the jurisdiction will have recourse to services, ensuring they can exercise their fundamental right to education.

The aim was to determine what structural gaps exist in the delivery of education opportunities for all children particularly children with disabilities and what inputs would be needed (sustainable, replicable, scalable) to meet their needs for basic education in a given jurisdiction (it is understood that some children with disabilities would need health intervention in order to be able to access education).

The key components of the project are mapping, screening, implementing interventions and forming DPOs.

The aim of forming DPOs was to create platforms to facilitate capacity building and training for persons with disabilities. Besides advocacy and sensitization, DPOs were to create awareness on legislative rights and conduct access audits and training programmes for parents and teachers.

Methodology

Shiksha Sankalp addressed this issue in an action research mode. The methodology was a combination of quantitative and qualitative data collection and need-based analysis was critical as an outcome: both elements being fully robust and subject to peer review. The project was framed within the constitutional and other legislative provisions of the Right to Education (RTE), persons with disabilities (PWD) and other relevant legislations. The principal components are represented in Figure 8.1.

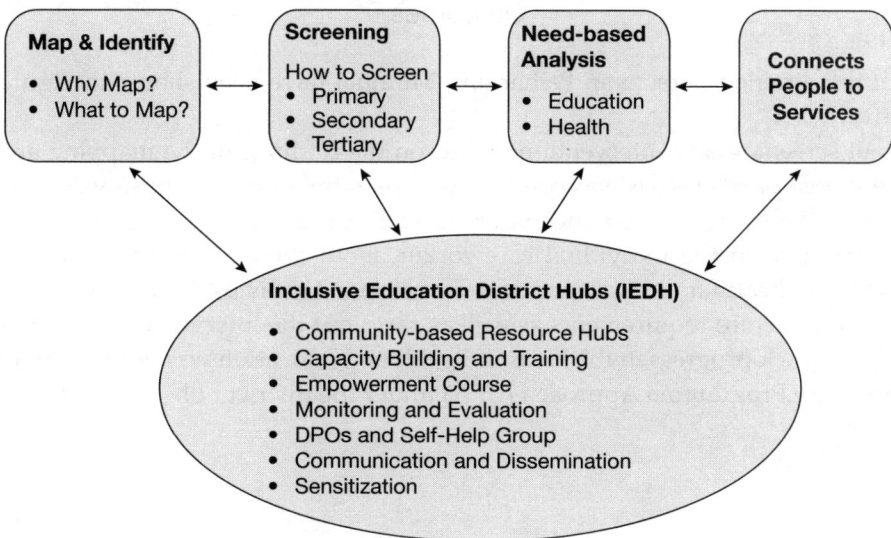

Figure 8.1. Making Districts and Schools Inclusive

Source: Shiksha Sankalp, an Indo-German project: Making Districts and Schools Inclusive.

1. Mapping for identification of children with disabilities:

    i.   Two project areas were chosen. The first is Colaba 'A' Ward, being the political and administrative jurisdiction in Mumbai city, representing an urban location with a cross-section of society. The second jurisdiction is Pelhar, representing a rural/tribal area. The sites were chosen on the basis that data from these locations could be tracked within the national educational data base—Educational Management Information System (EMIS) or District Information System for Education (DISE)—at the National University of Educational Planning and Administration (NEUPA).

    ii. Mapping for identification had three components:

         a. Identification of all children with disabilities in the jurisdictions using a household enumeration tool.
         b. Mapping of existing institutional health and educational resources in the jurisdictions to understand the capacity of the existing resources.
         c. Screening for validation of identified children with disabilities at three levels, namely primary, secondary and tertiary.

2. Health screening: To identify health and rehabilitation needs of screened children with disabilities.
3. Education screening: To identify educational needs of screened children with disabilities.
4. Gap analysis and development of intervention strategies: Based on the findings of the mapping exercise and gap analysis, strategies were developed for creating a nucleus (hub or composite support unit for continuum of support) through the Inclusive Education District Hub (IEDH)[13] that supports the health and educational needs of children with disabilities(CWD)/PWD.

Outcomes

Mapping of the disabled persons in Pelhar and Mumbai have been shown in Figure 8.2 and 8.3, respectively.

Results of screening and intervention: Based on the findings of the mapping and screening exercise, *a need-based analysis* was conducted to plan the intervention services which were at three levels—the micro, mezzo and macro model—propagated by SSI. A matrix[14] giving detailed information to the individual caseworker about the various types of intervention needed in areas of health and education was developed. This is useful to plan, organize and budget the infrastructure requirements as well as carry out the interventions in a timely manner. A system to track progress in the areas of health and education was done using care pathways and the Care Programme Approach (CPA) under the district hub.

---

[13] Dr Mithu Alur introduced the concept of IEDH for the project.
[14] Matrix approach for the project was developed by Mr Sathi Alur and Ms Kalpana Kumar generated the need-based analysis. It is available in the library.

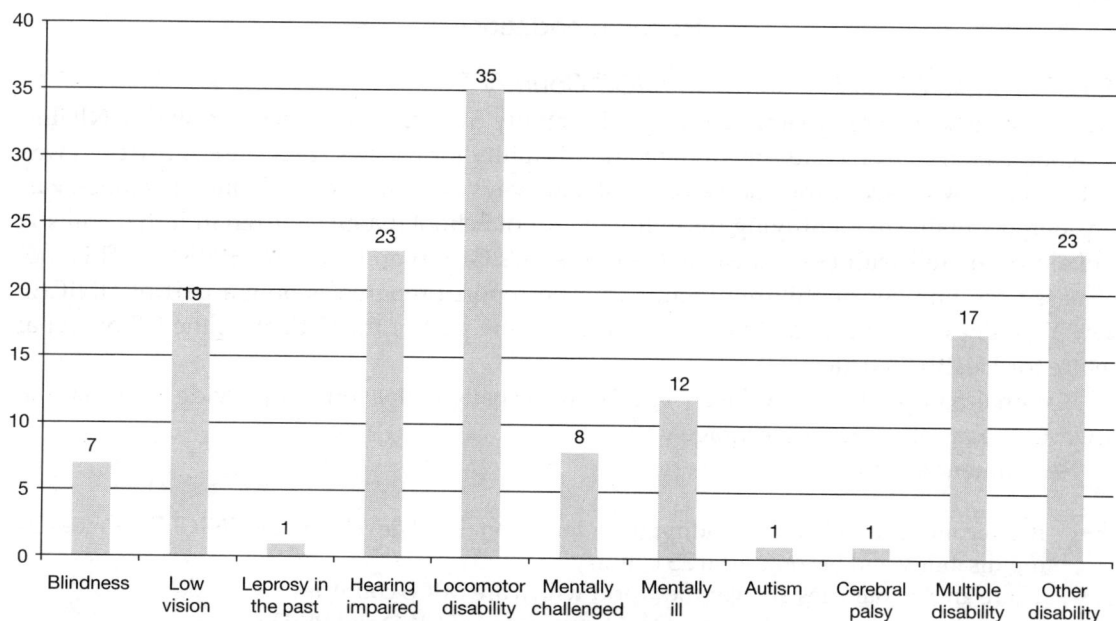

Figure 8.2. Stratification of the 147 Disabled Persons Mapped in Pelhar

Source: Shiksha Sankalp, an Indo-German project: Making Districts and Schools Inclusive.

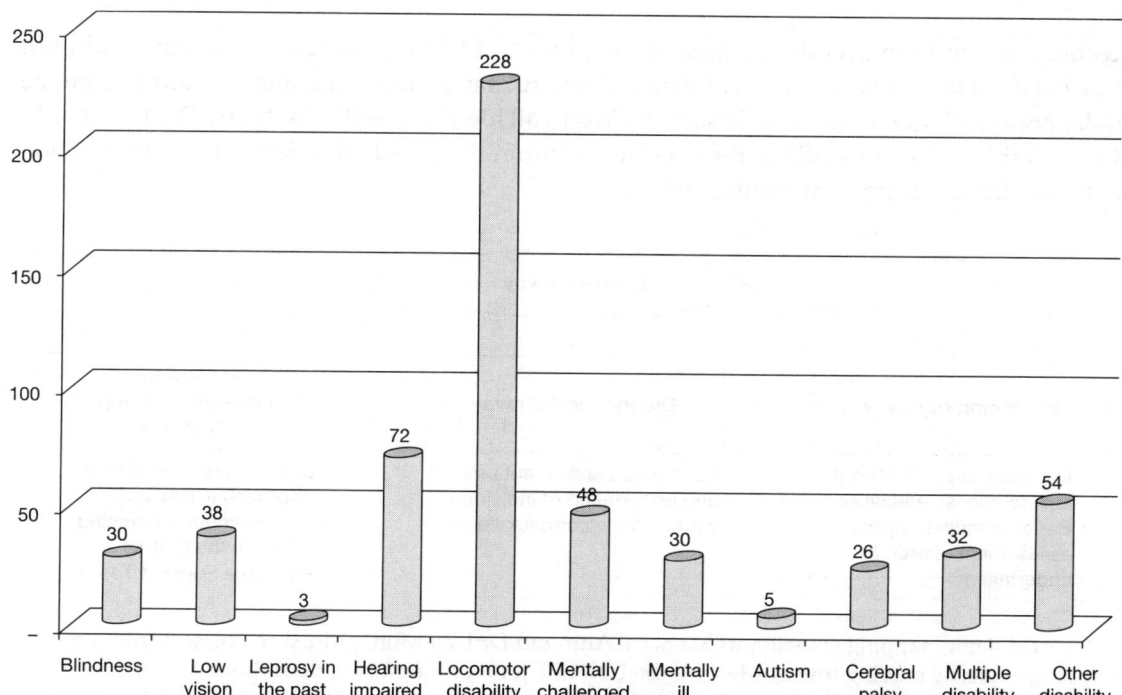

Figure 8.3. Stratification of the 566 Persons Mapped as Having Disability Mapped in 'A' Ward of Mumbai

Source: Shiksha Sankalp, an Indo-German project: Making Districts and Schools Inclusive.

Recommendations

Mapping: India Should Become an MICS Country[15]

The UN Statistical Commission's Group on Disability Statistics (in association with UNICEF) developed a module on child functioning and disability for use in survey and censuses. It was part of the UNICEF's Multiple Indicator Cluster Surveys (MICS). The tool being developed was considered suitable in identifying disability in Out of School (OOS) children in India. Shiksha Sankalp partnered with UN Statistical Commission's Group on Disability Statistics. This tool increased the number of children identified. The report prepared is now a part of UNICEF New York's best recommended practice. It is also now part of the Q Bank at the US National Centre for Health Statistics.

National Sample Survey Office (NSSO) and census endeavour to provide information, however the numbers and percentage vary.

Recommendations:

- It is recommended that India adopt the international tool developed by UNICEF for measuring disability and become a MICS country.
- There are 15 countries all over the world which are MICS countries.
- It is crucial to administer the correct tool for mapping of CWD and PWD.

Development of a District Hub[16]

Keeping in mind the overall objective of the project, IEDH was developed which would not only have the key responsibilities of data collection, management and analysis but also be the nodal point to disseminate need-based services to all identified with disability. The hub would direct all the PWD and CWD to the specialists within the jurisdiction for further intervention and remediation using a care pathway.[17]

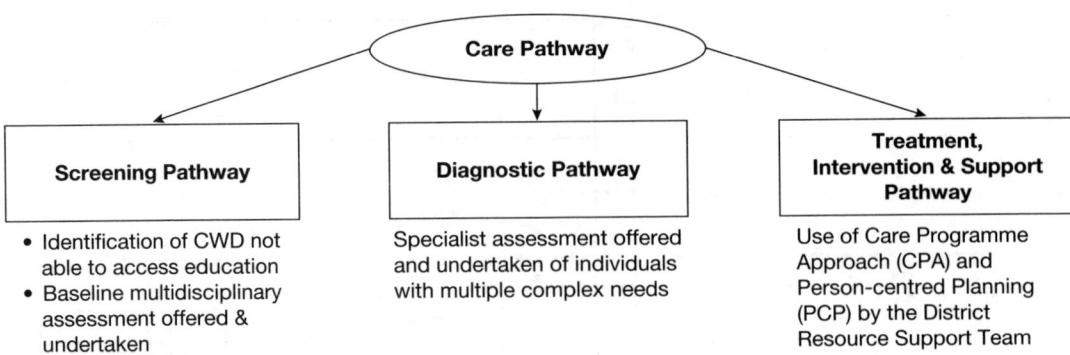

---

[15] World Bank mapping consultants Mr Sathi Alur and Dr Dan Mont guided the project from the first mapping exercise, moving towards testing the UNICEF tool for measuring disability.

[16] Source: Developed by Professor Zenobia Nadirshaw, Dr Alur and the Shiksha Sankalp team.

[17] Professor Zenobia Nadirshaw, consultant, helped design the intervention plan and coined the term care pathway for the project.

The IEDH model needs to be scaled and replicated by the government and incorporated into every state's inclusive education policy. The existing BRCs and DRCs should be strengthened, expanded and upgraded to become IEDH, with personnel forming a district resource support team (DRST) headed by an inclusive education and health needs coordinator (IEHNCO).

h. Developing a Code of Practice for Inclusive Education: Culturally Appropriate Policy and Practice (CAPP)

To create a mechanism of implementation of inclusive education dealing specifically with children with disabilities, a code of practice, called CAPP, emerged from all the research studies done.[18]

CAPP I, II and III was a multifaceted research project, which combined a number of different research approaches, involving teamwork by a multidisciplinary research team located in three countries (India, Canada and UK) and developed, in the process of work, some innovative new research tools using multiple research methods. As an action research project, the team developed and ran six day care centres in some of the most impoverished areas of Mumbai, hiring and training staff to work on the front lines of inclusion. The methodology designed for the field consisted of questionnaires, structured and semi-structured, house-to-house surveys, participatory observation, focus group discussions and meetings and home visits. Triangulation and rechecking among the researchers helped to avoid bias. Two separate teams were contracted to track the changes, quantitatively and qualitatively, for the UNICEF research (the result of which is CAPP II). The gathering of results through multiple techniques proved to be a rich and fruitful research strategy. As the demonstrations were in process, all the people involved—children, parents, AMWs, specialists, and researchers—learnt a great deal. The continual discussion and feedback generated by the research produced not only findings, but encouraged respondent reflection and generated a sense of input and ownership in the project. The dual research strategy collected both objective 'hard' data that showed statistics about the changes participants underwent during the project and qualitative data, simultaneously collected and analyzed by a separate team, which included responses and inputs from the various stakeholders.

[18] CAPP I, II and III is based on research studies done by the Inclusive Education Coordinating Committee or IECC, NRCII, making it culture- and context-specific to India. The stories and studies of certain events and children are based on real situations experienced by school heads, teachers, children and families experiencing inclusive practice in India. These have been drawn from the research studies that were carried out by the researchers. Details of the researches are available in the NRCII library, Mumbai, entitled 'A Journey From Segregation To Inclusive Education, the Final Report'. The researches were carried out under the guidance of Professor Gary Bunch, Dr Urvashi Shah and the authors were Varsha Hooja, Shabnam Rangwala, Anita Prabhu, Damayanti Thapa, Sharmila Donde, Dhaya Srinivasan, Sangeeta Jagtiani, Pranita Prabhakar, Swapna Deshmukh and Gulabjan Sayed. We would also like to acknowledge the administrative support we received from Cam Crawford (the Roeher Institute), Ami Gumashta (NRCII) and the technical support we received from Lucas Baretto and Manish Kapdoskar.

What Are These Manuals About?

The manuals provide for the implementation of inclusive practice, methods and strategies that can be introduced with simple modifications in any school, classroom or community moving towards inclusive education.

The manuals emphasize the importance of the preschool years, the first five years, when any child is able to learn the most. This holds true for 'all' children, including children with disabilities. In fact the consequences of neglect at an early age are especially disastrous for disabled children, as they are at high risk of developing secondary handicaps.

Who Is This Manual for?

Training in the community at various levels to see the importance of children with disabilities being included in it. The training needs to have a top-down, bottom-up approach on a macro, mezzo and micro level where all levels of people are sensitized to the needs of disabled children.

At the macro top level of training are the policy-makers at the national, state and municipal level, officials and administrators in all the three sectors of health, education, and welfare.

At the mezzo level, the manuals provide instructions for the policy implementers, professionals, paraprofessionals, community workers, teachers, therapists and master trainers.

At the micro level, the manuals provide training for anganwadi workers, parents and families in the community.

See for more details on instructional resource material in Annexure I: Developing a Code of Practice for Inclusive Education; CAPP.

Lessons Learnt

- The qualitative research yielded rich data for best practices and showed that a climate for inclusion existed but the 'how' of inclusion needed to be demonstrated and special education had to be demystified.
- Teacher training was a critical factor and active participation of the government and the school authorities was needed to address access and training issues.
- Shifting the onus from specialists to the community empowered the workers so that they could handle most situations.
- Strengthening the community and building support from within helped the community take ownership. This process I have called the *Whole Community Approach* and this is critical to creating an inclusive environment.

The Approach to Inclusive Education: Key Principles of Inclusive Education Emerged and Were Introduced

These are:

- Ecologically appropriate curriculum
- Differentiated curriculum

- Multiple ability teaching
- Multiple intelligences
- Learning styles
- Community involvement
- Cooperative and collaborative learning
- Least restrictive environment

Ecologically Appropriate Curriculum

An ecological inventory is designed by listing all the common activities and materials used by children in a particular environment: what they touch, smell, feel, see, what are the activities they are attracted to.... From this, a context-specific curriculum is drawn up which is culture-specific to their social mores; from this emerges an ecologically appropriate curriculum. *An ecologically appropriate curriculum provides a holistic approach within the framework of connecting knowledge to life outside the school.*

Differentiated Curriculum

A differentiated curriculum is one where content, activity and products are differentiated according to the needs of each child such that the curriculum matches the child's abilities. Each child learns at a different pace by keeping pace with his or her ability. Differentiation of each child's needs makes the learning and teaching flexible.

Mixed Ability Teaching

- Students with differing levels of need can all attend regular classes. It means teaching groups of children with different abilities in the same class using group work, differentiated curriculum, cooperative learning and collaboration.
- This allows children to progress according to individual rates of learning, instead of *one standardized manner.* Teachers are encouraged to see children as unique individuals, plan for a wide range of abilities, and adjust to individual needs, enabling slower children to catch up with their classmates ... again this individualizes teaching.

Multiple Intelligences

- There is increasing understanding on the part of educators and researchers of the importance of all of these intelligences for a child's development and academic success. Opportunities for children to express themselves creatively in multiple media—visual art, music, drama and dance—is particularly important for children from linguistically and culturally diverse backgrounds.

Learning Styles

- Learning styles is perhaps the most vital development in education today. Learning styles definitely calls for the learner-centred approach to teaching. We all may need different strategies, and bring different gifts to the table of learning, but the quality and the style of our learning is not less because we learn differently than does someone else.

Community Involvement

- Creating a community of learners, in which all members see themselves as both teachers and learners, enables children, teachers, and parents to develop shared understandings about what is important to know and why it is important.
- Community-based programmes grounded in the community's cultural mores are likely to play a major role in inclusion.
- An inclusive community recognizes cultural variations such as income level, education, geographical origin and opportunity.
- It is considered a good practice to give attention to the individual child, the family and the community.

Cooperative and Collaborative Learning

- Collaboration with other teachers and relevant staff for support to meet the individual needs of the students is important. Teachers, parents and others can collaborate in determining and meeting the needs of any student.
- Peer tutoring like peer teaching and child-to-child learning. Small group teaching helps in building a support system and effective teaching. It leads to cooperative learning, which occurs when children share responsibilities and resources as well as when they work towards a common goal. Problem solving and negotiations help learners resolve conflicts and make decisions.

Least Restrictive Environment

Students with special needs spend their leisure time in heterogeneous environments in the community. If they are to develop skills to function in that community, they may need to spend as much time as possible in regular school setting. Special schools may be seen as restrictive as they limit the opportunities to access experiences available in regular schools or classrooms. Inclusive settings offer more opportunities for interaction with peers than segregated settings.

Parents are the main educators of their children in the earliest years and a major task for official agencies is to support parents in promoting the development of their young children with disabilities.

Remembering Lotika Sarkar

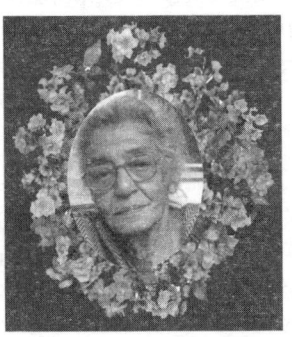

'Trailing clouds of glory did she come and go …'

Amidst all this work, we lost another strong supporter of the movement, my aunt who had been vice chairperson of SSI for over 25 years.

What People Said About Lotika Sarkar

Lord Anthony Lester, Member of House of Lords, said of her: 'Lotika (Monu) changed my life when I met her and Chanchal at Harvard in 1960–61. She urged me to become a barrister and use law as an instrument of social change and I took her advice. Her grace her humour, her beauty and intelligence matched her selfless devotion to her students and to the dispossessed women in the villages of West Bengal. All attempts to wean her from cigarettes and black coffee failed and she proved that it was possible to live a long and fulfilled life despite these petty vices! We loved her and will always remember her. We will not see her like again except in heaven.'

Usha Ramanathan said: 'After four years of sharing a home and being witness to her inexhaustible charm, cheer, comradeliness, compassion, concern, quiet—very quiet—dignity, trust and fairness, we know why the applause will never stop. *Mutual respect, no hierarchy, unacceptance of nonsense and a deep sense of fairness. No pre-judgement, no prejudice, but excellent judgment, that was Lotikadi.'*

Mithu Alur said: 'It was during the last four years that I was also able to take her out several times. She loved her gin and tonic, her cigarette which she would have clandestinely and whisper, "don't tell Usha!" It was this love for fun, the humour, the quick wit, the eye for detail … tell me what's the latest about the work.… Her camaraderie, her stiff upper lip when she was severely ill and dying and you asked her how she was … always "I am fine!"… my mentor, my intellectual guide, my friend,… yes my guardian while in college …'

'All this and so much more will be missed …'

'But today I rejoice in the fact such a person touched our lives and pay my tribute to her valuable contribution in nation building. It is indeed more a feeling of great inner pride and privilege that this extraordinary person touched our lives and influenced us in some ways.'

Domain IX

Policy and Macro-level Change: Legislation and Policy

a. Moving from Charity to Rights: ADAPT Rights Group (ARG)

Malini Chib was by now finishing her first Masters in gender studies at the Institute of Education (IOE), University of London, 2002. Simultaneously, she began her activism at home in India during her vacations. She decided to establish an organization ARG which was to study 'rights and entitlements of people with disabilities'. The message was that charity was no longer needed. Today, the social model and the rights model prevailed. Today all disabled people advocate 'nothing about us without us'.

ADAPT (Able Disabled All People Together) aimed to bring a wider social and public recognition to the human rights violations people with disability faced in all aspects of their lives. ADAPT was distinctive from most other disability advocacy organizations as it includes as equal members both those with and without disabilities. In keeping with the title of ADAPT, Malini, who was the chair, said, 'This is a model culture specific to India where many members of our family have come forward and worked with us in establishing the disability movement. It is

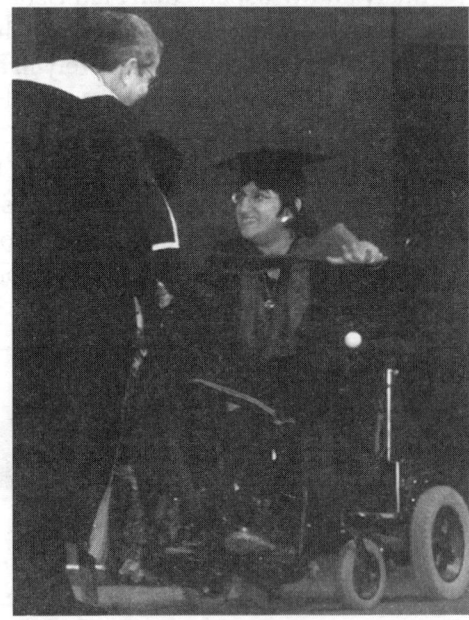

Malini Chib at the Convocation of her Masters' in Gender Studies

not like the West. Being used to large joint families, we the disabled are not ghettoized but have been working together with many non-disabled people and members of our families.' Anita Prabhu was appointed the co-chair; Nilesh Singit was a leading founder member with others like Neenu Kewlani and Sunita Sanchetti. The group began networking and formed a strong bond with Ketna Mehta and her team of The Nina Foundation. Legal luminary Jamshed Mistry took leadership as legal advisor.

From a Medical Model to a Social Model

The formation of ARG was one of the outcomes of a conference organized by Malini Chib and a group of others and convened in Mumbai in November 2000 on the theme of 'Citizenship and Barriers'. The conference explored the transition from a medical to a social model of disability and approaches to citizenship rights that could help bring this model into practice, with an emphasis on moving beyond basic civil and political rights to social and economic citizenship rights as well.

In opening the conference, Malini Chib set the tone and focus:

> Ultimately it is society that has to make the necessary changes and provisions to include disabled people as citizens. All policies should be changed in order to accommodate all citizens, regardless of their diversity. Disabled people and other oppressed groups must be more assertive and empowered to voice their opinions. These groups should be able to feel that they can make decisions, which will be on the policy level, which will affect other generations of citizens. It is only when the civil/legal, political, economic and social structure of society changes and includes all its citizens, then only can citizenship be enjoyed by those who remain marginalized. (Chib 2000, cited in Alur and Bach 2010)

We would also need to build a form of social solidarity where others could identify with, or at least care about, the realities and voices of disabled people.

ARG's mission was:

- To influence public policy. To ensure that disabled people work in partnership on critical issues.
- To provide a forum for leaders of the disability movement to work together.
- To work on issues of employment and accessibility.

From Charity to Rights

Until deep-rooted attitudes change, unless we, the people, start acting and not just pointing fingers at the government and unless the disability advocacy groups emerge as a strong force, nothing will happen.

Many of the ARG members had received their education through the special schools of The Spastics Society of India (SSI). They knew only too well that there was life beyond graduation. Unless the National Resource Centre for Inclusion (NRCI-I) was also addressing the broader issues of citizenship and participation in society, as part of its drive for inclusive education, students would end up leaving inclusive school settings only to return to lives of isolation, loneliness and exclusion. A broader agenda for full citizenship took root in NRCI-I's work as a result of ARG's efforts.

Over the course of the next six years, ARG began to undertake over 20 audits of shopping malls, recreation centres, hospitals, cinemas, churches, museums, taxis, train, stations and buses. As they developed guidelines for accessibility and auditing, members of ARG made various presentations to professional associations (e.g. Indian Interior Designers' Association) and at conferences in India and internationally.

Several public interest litigations (PIL) cases were filed. On the non-implementation of the Persons with Disabilities Act, ARG decided to intervene in the litigation because it felt that the views of persons with disabilities were not being adequately addressed.

ARG intervened in a PIL case in 2003 against the state of Maharashtra for the non-implementation of the same act. The case focused on section eight of the Act which deals with non-discrimination and accessibility in transport and public places. Well-known disability-friendly lawyer, Mr Jamshed Mistry, Advocate of the High Court, joined ARG and began helping.

As a result of this litigation, three disabled-friendly buses were put into service on a trial basis by Brihanmumbai Electric Supply and Transport (BEST), Mumbai's bus company. The World Bank was planning to fund the purchase of the buses under the Mumbai urban transportation project. ARG audited these buses and informed BEST that none were disabled-friendly and made recommendations on how to make them fully accessible. As a result of their audit, ARG decided to add the BEST to their filing for the litigation. The court requested the general manager of BEST to incorporate their recommendations into the new buses purchased and also ordered that 30 disability-friendly buses should be procured for the city of Mumbai. It was a historic achievement for ARG and indeed for the disability rights movement and was widely reported in the media.

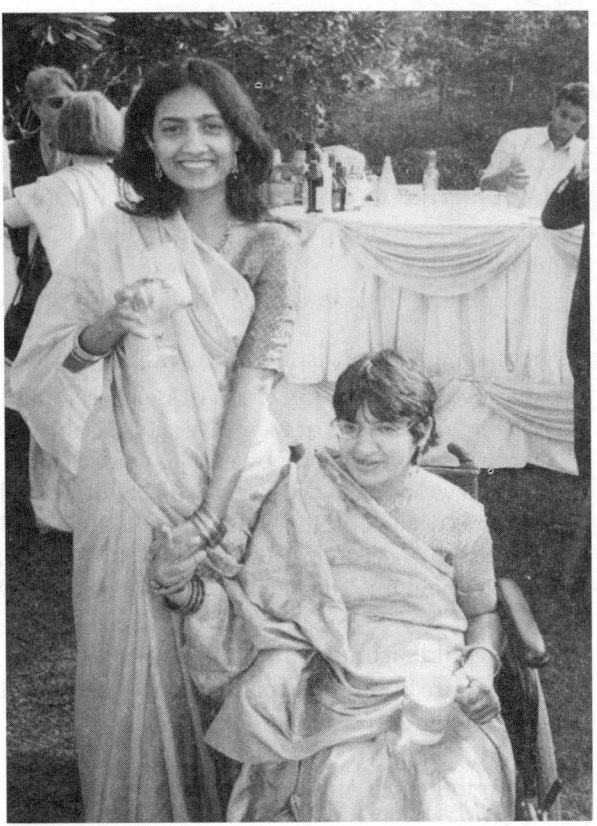

Karuna Nundy, Advocate Supreme Court, Advisor the ADAPT Rights Group with Malini Chib

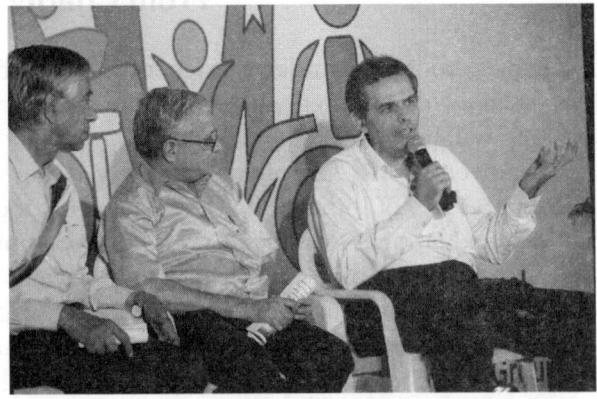

Mr V. Ranganathan, Chair, Heritage Committee, Mr S.M. Khened, Director, Nehru Science Centre and Mr Jamshed Mistry, Legal Advisor, ADAPT, during International Day of Disabled at Azad Maidan, Mumbai

ARG next brought to the court's notice that the High Court itself was not accessible. With no ramps and no accessible washroom, some of the ARG members who used wheelchairs would not be able to attend the hearings for the case. When this was pointed out to the Chief Justice, he ordered a ramp and an accessible washroom in the premises of the High Court. Later in the case, the court passed an order stating that all government buildings in the state of Maharashtra should be made accessible including ramps, accessible washrooms and accessible signage as needed.

How Inclusive Are We? Empowerment Course

Malini, also a strong proponent for empowering persons with disabilities, introduced the social model of disability through empowerment programmes for persons with disabilities, their families, professionals or 'allies', in 2004, in collaboration with Richard Rieser and DEE (Disability Equality Education), UK. This unique course was facilitated entirely by disabled advocates.

The empowerment course aimed to strengthen the voices of people with disability and their families. It was entitled 'Does inclusion matter... How inclusive are we?' The course focused on developing a rights-based approach to empowering people with disability. It emphasized the importance of appropriate nomenclature and etiquette, with a special focus on topics that impact adults with disability (e.g. employment and relationships).

ARG also played a key role when disabled people were left out of the Mumbai Marathon. ARG approached the charity commissioner and SSI Patron Shri Sunil Dutt, who was then minister for sports and youth affairs, to ask the marathon be stopped from taking place in the face of this exclusion. ARG also took the matter to the press. NDTV flashed the exclusion of persons with disability as their ticker continually. The High Court intervened,

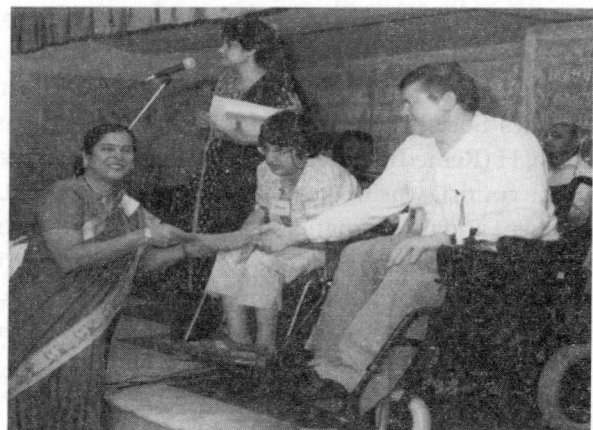

Mr Richard Rieser and Ms Malini Chib giving away Participant Certificates in the Empowerment Course

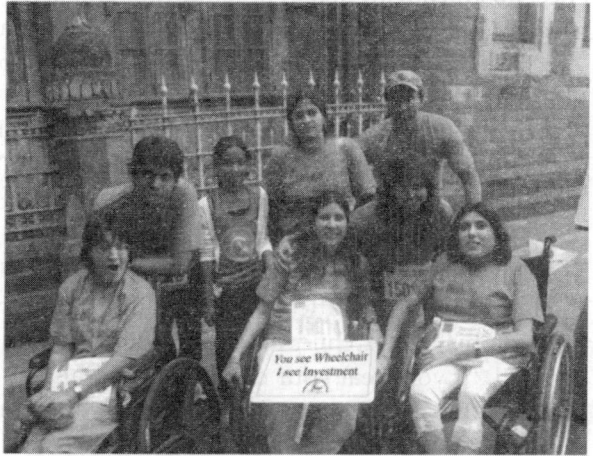

Members and friends of ARG, participating in the Mumbai Marathon with Nagesh Kukunoor, our Ambassador for the Marathon

the minister stepped in and for the first time in Indian marathon history people using wheel-chairs were allowed to participate. Press reports called the ARG 'The Real Heroes'.

b. Workshops, Seminars and Conferences

From 1972, there were numerous workshops, seminars and lectures conducted by various specialists from abroad for professionals working in the field of cerebral palsy (CP). These workshops have been well attended, very well received and have helped greatly in the spread of know-how in the field. Proceedings of many of the conferences were published.[1]

National Coordinating Council

In August 1982, The National Coordinating Council was formed by SSI, together with the Spastics Society of Eastern India (SSEI), the Spastics Society of Northern India (SSNI) and REACH (Remedial Education Assessment Counselling Handicapped), Calcutta. The objective of the council was to create a platform for presenting a concerted and united front to the government and to international agencies on matters of common interest and to establish a bank of experts from various regions for sharing of expertise. The faculty was involved in a number of such sessions, throughout the year, in Baroda, Trivandrum (now Thiruvananthapuram), Delhi (now New Delhi), Chandigarh, Madras (now Chennai) and Bombay (now Mumbai).

Changing Attitudes Towards the Handicapped: 'Does She Take Sugar in Her Tea?'
While considering changing attitudes towards persons with handicap, the group identified various types of attitudes on the basis of a questionnaire circulated by Mr Leslie Gardner.[2] Major negative attitudes encountered such as rejection, pity, patronizing, revulsion, indifference, hostility, fear, denial of handicap, embarrassment and guilt were listed. The group proceeded to analyze the attitudes lying behind remarks such as the following:
    'Does she take sugar in her tea?' Where people do not ask the disabled person the questions but the person with him/her.
    'Just because my legs are wobbly, people think my mind is wobbly too.'
    'I treat the handicapped as completely normal.'
    'It's much better for the handicapped to live with their own kind in some home or institution.'
    'He hears when he wants to.'
    The group agreed that an aggressive retaliation would be counter-productive. Tackling the incident with a little humour would be the better alternative! The attitude of the parent towards his or her child determines and shapes that of the community. To illustrate, a parent said, 'If you treat your child in a natural way and accept her as she is, the other person is compelled to do the same.' It was also felt that parents and those working in the field have not

---

[1] Available in the NRCI library.
[2] Leslie Gardner was the principal psychologist of the Spastics Society of UK and played a key role in setting up the Psychology Department as well as the first Teacher Training course (TTC) with help from British Council.

concentrated sufficiently enough on informing the community and that there was a great need for better public relations. The workshop concluded with the clarion call of 'Let's not just sit and talk but do something' (Khare 1982).

National Seminar on Vocational Rehabilitation, 1990

In 1990, a national seminar was conducted at National Job Development Centre (NJDC) in Chembur, Mumbai. The major areas focused on were 'Models of Vocational Rehabilitation', 'Strategies for Placement', 'Breaking down Social Barriers' and 'Need for Legislation'.
    The objectives of this seminar were:

1. To create a platform for an exchange of expertise, technology and know-how in the area of vocational training and placement of the disabled by those who are making major contributions in this field;
2. To create awareness at a national level of the effect of societal attitudes towards disability and to evolve means of breaking down the barriers which serve as deterrents in their process of achieving independent livelihood;
3. To create awareness of the current state of employment opportunities provided for the disabled;
4. To plan strategies to change employment opportunities for the trained disabled workers.

Certain very practical and useful proposals arose during the proceedings, including the need for a federation of non-governmental organizations (NGO)s to work in unison towards not only establishing a meaningful dialogue with the government and the corporate sector on major issues but also towards achievement of common goals; working to ensure that the disabled be given rights to equal opportunities in gaining fundamental rights of education, occupation and economic independence; breaking down barriers between disabled employee and prospective employer; employer education; and emphasis on public awareness about the potentials of the disabled worker. There emerged a great need for trained professional service personnel to professionalize vocational rehabilitation. Furthermore, it was reported that there was a lack of awareness at the national level and it was learnt that efforts should be targeted towards educating the lay public about abilities of the 'differently abled' (Annual Report 1990–91).

National Networking Seminar on Vocational Rehabilitation and Employment

In 1992, another set of seminars of networking with other seemingly different groups was conceptualized. The seminars were planned as a regular event to focus on issues of awareness, employment and independence of the differently abled people of the country (Annual Report 1991–92).
    We extended the definition of disability for this seminar to include socially disadvantaged groups which remain marginalized due to the stigma attached. For the first time in the country, various groups working for employment of the disabled, cancer and leprosy affected, drug dependents and destitute women were brought together on a common platform to discuss

---

[3] The proceedings of National Networking Seminar on Vocational Rehabilitation and Employment, 1992, and the National Seminar on Vocational Rehabilitation, 1990, have been published in full and are available with SSI.

issues relating to job retention, training, job reservation, financial support and so on.[3]

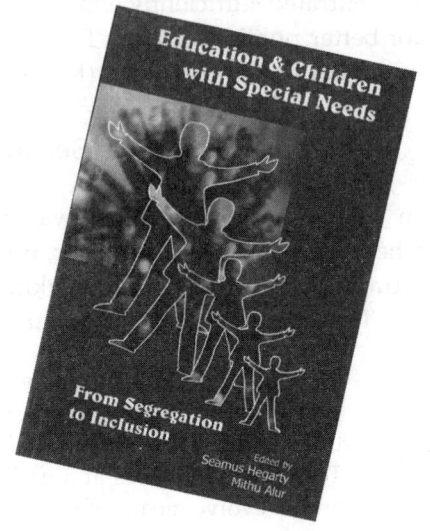

The seminar in Delhi was inaugurated by the then vice president, the Honourable Dr Shankar Dayal Sharma and in Calcutta by Swami Lokeshwarananda of the Ramakrishna Mission. Both seminars received a spontaneous response from government officials, parents, achievers, decision makers in the private and public sectors, trade union representatives as well as the workers from the represented groups.

Although employment was the primary focus, through the deliberations, many issues common to all groups emerged quite clearly. Attitudes and awareness, difficulties of access and transport, role of government and private sector, training and employment and finally the trade unions and legal issues were discussed as well as models of vocational training and employment.

Inclusive education was driven home by an achiever who said, 'I may be different, but aren't we all?' The messages that came through were 'We can ... if we think we can!' and 'Let children be children. Together'.

We received an extremely heartening response and very active and enthusiastic participation. The seminar was well covered by the media.

In November 1992, the third in this series of seminars was held at the National Centre for Cerebral Palsy (NCCP), Bombay. Shri Rusi Lalla, of Tata Sons, and Shri Nana Chudasama, sheriff of Bombay, were the guest speakers at the inauguration, along with our patron Shri Sunil Dutt, the then Honourable Member of Parliament.

This seminar was well attended throughout, as had been those in Calcutta and Delhi, and helped to forge new links between the different organizations working in Bombay. Proceedings of the seminar entitled 'Integrated Education for Children with Special Needs – A Matter of Social Justice and Human Rights, 1997', held in Mumbai, New Delhi and Jaipur, was published by SAGE, New Delhi, in 2002. It was entitled *Education and Children with Special Needs—From Segregation to Inclusion* and edited by Seamus Hegarty and Mithu Alur. Seamus Hegarty is a leading voice from UK and Europe who was connected to the organization and supported it right from its inception. Many of those who had made presentations in Calcutta and Delhi were a part of this seminar too, with new inputs from Bombay, Madras and Bangalore, together with a group of Bombay journalists including Rahul Singh, Kamlendra Kanwar, Dilip Thakore and M.V. Kamath.

Network Seminars on Inclusive Education

For the first time in India, another major series of three conferences on inclusive education was initiated by the society and co-sponsored by the ministry of human resources development (MHRD), Government of India and the National Centre of Educational Research & Training (NCERT), New Delhi. These conferences were held in Mumbai, Delhi and Jaipur in 1997.

Again, the aims of the conferences were to focus on equalization of opportunity and main-streaming children with special needs in India. International perspectives in mainstreaming, as well as in India, were discussed. The final core objective was to develop a policy strategy of inclusion *relevant in the Indian context*.

The target audiences for these conferences were people with special needs; parents of people with special needs and their siblings; principals, professionals and staff at normal schools, special schools and at integrated schools; District Primary Education Programme (DPEP) policy-makers; education policy-makers; disabled activists; the media and the government.

Issues that impede practice, curriculum changes, teacher training, resource teacher support, physical modifications of environment were discussed. The conferences examined the intervention and inclusion techniques in industrialized countries. The delegates deliberated on methods of developing an appropriate environment for evolving paradigms which are culture-specific.

The overall goal was to ensure that participants, including government officials, policy-makers, professionals, people with disabilities and their families all have the opportunity to acquire new knowledge, to share experiences and to develop renewed vision for the future, thus making the goal of education for all a reality (Annual Report 1996–97).

The outcome of all this discourse and deliberations helped in focusing the issue on a national level. Senior government officials agreed that although considerable work has been done over the years both by the Government of India and the voluntary sector, with substantial increase in the allocation of funds over different plan periods, a great deal needed to be done to include disabled people into the mainstream. The special education system has done pioneering work in the field of education of children with disabilities. However, it has a limited impact owing to limited coverage, lack of qualified teachers, a sheltered environment, limited funds and so on. To overcome some of these problems, the ministry of welfare launched the scheme for Integrated Education for the Disabled Children (IEDC) in 1974. The implementation of this scheme was transferred to the Department of Education in 1982 from the ministry of social justice to MHRD. A great deal more needs to be done.

The former secretary for education in India writes:

India has witnessed a phenomenal expansion of educational opportunities in the post-independence period. However, disabled children have not benefited substantially from this growth in educational facilities. It is however faced with several problems like limited coverage, lack of qualified teachers and a sheltered environment. It was to overcome some of these problems that the Ministry of Welfare launched the scheme for IEDC. (Dasgupta 1997)

Important commissions such as the Sargent Report (1944) and the Kothari Commission (1965) had explicitly recommended that the child with special needs was to be included in regular mainstream education, but this had not been complied with.

With the introduction of District Primary Education Programme (DPEP), the scope has been widened to addressing the equality issue. Guidelines have been issued for providing integrated education to disabled children. Integration of children with special needs in DPEP districts was discussed. Changes in identification practices and active collaboration with NGOs were stressed.

Different paradigms of integration in rural areas were examined and suggestions for convergence between NGO sectors and government departments were also stressed.

Nature of services required by disabled children were discussed and the following stratifications were suggested:

- Children with mild disabilities (45 per cent) could be handled by general classroom teachers with a sensitization of one week.
- Children with mild/moderate disabilities (30 per cent) need counselling and assistance from time to time.
- Children with moderate/severe disabilities (15 per cent) need periodic help in academic areas.
- Children with more severe disabilities (10 per cent) require direct attention/preparatory assistance from special teachers.

Equalization of opportunities, changes in attitudes and removal of architectural barriers were reiterated. The need for avoiding labelling and the real meaning of equalization of opportunity was stressed. Barriers impeding integration and different methods of overcoming them were discussed.

The whole school approach and modification to curriculum were stressed. The other issues discussed included teacher training, career structure, belief systems, community/national ethos, and emotional, and spiritual commitments.

Education for all cannot be fully achieved unless special education moves on to a new phase of development. This entails action at system level and at school level. Action at system level must encompass legislation, administration and the allocation of resources for educational provision; early childhood education; acknowledgment of parental rights; professional development; and research and development.

It was reiterated that the government should make a budgetary provision for support to inclusive education in all sub-sectors of education. The state Plans should also make provision for this component as a part of education reform. The investment should not be perceived narrowly in terms of the number of special educational needs beneficiaries, but should be considered in a broader frame as it will improve quality of education for *all* children.

The guiding principle at school level is the creation of one school for all. This requires action in respect of academic organization of the school; curriculum planning and pedagogy; in-service training; and parental involvement.

The National Conferences Adopted the Following Resolution

It is the unanimous view of the participants of these national network seminars on inclusive education for children with special needs held in Bombay, New Delhi and Jaipur, and parents of various organizations, that education of children with special needs should be an integral part of the general education system of the country as it is in mostly all other countries and should be exclusively under the Department of Education and MHRD. This is because education is a fundamental right of every child as specified in the Constitution.

To provide a nucleus for the concerted and coordinated expansion of inclusive education in India, Mithu Alur took the initiative to announce the formation of NRCI, located at the Bandra centre of the society.

Move Away from Colonialism!

International Inputs: North South Dialogues I, II, III, IV

On the international level, four international conferences entitled 'The North South Dialogues on Inclusive Education' were held to share experiences in inclusion from both the northern and southern paradigms. The doctoral research (Alur 1999) had indicated that India did not have a comprehensive policy for children with special needs. The North South Dialogue (NSD) was initiated to build a partnership between organizations in India and abroad to learn from each other, exchange ideology and support each other in this journey of inclusion. It was essential for international professionals to be sensitive to differences and diversity of each region and to the fact that inclusion needs to be culture- and context-specific.

The objectives of the NSD were to examine models of inclusive education which were context-specific to regions in the North and in developing countries in the South as well as to get policy-makers and bureaucrats to attend and learn. The main aim was to put across the stand that every region can do inclusive education but differently from the West and that each model has to be context- and culture-specific to that region. The conferences have been well documented in two publications (Alur and Booth 2005; Alur and Bach 2005a).

The barriers to inclusion are stubborn and multi-varied and it is important to recognize the distinction between laudable rhetoric and actual practice. Exaggeration and unqualified assertions are a style of presentation that encourages moral panic (Barton and Armstrong 2007).

Too often there is an unacceptable disjuncture between the public rhetoric of representatives of government or institutions and actual practices or outcomes.

Human service industries and professional practices involved are fundamentally disabling.

The question of rights is central to the whole issue of disability. Demands for a greater empowerment of disabled people are essential. Disabled people need to be listened to and involved in key decision making. Achieving these objectives and establishing more informed perspectives necessitates difficult struggles (Barton 1989).

To discuss the issues of inclusion, role of professionals in the process, social model of disability and worldwide trends in the field of intervention for the disabled, it was necessary to provide a common platform for professionals and policy-makers in the field of education, welfare and rehabilitation. After months of work and discussions with colleagues in India and abroad, we took the initiative towards organizing three major conferences in India together with the ministry of education.

The North South Dialogue I on Inclusive Education 2001, Mumbai
Eminent speakers from Canada, the UK, Brazil, South Africa, Bangladesh, Hong Kong and Chile, as well as representatives from the World Bank, United Nations Educational, Scientific and Cultural Organization (UNESCO), United Nations Children's Fund (UNICEF), Canadian

International Development Agency (CIDA), Government of India and civil society organizations across the country shared their experiences of diverse cultures, contexts, resources and policies.

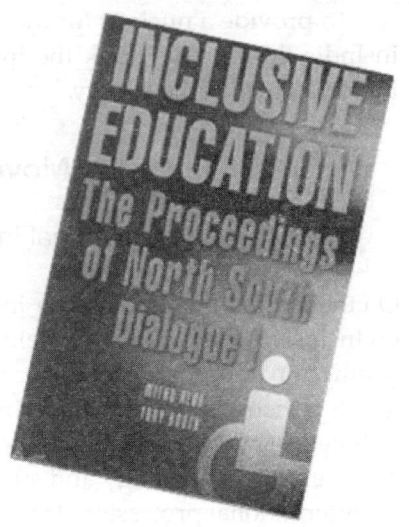

Governmental attitudes: 'I was on the interview panel for an applicant for the Indian Administrative Service (IAS). He was a young man, intelligent, capable—he had become deaf when he was 11 years old due to some medicine prescribed improperly. We had to interview this applicant with the aid of a computer. His answers were excellent and he was an above average applicant. We placed him very high on the marks that he got, but then the government stepped in saying, 'No, our rules say he has to be cleared medically'(Desai 2005, cited in Alur and Booth 2005).

As a result of the first NSD, an All India Regional Alliance (AIRA) for inclusive education was established and it was decided to coordinate with the National Council of Teacher Education (NCTE) to include a module on disability in the general teacher education programmes. The Third Amendment to the Constitution of India on the subject of education was enacted by Parliament in December 2001. A clause and a positive statement were added to include children with disabilities (Alur and Booth 2005).

Martin Luther King, the great human rights leader from the North who led several civil rights battles for many years in USA, said, 'The arm of history is long, but it inevitably bends towards justice. It is my beacon of hope in the work we do' (Rioux 2005, cited in Alur and Booth 2005).

The general intervention approach is that children have a right to go to school, but the problem for disabled children is that the access to inclusive education depends a lot on individual school districts, the province you happen to live in, the school that is in your neighbourhood—all these factors can prevent a child from getting an inclusive education. In some cases, children do not get an inclusive education and in some cases the children do not get education at all. To address this, people go to human rights groups or courts but it's a very time-consuming process (Crawford 2005, cited in Alur and Booth 2005). A view of inclusion that is solely concerned with students categorized as 'having special educational needs' retains all the difficulties associated with that label (Booth and Ainscow 1998; Slee 1993).

The attempt to make students fit in with an unchanged inflexible system catering for an imagined homogeneous group of students is assimilationist. It displays the same lack of respect for learners as a lack of attention to differences of language and culture, where learners are expected to aspire to a single standard of educational fitness and those who cannot shed their difference are seen as having an enhanced distinctiveness and may be subject to increasing rejection.

A transformative view of inclusion in education, then, involves a series of unending processes. It can be seen as the processes of increasing the participation and reducing the exclusion of learners from, the cultures, curricula and communities of local learning centres. It requires the retention of the link between these processes of inclusion and exclusion and I have experimented with calling this enterprise inclusion/exclusion. It requires the restructuring of the cultures, curricula, policies and practices in schools so that they support the learning and participation of the diversity of learners in their locality (Alur and Booth 2005).

Meaning of Sustainability:
The word 'sustainability', because of its usage in economics, leads us to think of the availability of material and financial resources that allow and ensure the permanence of certain actions. To many, it seems we are immersed in a world in which relationships between the markets have prevailed over human relations, even a time of globalization which is supposedly concerned with the 'global' as synonymous with collective, common, general or equal (Ibid 2005).

For inclusion to be more than empty rhetoric, it was imperative that discussions at all levels (global, regional, national and local) move towards a practical realization of inclusive policy.

North South Dialogue II on Inclusive Education 2003, Kochi—From Rhetoric to Reality Kochi Declaration

The second NSD aimed to do this: it aimed to discuss models of implementation of inclusive practice in the North countries that had relevance to the South; to explore difficulties of exploring policy both in the North and South; and to conduct comparative analyses of the process of implementation. The target audience included eminent professionals and representatives from North and South countries, government officials at state and central levels, NGOs, activists and others dealing with educational services. It was historic and will be remembered for the Kochi Declaration which was unanimously passed by the 170 delegates present, stating that all development initiatives must be 'disability sensitive'.

We, delegates convening at the North South Dialogue on Inclusive Education, an international conference at Kochi, Kerala, India, to advance a global agenda for inclusive education that is consistent with international commitments to education for all in the Dakar Framework for Action (2000) and the Salamanca Statement: A Framework for Action (1994), affirm the following:

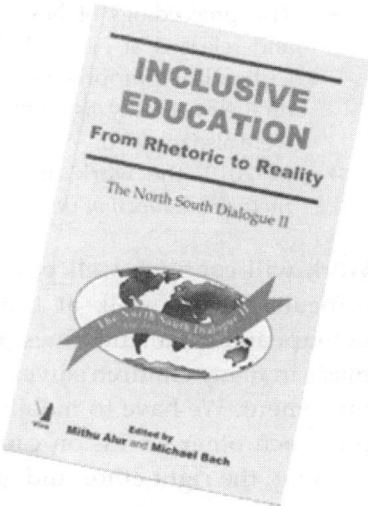

- Segregation is a violation of human rights. All children, including children with disability, have a fundamental human right to be included in mainstream local schools.
- *Education for all* will not be achieved without inclusion: inclusion will not be achieved outside *education for all*.
- By inclusion we mean quality education for all, based on the principles of equal opportunities and access.
- To achieve inclusion, the systemic barriers people and learners face in accessing education—as a result of differences arising from religion, race, gender, poverty, class, caste, ethnicity, language and disability—must be removed.

- The Dakar Framework for Action, signed by 164 governments in 2000, to ensure access to resources for education for all, must be extended to encompass inclusive education.
- Government responsibility for education policy and provision must not be fragmented or disjointed. A single department should be responsible for the *education of all children.*

(Alur and Bach 2005a)

The North South Dialogue III on Inclusive Education, 2005, New Delhi: Towards a Global Alliance

The third dialogue was aimed to further the international alliance and lend support to individual campaigns to end exclusion of certain groups from the sphere of education. In many cases those most affected by exclusion are people with disabilities. Other forms of discrimination occur on the basis of religion, creed, race, gender, poverty, class, caste, ethnicity, language, armed conflict, natural disaster, sexual orientation and other factors. Disabled people and other adults and youth facing marginalization, their families, practitioners, academics, government representatives and other likeminded allies welcoming diverse perspectives and supporting inclusion were the target group. It was determined that disabled people, their families and other segregated groups must play an active role in the struggle for inclusive education.

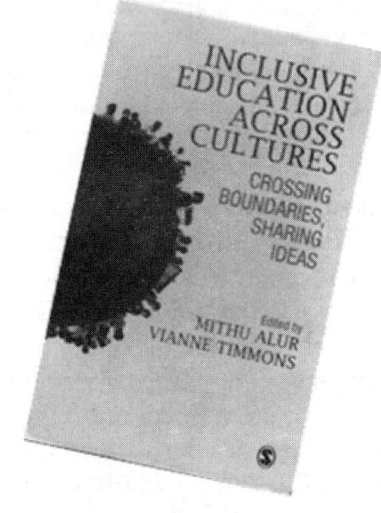

- In 2009, the conference proceedings were published as *Inclusive Education Across Cultures—Crossing Boundaries, Sharing Ideas*
- The proceedings of NSD I and NSD II were published and released at NSD III. Additionally, three volumes of Culturally Appropriate Policy and Practice (CAPP)—based on their necessity, as mentioned in the previous domain—were also released.
- In 2010, the work of NRCI entitled *The Journey for Inclusive Education in the Indian Sub-Continent*

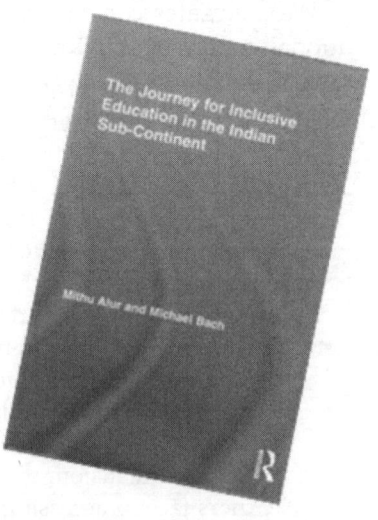

Work will continue well past our lifetimes. We find it a difficult path to walk at times, facing lots of barriers, detours and even landmines. We want to see a difference made in many children's lives and this means a large scale movement. We have to mobilize, work together and support each other. Inclusion can be a success when during training, the right ethos and attitudes are developed by school systems. Finally, in all our deliberations over these issues, we need to remind ourselves that meeting these demands with all the changes they involve will be beneficial for all people. We strongly believe that we cannot perpetuate the divide we so often see between academia and the community, parents and teachers, disabled children, adults and practitioners. It is time to cross those boundaries, share ideas, explore others' views and experiences and remain together (Alur and Timmons 2009).

The North South Dialogue IV on Inclusive Education, 2012, Goa: Implementing Tools of Change for Inclusion

NSD was conceptualized by Dr Mithu Alur with the primary aim of exploring models of inclusion in education. Against the backdrop of the development of inclusive educational practices worldwide, it was important to look at culture- and context-specific challenges of countries and regions (Bordoloi 2004).

This conference was historic as it celebrated 40 years of our service in the field of disability as well as the completion of 10 years of our association with the Women's Council, UK, for the CII (Community Initiatives in Inclusion) course, a project supported by the Centre for International Child Health, London. This three-month course trains trainers and partners of community disability services and has had students from 22 countries in attendance since its commencement a decade ago.

As all the dialogues have done, the fourth dialogue also focused on the difficulties of the developing countries (the South countries) facing huge systemic barriers in including Children with Disabilities (CWDs), leaving millions of children out of schools. Other marginalized groups out of school such as the girl child, children from socially disadvantaged groups (like Dalits, children in the work force and street children) and any child marginalized due to class, caste, gender, religion or ability will also be addressed. Our colleagues and friends from the Western countries joined us, contributed and participated.

There was a huge chasm between policy enactment and transformational change at the ground level. This and other related issues were addressed as 'Tools of Change' in the Southern countries and Asia-Pacific region. Different models of intervention in the developing countries from Nepal, Tajikistan, Sri Lanka, Bangladesh, Cambodia, Indonesia, Mongolia, and Vietnam were also showcased. Experiences from the developed countries were shared.

Importance and Intention

Disability and inclusion of the disabled has so far not become a mainstream issue in India, unlike in the West. This conference was a key event in making that possible and in helping everyone working in the sector to streamline their activities and their fight against seclusion of the disabled and towards their right as equal members of society.

Delegates from 22 nations brought together the 'evolved' Western countries like the UK, USA, Canada and Australia with those who are fighting unimaginable oppression like Vietnam, China, Tibet and Cambodia.

Many study papers and heart-warming stories of the struggle and triumph of the disabled were shared at the conference.

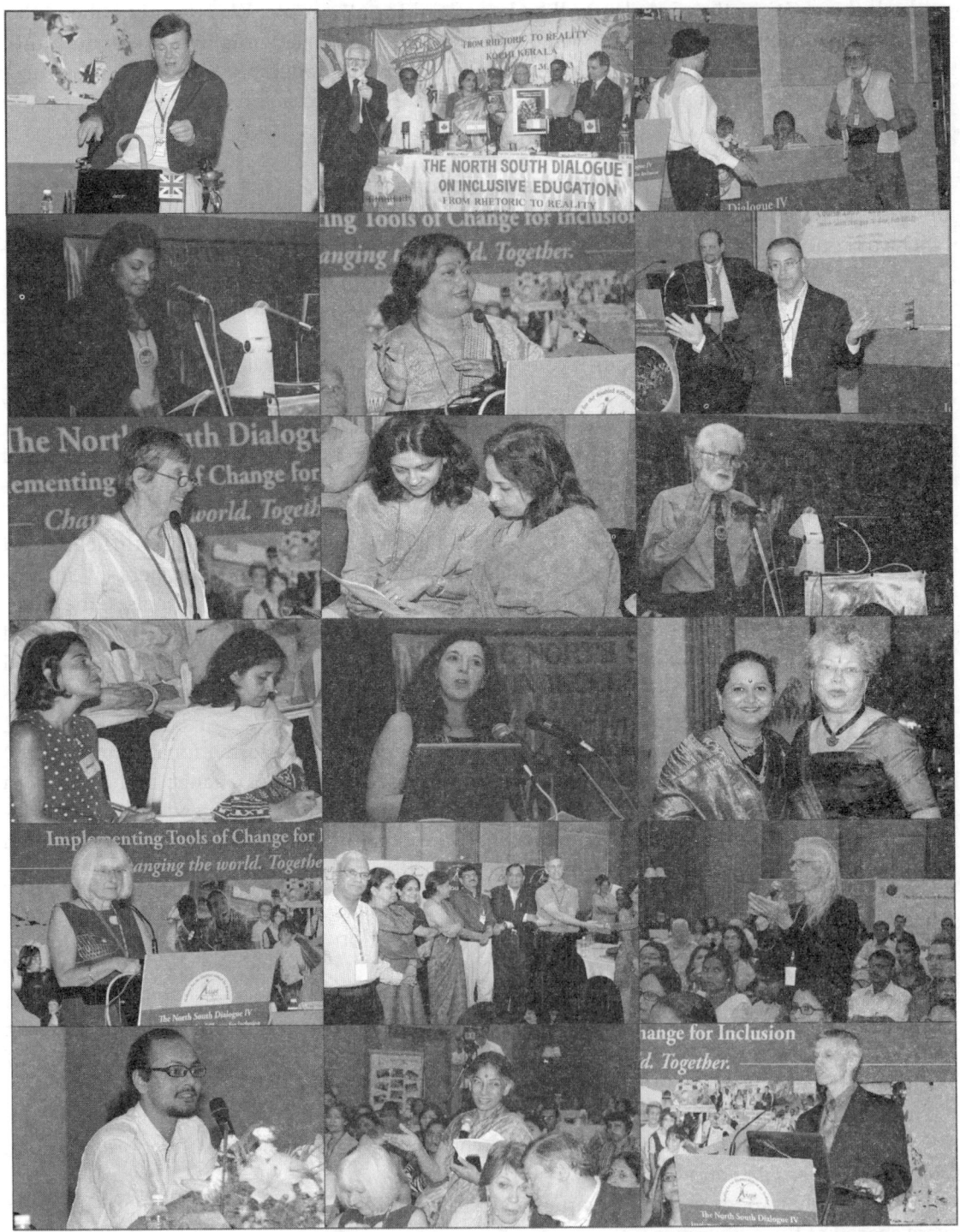

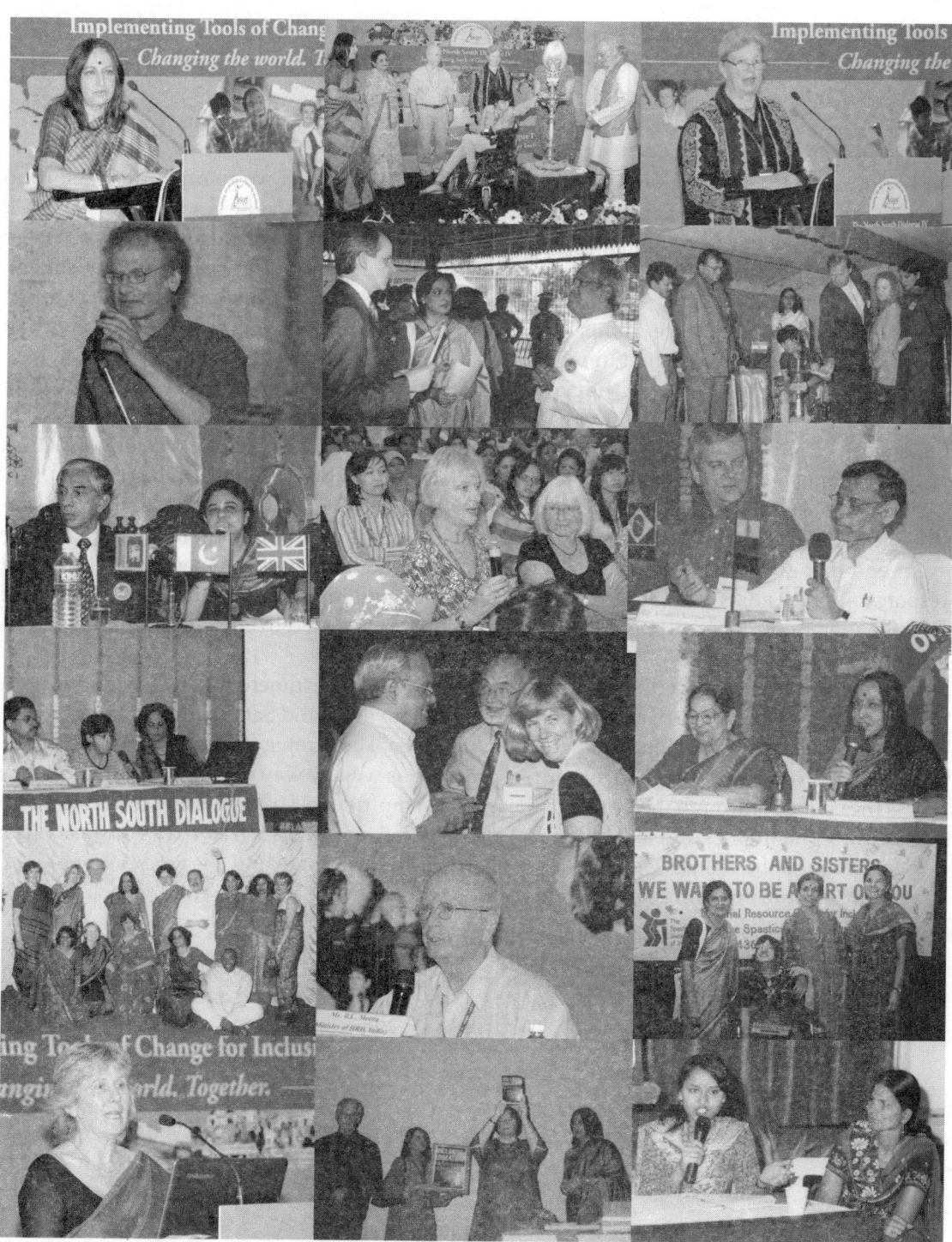

c. Engaging with Government: Striving to Make India a Disability-friendly Country

What of the Government? How Did We Engage with Them?

As I wrote at the beginning of this book, in the early 1970s when we returned to India from UK, I was devastated to find nothing had really changed since we had left seven years ago. CP was not one of the government's 'officially recognized' disabilities. People affected by CP were invisible—the forgotten millions—and their needs were not known. The system excluded them.

After having experienced state-of-the-art services in UK, we again faced a barrage of opposition, barriers and ignorance. If this was the abysmal lack of knowledge and awareness that prevailed in the country, my first thought was: 'What about other Malinis ...?'

Writers have argued that a wider value system underlies policy discourses. The values held by society are reflected in the broader historical, socio-cultural, ideological and political framework of any society. It is important to define and analyze the overall system, in which any programme gets embedded, before planning a solution (Barton and Tomlinson 1984).

Earlier I had believed that we or civil society must do everything; that disability is a private individual tragedy. Not anymore. I now believe that it is a public problem not a private event and that government, as the main trustee of a nation, must play a major role in bearing responsibility for all its citizens. Education is a fundamental right for all children, regardless of class, gender, minority group or ability. Consequently, we needed to engage and participate in governance at a national level.

So I began the next part of the journey, engaging with government together with our partners from all over the country and from Bombay with my husband Sathi Alur and team, whom I call the pioneers, who helped change policy in India The strategy used was more engagement, interaction, persuasion and, of course, pressure as well by way of lobbying and advocacy across the country, through the power of the media, a multi-level strategy using multiple methods. Being a practitioner and an academic, I also showed and demonstrated how inclusion can be done through the centres we ran. Plenty of articles were written and TV programmes aired.

In this section, I examine some of the methods which led to a shift in entrenched attitudes.

Areas targeted:

- Political Change
- Educational Change
- Legislative Change
- Structural Change

Strategies used:

- Regular interaction with key politicians, parliamentarians and policy-makers of all political parties,
- Critiquing of policy measures and documents,
- Sharing constructive suggestions with the government,

- Practical activities to operationalize existing as well as new initiatives,
- Creating a lobby for the implementation of laws that have been passed,
- Interaction with the media,
- Most importantly, addressing the imperative need for financial allocations without which no policy can be implemented.

After the initial struggles, as I wrote at the beginning of this book, I got an appointment to see the prime minister, the late Indira Gandhi. She was very sympathetic and agreed to support me in this venture at the first meeting. She had been well briefed by friends of mine who had been at the university with me. I was asked to speak to her for not more than 10 minutes. My aunt Dr Lotika Sarkar, who had worked extensively for the upliftment of women, advised, 'Don't ask her for anything, just for her blessings.' Mrs Gandhi spent half an hour with me asking details about Malini. She also gave me the names of a dozen leading citizens. Nargis Dutt, a leading actress was one of

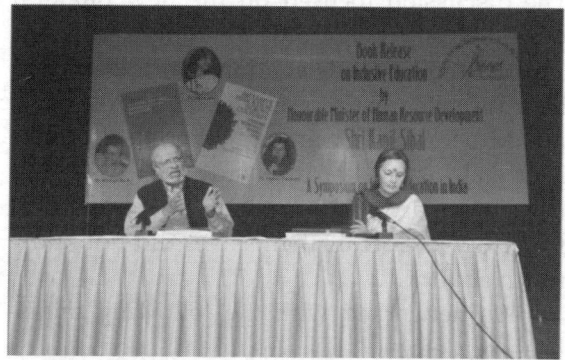

Shri Shyam Benegal and Mrs Brinda Karat voice their support for the structural change required to bring the education of children with disability into the Ministry of Human Resource Development from the Ministry of Social Justice and Empowerment

them. Nargis, as I mentioned, was very taken up with the cause and became the first patron. This certainly helped to bring disabled people out of the gloomy and dreary image and gave the cause a touch of glamour. After her death, her husband Sunil Dutt took it up and was very committed to the cause for over 23 years. The interaction with government was much easier with the patrons not only being Members of Parliament but also being well-known film stars and much loved public figures. Moreover, the fact that we were strictly apolitical and worked with all parties and all governments, gave the cause a head start. Other parliamentarians came forward to learn about the subject and raise questions about inclusive education in Parliament, including Mr Shyam Benegal, Brinda Karat, Priya Dutt, Milind Deora, Supriya Sule, Tarun Vijay and many others.

I had several meetings in Delhi with various leaders of different parties. The first stage was making them aware of the problems and the gaps. One of the politicians, whom we had invited, had a disability himself and he actually said, 'I will come but you will not mention anything about my disability!' Stigma indeed!

Meetings with senior cabinet ministers, bureaucrats and policy-makers were held. We lobbied and networked at the highest

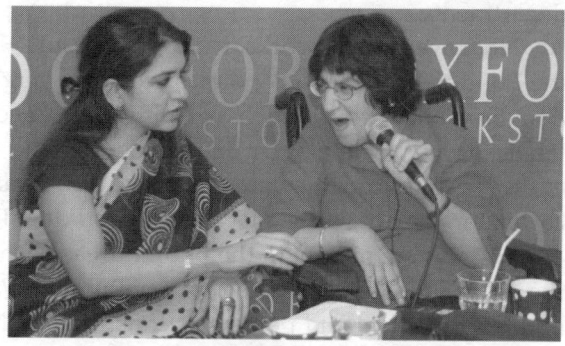

Shaina NC with Malini Chib at Oxford Book Store

government levels in New Delhi, pressing for the human rights model on disabilities and for educational practices and rights that, in effect, leave no child out. I met with the then Union finance minister, Mr Jaswant Singh, of the BJP. The discussion focused on the new bilateral positions on foreign aid. Mr Singh, in reply, assured the NRCI delegation that they would be put on the list of credible NGOs. We also met Mrs Sushma Swaraj, the then health minister, and asked her to ensure that disability became a part of the training of the medical fraternity as doctors themselves did not know much about CP.

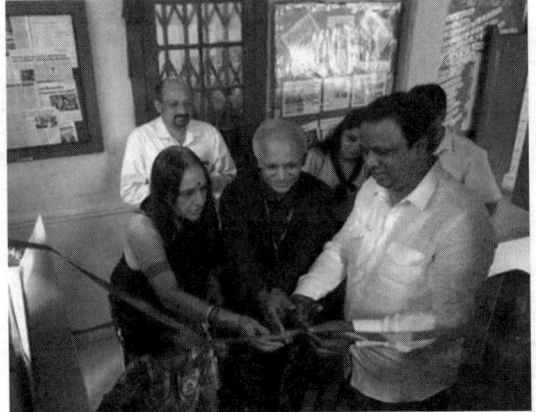

Stair-lift inauguration by Mr Ashish Shelar, MLA & President, Mumbai Unit of BJP, Mr S. Kulkarni, GM Material Dept., HPCL, ADAPT Project Lead with Dr Mithu Alur at the CSE Colaba

We networked with the following ministries regularly:

- Ministry of human resource development
- Ministry of social justice and empowerment
- Ministry of women and child development
- Ministry of health
- Planning Commission
- Census
- Election Commission

To name a few, we had meetings with Meera Kumar, Murli Manohar Joshi, Montek Singh Ahluwalia, Kapil Sibal, minister human resources development, and even apprised two presidents about disability! At the state level, we met up with the chief ministers, governors, chief secretaries and secretaries of various departments.

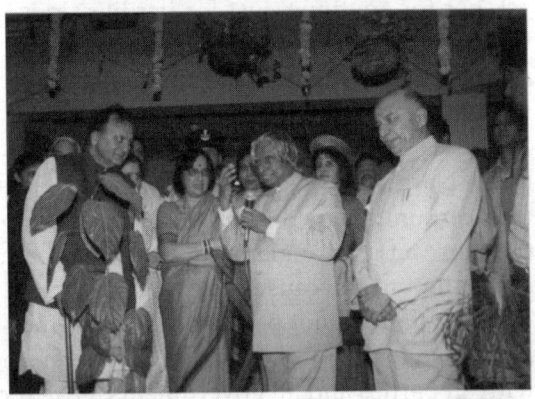

Honourable President Abdul Kalam visited us and wrote a special poem for our children and parents

No government works without pressure. The policy process is a political process. At the London School of Economics we were taught that NGOs needed to get into the political domain. Other groups such as Dalits and scheduled castes (SC) have had powerful political lobbies from the time of Dr B.R. Ambedkar and Gandhi. Although disabled persons are a part of these groups too, they are powerless as a group. The disabled have had no one single political leader, they have been left behind and depoliticized.

Numbering mainly in the poorer areas of the country's rural, tribal and urban slum areas, the disabled people have no representation in Parliament. The political system clearly did not address this silent and powerless constituency. Nobody has heard their voices—they were not on the agenda of any political party.

Political Action: A Civil Rights Campaign

We began a campaign for civil rights called The Disabled Vote and promised it to any party that would bring out disability in their political manifesto. Political strength will only come in with representation in Parliament by disabled people.

We first created a political charter, outlining four major demands of people with disabilities.

- Disability issues should be included in the political manifesto of all political parties as well as in their common minimum programme.
- A national disability advisor working under the jurisdiction of the prime minister, within the prime minister's office, would help bring about effective public–private partnership and monitor implementation of all programmes for the disabled.
- A commitment must be made that 10 per cent of the Member of Parliament's budget or the MP Lad Fund is spent on disabled people for their education, health and programmes benefitting them.
- Disabled peoples need to be heard in Parliament.

Posters talking about the 100 million people out of the purview of services were sent around the entire country. We aimed to appeal to voters to vote for the party, which supported disability issues. We managed to create a groundswell that could 'swing' the vote. To continue building the groundswell, we used the upcoming elections to our advantage and organized a solidarity march, culminating in a public meeting on 9th of April, 2009. A meet was organized to announce the solidarity march as well as sensitize the media on the civil rights campaign.

Solidarity March for the Civil Rights of the Disabled

One afternoon on the 9th of April, 2009, over 3,000 concerned citizens of Mumbai comprising families and persons with disabilities, well-wishers, members of DPOs (Disabled Persons Organisations) and NGOs came together in a show of solidarity for disability issues. A group of about 500 citizens assembled at the Azad Maidan. Offering their support to disability issues were sheriff of Bombay, Dr Indu Shahani; Members of Parliament, Shyam Benegal, Priya Dutt and Milind Deora; Independent Lok Sabha candidate from South Mumbai Meera Sanyal; Mona Shah, another independent candidate from South Mumbai; Supriya Sule from NCP; Shaina NC, and Advocate Ashish Shelar from the BJP; and Dr Pravina Shah all announced their support. Dr Indu Shahani pledged to make Mumbai a disability-friendly city. She offered Dr Alur the help of her 'Sheriff's Brigade'—a group of socially active students—to assist in ensuring that the polling booths for the Lok Sabha election were accessible. In an effort to ensure that every citizen of Mumbai is given an opportunity to exercise their right to vote, we collaborated with Mr Debashish Chakrabarty, secretary and chief electoral officer, Maharashtra and Dr Indu Shahani to ensure that election booths in the city of Mumbai were accessible for persons with disabilities (PWDs).

All this activism resulted in widespread awareness about the political charter of, by and for the disabled. It was at once disseminated across the Internet and sent out to various media agencies for spreading awareness among the disabled voters about the importance of taking a stand and demanding one's rights.

Similar meetings on lack of accessibility in Bombay and transport and employment problems were held. Leading celebrities like Shonali Bose, Kalki Koechlin, Nagesh Kukunoor and

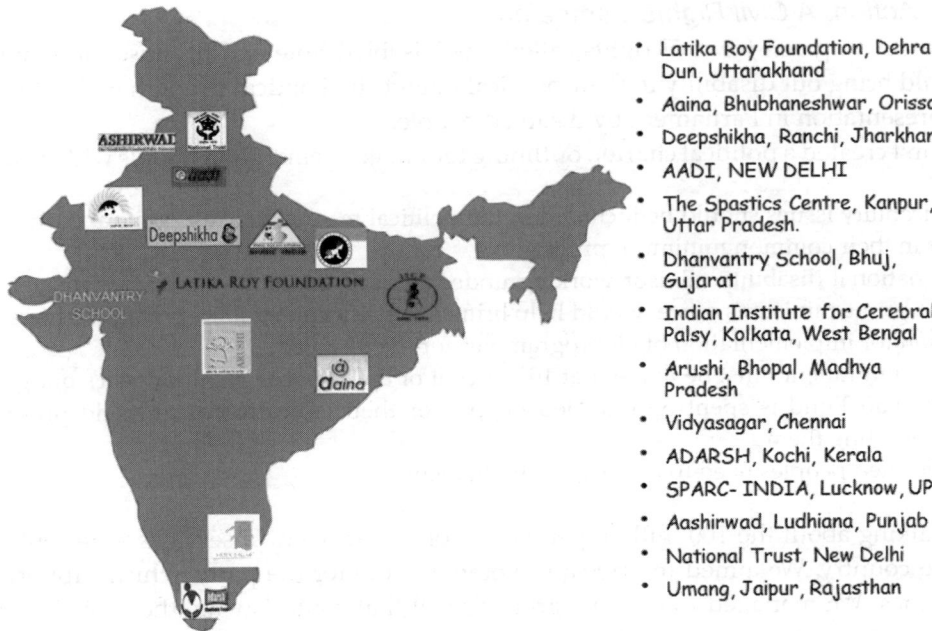

- Latika Roy Foundation, Dehra Dun, Uttarakhand
- Aaina, Bhubhaneshwar, Orissa
- Deepshikha, Ranchi, Jharkhand
- AADI, NEW DELHI
- The Spastics Centre, Kanpur, Uttar Pradesh.
- Dhanvantry School, Bhuj, Gujarat
- Indian Institute for Cerebral Palsy, Kolkata, West Bengal
- Arushi, Bhopal, Madhya Pradesh
- Vidyasagar, Chennai
- ADARSH, Kochi, Kerala
- SPARC- INDIA, Lucknow, UP
- Aashirwad, Ludhiana, Punjab
- National Trust, New Delhi
- Umang, Jaipur, Rajasthan

All India Regional Alliance for Inclusive Education

This figure is not to scale. It does not represent any authentic national or international boundaries and is used for illustrative purposes only.

Dia Mirza lent their support. The events were very well covered by various TV channels such as NDTV, Zee TV, Doordarshan, and in the press by the *Hindu, DNA, Hindustan Times, Times of India, Indian Express* and in the leading vernacular papers such as *Lok Satta, Lok Mat* and *NavBharat Times.* This charter was shared with all political parties, disabled rights groups, other NGOs, parents, well-wishers and supporters.

There was an overwhelming response. Thousands of signatures of support were obtained in support of the charter. Citizens agreed to cast their vote in favour of the party that supported disability. The charter was also forwarded to members of AIRA, a group I had convened earlier, consisting of organizations from across the country to further the inclusive movement in the country. AIRA consisted of organizations from across the country committed to 'education for all', who advocate on policy issues and promote local inclusive education initiatives in their respective regions. Many of the SSIs from across the country are our regional partners; each of them liaised with a network of individuals (parents, students, volunteers and well-wishers), NGOs and government departments.

Members of the ADAPT Rights Group conducted access audits with the Sheriff of Mumbai, Indu Shahani's Student Brigade, visiting all polling stations across the city. Parents and staff audited their own polling stations, the results of which were analyzed and forwarded to the chief electoral officer. Mr Chakraborty agreed to depute students from the National Sample Survey (NSS) and National Cadet Corps (NCC) to help people with disabilities and their families if the polling booths are inaccessible or not on the ground floor.

Expressions of Solidarity across the Nation

AIRA partners, too, participated in solidarity marches, held press meets, approached those in power with memorandums based on the political charter and conducted similar audits. These are some reports:

Delhi:
Leading advocates like Javed Abidi, Vandana Bedi, G. Syamala, Radhika Alkazi and many others joined us in our appeal to Mrs Sonia Gandhi, Dr Manmohan Singh, Mr Kapil Sibal and participated in the media campaign

Chennai, Tamil Nadu:
SSI Vidyasagar, Chennai, working under the leadership of Usha Ramakrishnan and Rajul Padmanabhan handed over the political charter to major leaders of the political parties over the election period. Activists from Vidyasagar's Disability Legislation Unit (DLU) checked out polling booths to see how accessible they are and arranged for voter identification for people with disabilities. The DLU has created a website on accessible elections and the charter was uploaded for wider dissemination.

Kolkata, West Bengal:
Ankur, the advocacy group of AIRA and partner of Indian Institute for Cerebral Palsy (IICP) along with the Human Rights Law Network (HRLN) and the Disability Action Forum (DAF) organized a press meet in Kolkata on 9th of April, 2009, at the Press Club in solidarity with the march held in Mumbai. The conference focused on all marginalized groups. Young adults with disability shared their experiences and spoke on inaccessible booths, their desire to be treated with dignity and about wanting to be a part of the change.

Jaipur, Rajasthan:
Mrs Deepak Kalra, director, Umang, AIRA partner in Rajasthan, led a delegation of disabled persons and media persons to the party offices of the BJP and Congress to demand inclusion of the four demands made by the political charter. The charter was handed over to the party Heads and the issue of barrier-free elections was also taken up. In addition, the memorandum was given to 100 persons at a meeting of the Muscular Dystrophy Association.

Bhubaneswar, Orissa:
AIRA partner AAINA used the occasion of World Autism Day on 4th of April, 2009, to address the consultative meeting of DPOs and civil society organizations arranged by the Association of the Blind. The points outlined by the political charter were discussed and added to their memorandum. Over a 100 activists and delegates marched in a rally demanding their rights. Subsequently, a delegation of 30 persons met with the general secretary BJD and representatives of the NCP, BSP, OPCC, BJP and CPI (M) and handed over the memorandum, asking that the demands be included in the manifestos as well as their programmes. The issue of accessibility in the voting booths was also brought up. This demand was also conveyed to the chief election commissioner Ms Alaka Panda.

Aashirwad, Ludhiana, Punjab:
Dr Neelam Sodhi, director, Aashirwad, AIRA partner in Punjab, organized a protest meeting along with members of the School For Deaf and Dumb, Vocational Rehabilitation Training Centre, Bhartiya Vikas Parishad and the Voice of the Handicapped. A memorandum was given to the parliamentary secretary Mr Harish Rai Dhanda. Dr Sodhi termed this meeting 'an extension of the solidarity march carried out across the nation for non-inclusion of the issues concerning "disabled" by the parties in their election manifestos'.

Irked over the indifferent attitude of the parties and their candidates who had failed to include even a single issue of the 'disabled' in their election manifestos, the members of NGOs said it pointed towards the insensitive approach of people's representatives towards the needs of the disabled. The NGOs present threatened not to cast their votes if their demands were not met with.

The prime minister's office forwarded our petition of the four demands to the ministry of law and justice and the ministry of statistics and programme implementation for appropriate action.

Outcome

The outcome was that four major political parties, the Congress, CPI (M), BJP and the NCP *included disability issues in their political manifestos.*

Reformative Action in the Educational Sphere

In March 2005, Shri Arjun Singh, Honourable minister of human resources development, announced a policy which will remain a landmark in the lives of disabled people. The statement was entitled 'Inclusive Education for Children and Youth with Disabilities' (IECYD). It shifted the responsibility for the education of children with disability from the ministry of social justice and empowerment to MHRD, a critical structural change that we had been working towards for three decades. India was earlier among the minority 4 per cent of countries in the world that had not affected this shift.

The Honourable minister stated in Parliament:

Under this plan, the first level of intervention will be through the Integrated Child Development Services (ICDS) programme. As Members of the House are aware, the ICDS programme reaches out to all children in the age group of 0–6 years. The *anganwadi* workers will be trained to detect disabilities at an early stage by the Department of Women and Child Development, which will use the training modules prepared for this purpose by the National Institute of Population Control and Community Development (NIPCCD) and other such agencies with the inputs of the ministry of social justice and empowerment. ICDS workers will be trained to motivate parents of children with disabilities. The ICDS programme itself will provide for supplementary material to be used in the centres. We look to the collaboration of the state governments in strengthening this new dimension to the ICDS programme.

We had played an important role in developing IECYD. As a result, we were asked by MHRD to hold consultations, to develop an action plan for the statement to be delivered at the ground level. The consultations were organized by SSI in collaboration with their partners under the guidance of Mr K. Desiraju, joint secretary, human resources development. Both Mr Keshav Desiraju and Mr Sathi Alur played a critical role in drawing up the action plan after the minister's statement in Parliament.

The main objectives of the action plan were:

1. To ensure that no child with disability is denied admission in mainstream education,
2. To ensure that every child has the right to access an *anganwadi* and school and no child would be turned back on the ground of disability,
3. To ensure that mainstream and specialist training institutions serving persons with disabilities, in the government or in the non-government sector, facilitate the growth of a cadre of teachers trained to work within the principles of inclusion,
4. To facilitate access of girls with disabilities and disabled students from rural and remote areas to government hostels,
5. To provide for home-based learning for persons with severe, multiple and intellectual disability,
6. To promote distance education for those who require an individualized pace of learning,
7. To emphasize job training and job-oriented vocational training, and
8. To promote an understanding of the paradigm shift from charity to development through a massive awareness, motivation and sensitization campaign.

Consultative meets supported by MHRD were held at Kolkata and Bhopal on 23rd and 30th of September, 2005, respectively. The co-organizers of the consultative meet at Kolkata were the Paschimbanga Rajya Pratibandhi Sammilani, IICP and Mr Jayabrato Chatterjee, member, governing body, ADAPT and at Bhopal, Arushi fulfilled the same role.

The Kolkata meet was inaugurated by Shri Gopalkrishna Gandhi, governor, West Bengal. The other dignitaries who attended the inauguration were Shri Kanti Ganguly, minister of state in charge, Sunderbans, West Bengal; Shri Debaditya Chakravarty, principal secretary education, West Bengal; Shri Keshav Desiraju, MHRD, New Delhi; Mr Philip O'Keefe, World Bank, New Delhi.

AIRA partners from Orissa, Chennai, New Delhi, Mumbai, Jharkhand and Kolkata supported the Kolkata meet, whereas partners from New Delhi, Gujarat, Rajasthan, Bhopal and Mumbai supported the Bhopal meet.

The participants for both the consultations represented various NGOs around the country, government officials from the Department of Integrated Child Development, Department of Women and Child Development, the Department of Secondary Education, professionals, disabled activists, parents, principals, teachers and management of various mainstream schools in and around the cities.

The themes of the workshops were:

1. Every child matters: 'No Child Left Behind' is the goal;[4]
2. Pedagogic Change: Putting inclusive principles in teacher training;

[4]From a British and American Law

3.   Accessibility: Key element to inclusion;
4.   Participation and equal opportunity in education;
5.   Employment: A vital link to empowerment.

The aim of the consultations was to provide inputs for the action plan based on suggestions from the participants. The consultations were designed in the form of workshops, planned around the key themes of Shri Arjun Singh's statement, to enable all voices to be heard. The recommendations emerging from the consultations were forwarded to MHRD in 2005 and were incorporated into the action plan developed to operationalize the policy by the ministry of human resources development.

Presence on National-level Committees: Reforms in the Educational Sphere

The government reconstructed a high-level committee called the Central Advisory Board of Education (CABE) committee which has been resurrected in 2005, comprising State education ministers, educationists, activists, experts and some eminent high-profile people from civil society from across the country. Although not popular, they included me in the CABE! Our work at the national level was certainly further enhanced by my appointment over the years on various committees, which provided good opportunities of engaging with government on various issues of inclusive education, like the national curricula on teacher training. Smaller educational committees like the round tables on elementary education and education of the disadvantaged certainly showed that the government was serious about its intent to include children with disability into their programmes. Due to the fact that they are *not specifically included in the definition of the target groups of government schemes*, children with disabilities were getting excluded from the benefits in the government programmes. So my first task was to advocate for policy changes by addressing the existing lacunae. In a sub-committee constituted by Mr Kapil Sibal, minister, MHRD, that was to scrutinize definitions of all disadvantaged groups I managed to squeeze in the recommendation that a positive discrimination clause is inserted which specifies 'including the disabled' in all the ministry's schemes, cross-referencing and cutting across all sectors. This read as the following:

'Development of education of SC, scheduled tribe (ST), other backward classes (OBC), minorities, girls and the disabled and other disadvantaged groups'.

Census

We then tackled the census.

A question on disability had been last included in the 1981 census. The national census for the year 2001 ignored the disabled on grounds of inability and claimed that such a survey was beyond the scope and capacity of its operations. The call for inclusion of disability in the 2001 census became a primary policy strategy and our first major effort in policy reform. Frequent questions asked and statements made were: 'We don't even know the number of disabled in this country'; 'We haven't had a proper survey. Our entire census figures are completely insensitive as far as the disabled are concerned. What do you mean by disabled?' Phrases such as *'being considered a non-person', 'did not come into the purview of the masses', 'did not figure at all'* reinforced the invisibility factor.

Our patron, Shri Sunil Dutt, the well-known film star and Member of Parliament, had become temporarily disabled in a plane crash and led the crusade for inclusion of people with disability in India in the census. Our vice chairperson Mr Kamal Bakshi and Sathi Alur networked with the census Commissioner and put forth the concerns of the disability sector. We met with prime minister Mr Manmohan Singh and principal secretary as well to push the cause. A great deal of research was done by Shri Arun Shourie, Member of Parliament (who is also a parent of a disabled son Aditya). At a meeting with the deputy prime minister Shri L.K. Advani and the director general of census, previous questions which had had a large degree of failure were brought up. A particular question in the Indian census which had been a failure was: 'Are you a vegetarian or an eggetarian, if you are an eggetarian, do you eat ducks' eggs or chickens' eggs or quails' eggs'.

Mr Shourie asked why a question asking whether a family had a child who could not see, hear, move, or was different from other children, could not be included in the census. Fortunately Shri Advani and the committee agreed to include it.

Disability Was Now in the Census! It Had Taken Us Concerted Lobbying for Five Years

The landmark decision of including of disability as a category in the census was clearly a victory of intense and sustained NGO efforts. It received wide publicity in the print and electronic media.

The results of the census (2011) exercise, however, were deeply disappointing for the disability movement as it concluded that there were only 2.13 per cent or 21 million Indians with any kind of disability, a fraction of the estimates by a World Bank report (2007) prepared at the request of the Government of India which put the figure at between 4 per cent and 8 per cent of the population (around 40–90 million individuals). This conclusion was widely accepted as being caused by the questions being inappropriate and the lack of training of the enumerators. The focus of the question on disability needed to be on *functionality* rather than labelling *the type* of disability. A sub-question on the extent of disability was required to be included in the census. In order to gather accurate information on disability, enumerators needed to be appropriately trained and sensitized.

After an examination of international standards of questions for identifying people with disabilities, the sub-committee suggested that the Six Question Standard recommended by the Washington Group be incorporated as the standard for mapping disabled people in the country. A number of AIRA partners had also supported ADAPT's proposal that the Washington Group questions related to the identification of disability should be included in the forthcoming census of India. Mr Kamal Bakshi and I met with the census commissioner to explain the rationale behind the insertion of the Washington Group questions in the 2011 census. The commissioner explained that it was not possible to include the Washington Group questions in the main form due to the paucity of space in the census document. The commissioner suggested, however, that the census enumerators could be trained to ask the Washington Group questions while filling in the forms, thereby ensuring that the social model of disability was followed. He also requested us to rewrite and forward the relevant portion of the enumerator training manual, which would then be considered by the expert committee on the census. A rewritten training manual, using simple, straightforward and non-technical instructions and explanations for the enumerators, was worked out and forwarded to the commissioner along with an offer from ADAPT to train the enumerators in the state of Maharashtra.

Mapping: Counting the Numbers and Where They Are

Robust data was not available in the country about the numbers and whereabouts of the children with disabilities. Some mapping was being done by the ministry but there was a disconnect between figures shown and the figures on the ground. Our own experience with the state Sarva Shiksha Abhiyan (SSA) showed gaps in the information gathered. There are large discrepancies in the numbers of CWDs identified between the census data and schools-based records through the District Information System in Education (DISE) surveys, especially because a large number of children, especially disabled children, are out of school.

'A lack of robust data has been the biggest barrier in the implementation of services required for PWDs. Accurate figures are hard to come by and when available they vary depending on the definitions, source, methodology and the scientific instruments used in identifying and measuring an individual's degree of disability. According to a report by the World Bank, using data from the NSS, only 26 per cent of children with severe disabilities in India attend school. About 56 per cent of children with moderate disabilities attend school and even among children with mild disabilities that figure is only 68 per cent. The barriers that prevent children from going to school are many—inaccessible schools and transportation, lack of assistive devices and rehabilitation services, insufficient teacher training, and even teacher and parental attitudes, among others. In order to overcome these barriers, children must receive the services and supports they need.'

Identifying children with disabilities using survey and screening instruments is not an easy task. Some previous efforts in developing countries have had some measure of success and building on that knowledge UNICEF and UN Statistical Commission's Group on Disability Statistics have developed a new approach. These questions are incorporated into the Multiple Indicator Cluster Survey (MICS), which has become the international standard for monitoring childhood disability.

These questions serve as a screen for identifying children who have functional difficulties, but in order to clearly identify children with disabilities and assess their needs, a second stage assessment process is done. This becomes particularly important for linking children with identified needs to available services (Alur 2014).

The 2001 census indicated that there were 21.91 million persons with disabilities (2.13 per cent of the population) in the nation. Alternative estimates suggest a higher incidence of disability (4–8 per cent) which is around 40–90 million individuals. Data collected through mapping exercises and the census could address this lacuna. According to the 2011 census, there are nearly 260 million children in the 5–14 age group (i.e., children who are entitled to free and compulsory education under RTE). Our most recent study conducted in Mumbai using the MICS protocol has indicated a prevalence of 4.4 per cent with regard to childhood disability. Extrapolating this prevalence rate to the data reported in the 2011 census, there are approximately 11.4 million. Further, if one were to use the NSS/World Bank figures of inclusion/exclusion mentioned above, there could be as many as 6 million Children with Special Needs (CWSN) who are Out of School (OOS). About 73 per cent of these children are in rural India.

We again began working with the census commissioner on the method of definition of disability. We recommended certain questions that needed to be asked and worked out a simple module of training for the enumerators, so that they posed questions to the disabled with sensitivity and actually captured the right numbers. Shri Kamal Bakshi, our Honorary vice chairman and Sathi Alur, advisor, spearheaded this work.

Structural Changes

The Department of Women and Child Development was earlier within the MHRD. As a result of a structural change, a new ministry of women and child development was created. The agenda of this ministry includes early childhood care and education under ICDS. This ministry is revamping the ICDS and we were asked to send in a recommendation on the 'whole community approach' to inclusive education.

While I was invited to committees at the national level, several members of the ADAPT team, who have contributed to this book, were nominated to various committees at the state and district level. Varsha Hooja was nominated to the general council of the Ali Yavar Jung National Institute for the Hearing Handicapped (AYJNIHH). Dr Shabnam Rangwala is a part of the Rashtriya Bal Swasthya Karyakram (RBSK) under the National Rural Health Mission (NRHM), ministry of health, Government of India, contributing in the area of developmental disabilities. Deepshikha Mathur was on several university committees, including the Rehabilitation Council of India (RCI) Expert Committee on Cerebral Palsy and Locomotor Impaired. She was also on the Ad Hoc Board of Studies dealing with Special Education. Dr Sharmila Donde was invited to the SSA Committee for Teacher Training in inclusive education. Sangeeta Jagtiani was appointed member, Special Education Committee, Maharashtra State Board of Secondary and Higher Secondary Education. Reshma Tanna and Shabbira Moosabhoy were invited to the Annual Status of Education Report (ASER) Research Committee set up by Pratham. At the local level, Gulab Sayed was invited to committees in Dharavi.

We were approached by the Observer Research Foundation to be a part of the Change Agents for School Education and Research (CASER) round table set up by the Department of School Education and Sports, government of Maharashtra, to assist the Rashtriya Madhyamik Shiksha Abhiyan (RMSA) with proposals for Inclusive Education for Disabled Children at Secondary Stage (IEDSS). Seven members of ADAPT were co-opted on this. ADAPT launched a series of PILs. Members interacted with senior advocate Jamshed Mistry of the Bombay High Court and the outcomes of the PILs after ADAPT intervention were.

- 30 disabled-friendly BEST buses in the city of Mumbai.
- The High Court added a ramp and a disabled-friendly toilet.
- The backlog for employment for physically challenged or disabled persons has largely filled. The court directed the state government to ensure that the backlog will be cleared no later than six months from 21st of December, 2006.

Legislative Changes

On the legislative front, landmark legislation in India had been passed, beginning with the Persons with Disability Act in 1995. India had ratified the UN Convention on the Rights of Persons with Disabilities (UNCRPD). However, since it did not incorporate a number of rights recognized in the UNCRPD, there were many consultations to ensure that it did tally with UNCRPD. That exercise was done by many of us but the new amended act, unfortunately, is presently still a bill and has not gone through the houses of Parliament to become the new act.

The Right to Education Act (RTE)

In November 2009, the Government passed the RTE Act in Parliament… it was a historic moment 62 years after independence. The act made education a constitutional right and extended the right to universal education for all children in the disadvantaged areas but unfortunately *failed to include the disabled in its key definition.* We were very disturbed. It came as a bolt from the blue and we were left completely shell-shocked and stunned. Even after 40 years of demonstrating that children with disability could benefit from education, the disabled had been left out of the RTE Act! This was a massive oversight. It left the future of 30 million disabled children out of the purview of the act and their fate hanging in the balance.

Well, it needed us to strike again! Demonstrations, several trips to Delhi and extensive lobbying for the cause, included meetings with Mrs Sonia Gandhi and Mr Manmohan Singh, a high-profile exercise. We also went to the media. The matter was very well covered by Prannoy Roy from NDTV and other channels as well as the print media. All was not lost. As a result of these efforts, minister for human resources development Shri Kapil Sibal gave an assurance in Parliament that all disabled children would be included in the definition of disadvantaged groups through an amendment to the act. Mrs Sonia Gandhi herself made it a point to be present in Parliament and every time the minister talked of children with disabilities, she intervened and kept interrupting the education minister when he talked of disabled children… She kept saying: 'Children who are differently abled must be brought in.' An amendment of the RTE Act was passed which brought the words 'including disabled children' into the definition of weaker and disadvantaged groups within article 2(d) of chapter I of the RTE Act.

The clause now reads:

'Development of education of SC, ST, OBC, minorities, girls and the disabled and other disadvantaged groups'.

This statement meant that more than 30 million children would now have right to education. No child can now be denied admission in mainstream education on the ground of disability. This has taken us 40 years.

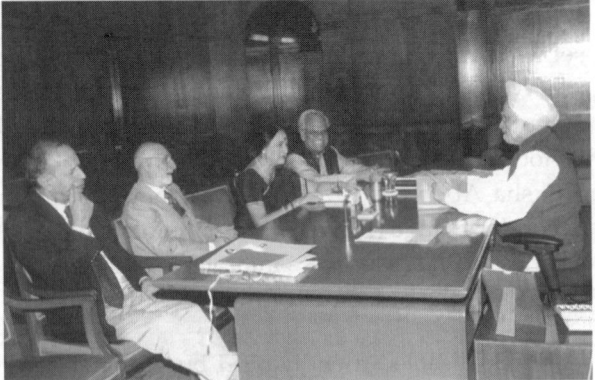

Dr Mithu Alur along with Mr Sathi Alur, Mr Kamal Bakshi and Dr Samiran Nundy, presenting copies of the books to the Honourable Prime Minister, Dr Manmohan Singh in Parliament House

We reached a record height when the prime minister received our books and the education minister came to a function and actually released the books.[5]

Show more sensitivity to disadvantaged groups, the prime minister Shri Manmohan Singh urged. He added:

What can we do to become a more humane and socially progressive society and thereby a more developed society? It appears to me we can begin by changing a mind-set that sees people of disadvantage not as the productive national resource that they are but as a marginal section of society at the fringes of our policy establishment.

With India being a signatory of UNCRPD, Manmohan Singh emphasized the statute casts obligations on all signatories towards enforcement of various rights of persons with disabilities.

He stated:

We propose therefore to comprehensively amend the Persons with Disabilities Act, in consultation with state governments and all stakeholders, so as to bring it in line with our obligations under the UN Convention.

Accessibility, too, he pointed out, was a major issue for persons with disabilities.

I would urge that our educational and healthcare institutions, our government offices, our banks and other places with public dealings ought to be made more user-friendly and accessible to the disadvantaged persons.

The operationalization of this law is now the need of the hour. Figure 9.1, below, is a graphical representation of the work that was done from 2000–14 in reforming public policy.

d. Media Coverage

Substantial resources, such as our library of over 7,000 books, as well as archived documents played an important role in dissemination and creation of awareness. The media played a critical role. Jayabrato Chatterjee assisted with the organization's brochures, press releases audio-visuals and media management. Noted filmmakers came forward to make films. The first film, called *Molly,* was made by Shukla Das and sponsored by Larsen and Toubro. A number of films have since been made. Radhika Roy made *Towards Independence.* Shyam Benegal directed *The Love We Give For Nothing.* Anand Adiverekar made a film on our community project called *Mil Julke* (Together We Can). Amol Gupte captured the children in their lighter moments.

---

[5] *Inclusive Education across Cultures: Crossing Boundaries, Sharing Ideas* by Dr Mithu Alur and Dr Vianne Timmons, published by SAGE, New Delhi, 2009; and *The Journey of Inclusive Education in the Indian Sub-Continent* by Dr Mithu Alur and Dr Michael Bach, published by Routledge, New York, 2010.

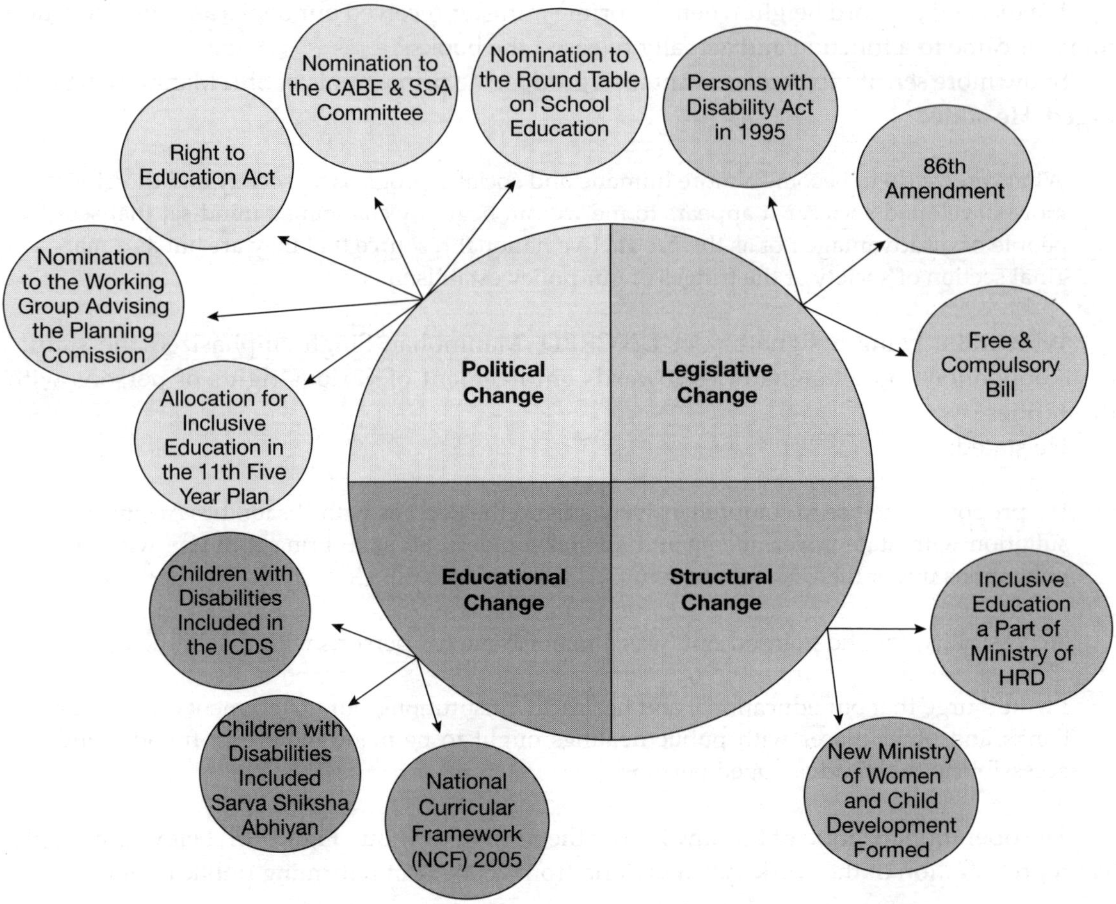

Nomination to the CABE & SSA Committee

Nomination to the Round Table on School Education

Persons with Disability Act in 1995

Right to Education Act

86th Amendment

Nomination to the Working Group Advising the Planning Comission

Free & Compulsory Bill

Allocation for Inclusive Education in the 11th Five Year Plan

Political Change

Legislative Change

Children with Disabilities Included in the ICDS

Educational Change

Structural Change

Inclusive Education a Part of Ministry of HRD

Children with Disabilities Included Sarva Shiksha Abhiyan

National Curricular Framework (NCF) 2005

New Ministry of Women and Child Development Formed

Figure 9.1. Graphic Display of the Work That Was Done from 2000 to 2014 in Reforming Public Policy
Source: Author.

Malini's first book *One Little Finger*, published by SAGE, has received rave reviews and much acclaim in India and abroad. After being released in New Delhi on the 3rd of December, 2010, on the occasion of the International Day of the Disabled, the book was subsequently launched in Mumbai, Kolkata, Jaipur and in The House of Lords, London. Audiences everywhere have been inspired and moved by Malini's account of her life, her philosophy and ideology and her incredible journey through many challenges, recounted with rare candour and poignancy. Through all the adversities she has had to face—lack of access to public places and people's attitudes ranging from negative to indifferent to annoyingly patronizing—what stands out is Malini's determination to forge ahead keeping intact her essential joie de vivre.

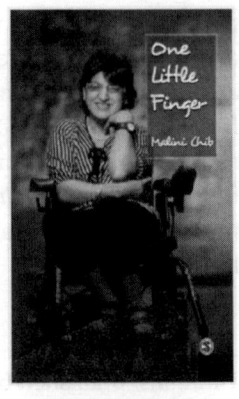

***One Little Finger* by Malini Chib**

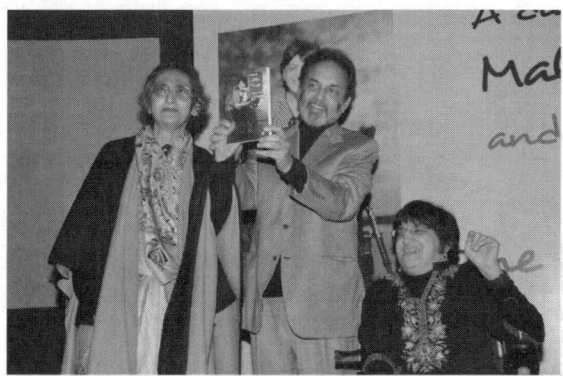

The late Mrs Mita Mundy and Dr Prannoy Roy release *One Little Finger* in New Delhi, on IDOD

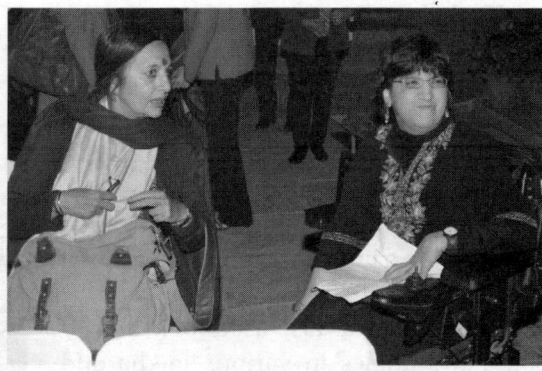

Mrs Brinda Karat, MP with Malini at the book launch in New Delhi

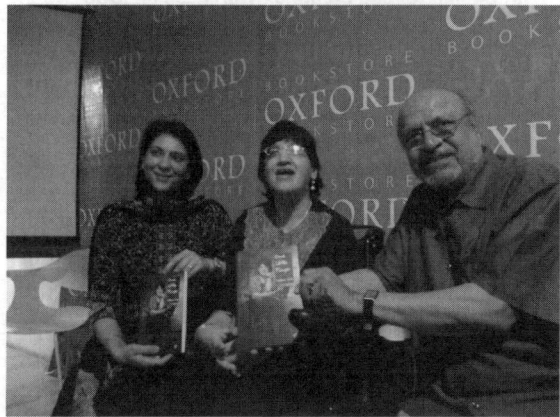

Mr Shyam Benegal (MP) and Mrs Priya Dutt (MP) with Malini at the book launch in Mumbai

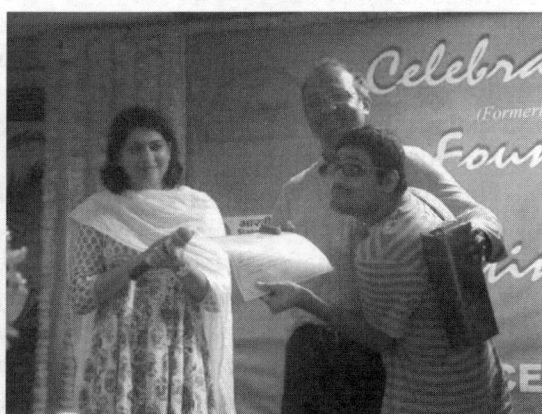

Mrs Priya Dutt and Dr Taral Nagda celebrate World Cerebral Palsy Day

Media Strategies for Tracking Change

A communication and media strategy was central in changing public attitudes towards people with disabilities and education. Designing the strategy was a challenge, especially as news in India is available in17 languages. Twenty-six per cent of the newspapers are in English; 32 per cent in the national language, Hindi. In Maharashtra, 7 per cent are in the state language, Marathi. Each state has its own language and local newspapers. A communications firm, Take 5, (through the offices of Anil Dharkar) was contracted through the project to facilitate communication with the English and vernacular print and electronic media. It was decided that a concerted effort was needed to initiate a shift in media focus from coverage of disability as an individual tragedy or 'curse' to the exclusion and discrimination that people with disabilities face. The strategies used enabled us to carry out an extensive networking effort. The information services, conferences, media coverage, PILs, self-advocacy efforts, public events and NSDs drew NRCI-I into contact with tens of thousands of individuals and organizations across diverse sectors, locally, nationally, regionally and internationally (Alur and Bach 2010).

To help make this shift we organized a 'Solidarity March' annually on
International Day of the Disabled (IDOD)
on the 3rd of December, which attracted
a considerable amount of attention. The
inclusion of film stars handing out leaflets,
highlighting our demand for education
for all, made a huge impact on the general
public (Ibid 2010).

This event was also used to tie in suitable news angles in various media and
provide information about the issue and
identifying sponsors/funding for future
events. There was a significant response

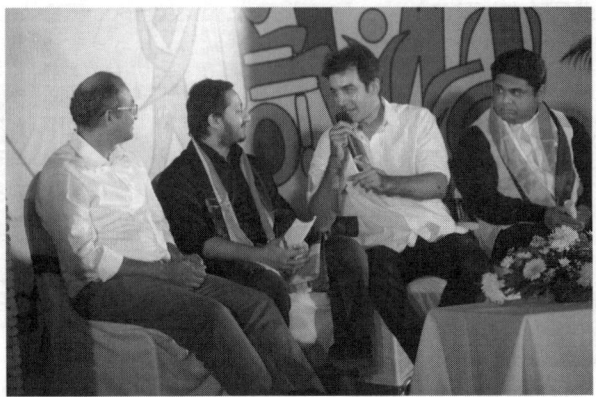

**Dr Taral Nagda, Mr Sudeep Pagedar, Mr Nikhil Chib and
Mr Sachin Kalbag creating awareness on IDOD**

from media with over 600 cc of coverage in the print media (15 English and seven vernacular
publications) and a further 10 clippings in the electronic media. Factsheets were disseminated
and sponsorship for the event was arranged. Media awareness of the concept of inclusion was
significantly enhanced.

Hosting and participating in public events have been a primary means for us to raise public
awareness. Tracking of media coverage of NRCI-I-related events showed significant increases in
coverage. Over 20 national and local newspapers and magazines in the print media published
over 480 stories during the project. In addition, there was wide coverage in the electronic media.
A total of 3,000 people participated in rallies held. Through conferences/seminars, workshops,
training and orientation programmes over 6,500 participants have been registered. 'Orientation
programmes on inclusive education' delivered to public, private and community schools, colleges, polytechnic institutes, education institutes, teaching staff and youth groups targeted 2,600
individuals. Eight major conferences were hosted over the five-year period, with a total of 1,400
participants. Internationally, in addition to the NSDs, we networked with multilateral and international agencies including the World Bank, UNICEF and UNESCO. A number of international
NGOs got involved as well as a growing network including government leaders and officials
from international institutions from Canada, Italy and the UK. This helped to build linkages with
universities and NGOs in Canada, Sweden, Australia, South Africa, the USA, Bangladesh as well
as DPOs around the world. Over the five-year project period, NRCI-I engaged over 25,000 people
in events it hosted and reached over 75,000 people in events in which it participated (Ibid 2010).[6]

We also had tremendous support from theatre personalities. Pearl Padamsee's swansong
was for us. She rang me up and offered the play *Betrayal* as part of our annual show. The show
was a grand success. Now her daughter Raell collaborates with us and conducts regular drama
classes for children.

The most recent film that put CP out in the public domain was *Margarita With A Straw*.
Directed by Shonali Bose, the lead actor Kalki Koechlin has delivered a stellar performance.
ADAPT was one of the co-producers of the film which has received many international awards.

---

[6] Name of the participants registered are available in the Library. Noted and published in *The Journey
for Inclusive Education in the Indian Sub-Continent*. Routledge Publications, USA.

Media Coverage done between 2010-2014

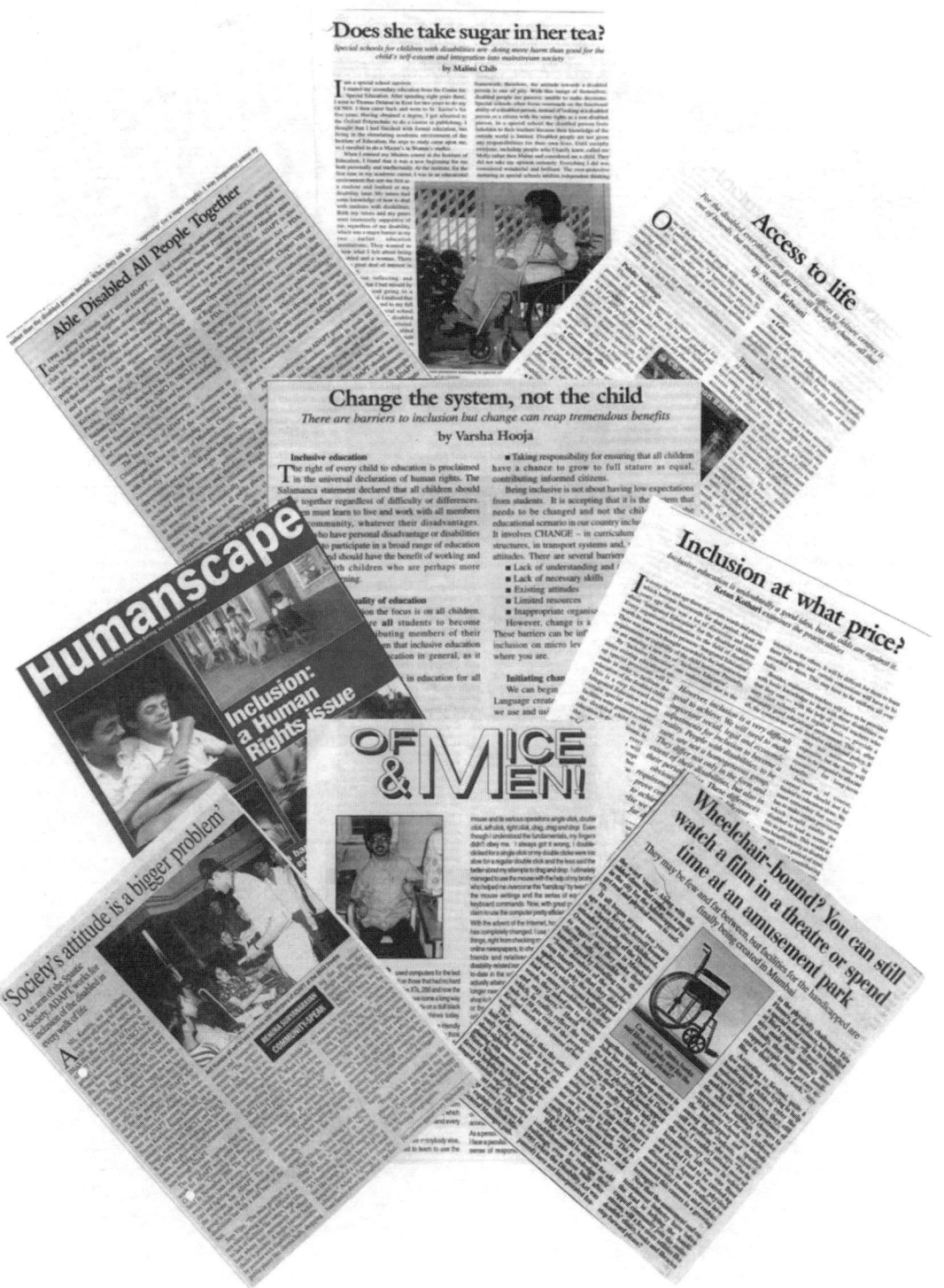

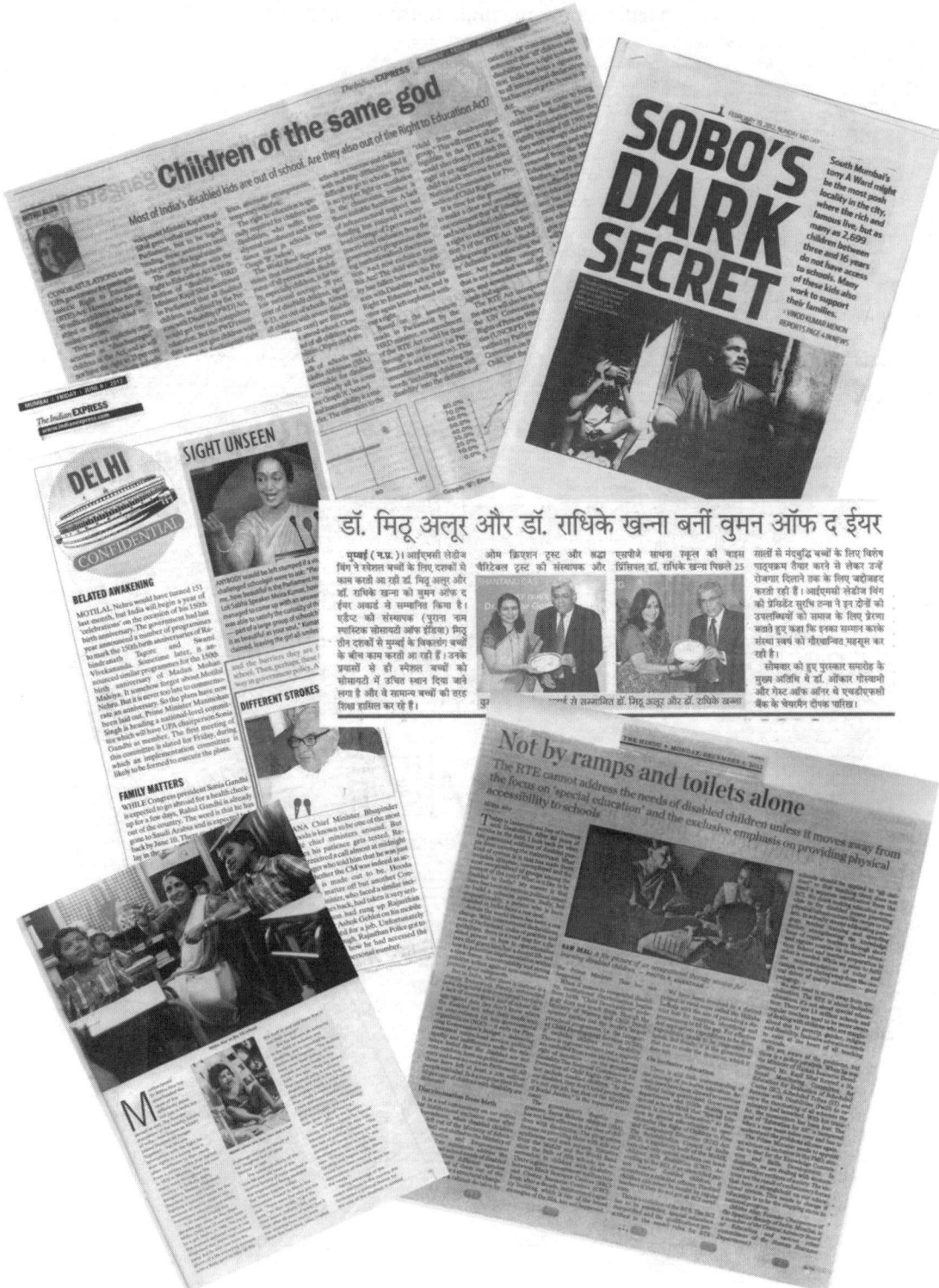

Children of the same god

Most of India's disabled kids are out of school. Are they also out of the Right to Education Act?

SOBO'S DARK SECRET

South Mumbai's tony A Ward might be the most posh locality in the city, where the rich and famous live, but as many as 2,699 children between three and 16 years do not have access to schools. Many of these kids also work to support their families.

– VINOD KUMAR MENON
REPORTS PAGE 4 IN NEWS

डॉ. मिठू अलूर और डॉ. राधिके खन्ना बनीं वुमन ऑफ द ईयर

DELHI CONFIDENTIAL

SIGHT UNSEEN

BELATED AWAKENING

DIFFERENT STROKES

FAMILY MATTERS

Not by ramps and toilets alone

The RTE cannot address the needs of disabled children unless it moves away from the focus on 'special education' and the exclusive emphasis on providing physical accessibility to schools

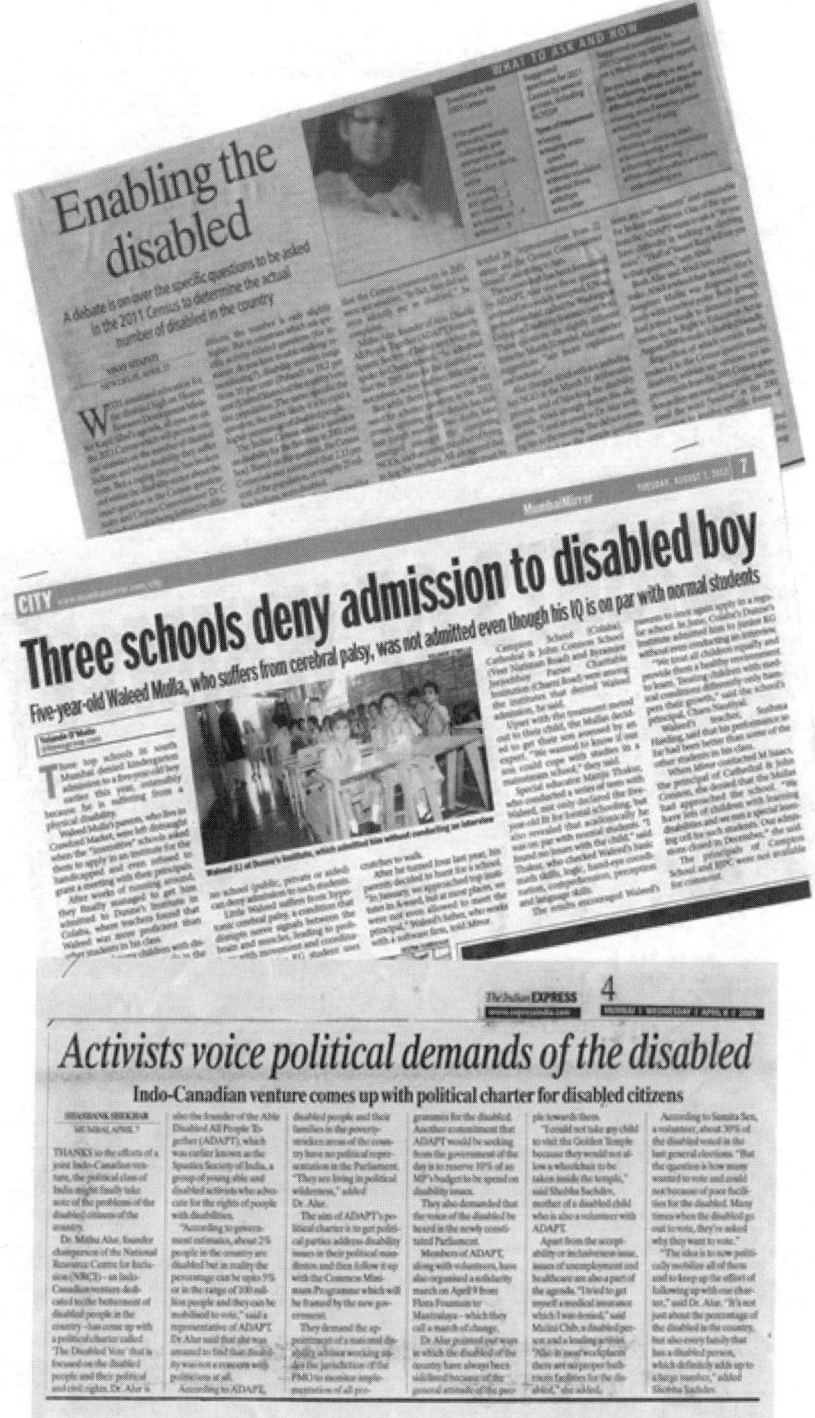

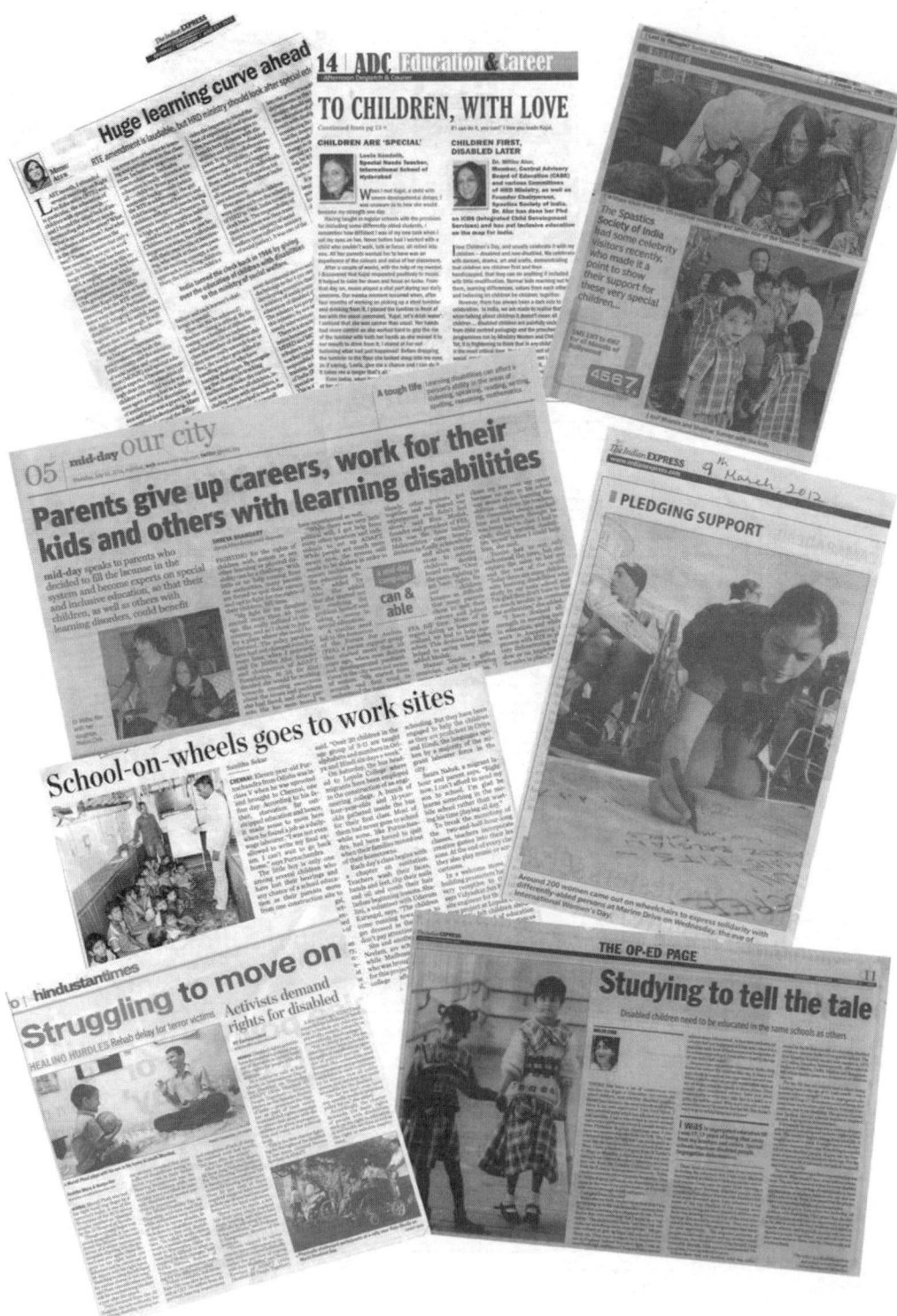

Shonali Bose writes:

'I have grown up immersed in the work of my aunt Dr Mithu Alur with SSI. I have witnessed the struggles, the pain, the hurdles, the triumphs and the enormous growth of this organization and movement.'

'But the first time that I truly engaged with the organization myself was in making my feature film—*Margarita With a Straw*—in which the protagonist has CP.'

'The film could not have been made without the enormous support of the organization.'

'We worked with the physio and speech therapists in understanding the mechanics of the condition so that our able-bodied actor could authentically perform the role. The school organized for her (our actor) to spend time with the youth so that she could experience their lives, their joie de vivre, their emotions and how they physically expressed themselves. They allowed us to use the institution to hold our auditions, do our editing and all the myriad work involved in making a massive feature film.'

'At all times they were open and supportive, never interfering in the creative process but just there to guide and make things happen. My fear was that they would want to intervene and make changes in the script as the story was about something very taboo—the sexuality of the disabled. Their whole-hearted support of the film made this journey very special.'

Remembering Mita

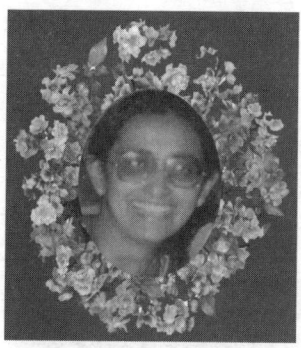

In August 2014, Mita—a stalwart supporter of the cause, a writer, an institution builder, a humanist, who loved the poor, the needy and the disabled—passed away, leaving a void which can never be filled. One of her doctors, Dr Srinath Reddy, wrote an obituary which I quote below:

A Woman of Silk and Steel

If I have to search for a reason to feel proud of belonging to humanity, in an era which Pope Francis aptly describes as one where the world is witnessing the 'globalization of indifference', I only need to recall the life of Sushmita Nundy (Mitadi).

I first met Mitadi as a patient in the All India Institute of Medical Sciences (AIIMS), Delhi, even though I knew of her earlier as the wife of Samiran Nundy, a renowned surgeon at that premier institute and also as the founder and head of SSNI. Apart from working as a cardiologist at AIIMS, I was also the associate editor of the *National Medical Journal of India* of which Samiran was the founder editor. I came to know him well professionally but had not yet met his wife in person.

It was in late 1988 that I first met Mrs Nundy. I had just returned from 16 months of stay in Canada after completing an MSc in epidemiology at McMaster University, having gone there on study leave from AIIMS. I learned then that Mrs Nundy had been admitted to the cardiology service of AIIMS a year earlier with chest pain. After investigations, she was diagnosed to have Syndrome X (angina with normal coronary arteries), a diagnosis with which doctors in London agreed. Her heart function was reportedly normal.

So it was a shock when she was brought to the hospital emergency, in late 1988, with severe congestive heart failure. This condition results from extensive damage to the heart muscle, often due to a severe heart attack and less commonly from other heart muscle diseases classed together as cardiomyopathies. On investigation, Mrs Nundy's heart problem was now diagnosed as cardiac amyloidosis, a type of cardiomyopathy. This condition is caused when the body produces an abnormal protein (amyloid) which gets deposited in the heart muscle. The heart becomes stiff, with restricted filling of blood and loss of efficiency in pumping it. As a result, there is fluid 'congestion' in the lungs, liver, legs and other parts of the body.

Clearly, the disease had begun insidiously a year earlier and had progressed to the advanced stage of cardiac failure. The diagnosis was confirmed by cardiac biopsy. Samiran's extensive professional contacts in the US and UK were used to confirm the pathological diagnosis.

This was gloomy news for Samiran and all doctors associated with Mrs Nundy's care. Chemotherapy, the only treatment for reducing amyloid production, is not effective in reversing the course of the disease. Supportive care, for treating congestive heart failure, was needed to reduce symptoms of discomfort but would not alter the dismal course of the disease. At least, that was the conventional wisdom of the time.

Samiran reviewed all available research evidence and consulted doctors at the Mayo Clinic who had the largest accumulated case series of cardiac amyloidosis. The average survival after the onset of congestive heart failure, even on the best available treatment, was six months and the longest recorded survival was thirteen months. It was at this time that I became the treating doctor for Mrs Nundy.

She was a revelation. Samiran had already disclosed to his wife all the facts about her medical condition. He was known to be always forthright in everything he did. In this case, his respect for his wife did not allow him to hide the truth even if it was so unpleasant. He also wanted to discuss the plans for their young children with her and to learn about the mother's aspirations for their future.

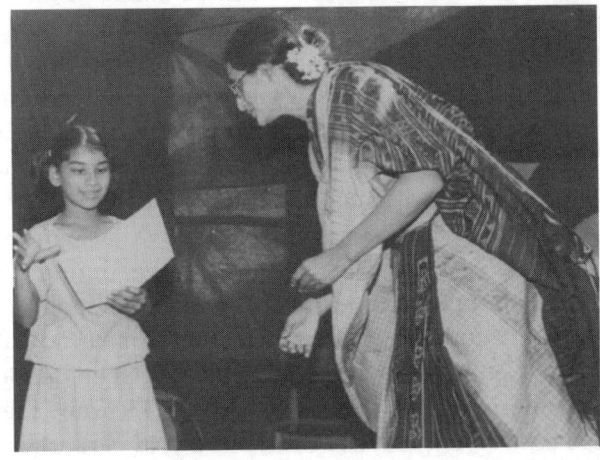

She told me about this conversation. I expected her to be depressed and despondent. To my great surprise, she radiated calm confidence. 'I am not going to die so soon,' she said, 'I will live to see my children grow up. I also have to continue my work with the spastic children who need care for their disability. I still have many things to do and I will surely live to do them.' It was not bravado or denial which sometimes patients display when confronted with an unpalatable truth. It was born from innate conviction that she could battle the disease with her will power and not let it defeat her purpose in life.

My respect for her increased each time I met her. She wanted me to give her the unalloyed truth about her clinical status and test results but in return infused confidence in me that she would beat the odds. It was always an engaging conversation about many things in life, with the unwavering thread being her unbounded optimism. I came to know of her love for classical Western music as well as her faith in Satya Sai Baba. By this time she had become 'Mitadi' to me.

In between periods of hospitalization, she continued to work, going to SSI, sometimes in a wheel chair. She tended to her own children with loving care. She lifted Samiran's spirits with her cheerful confidence. My wife, who had started working with SSI as a developmental paediatrician, gave me accounts of Mitadi's devoted and inspirational leadership which continued to guide the institution despite a disease that would have seriously disabled another person with a weaker will. Mitadi always greeted me with a warm smile and I invariably left her room a happier person than I was when I entered it.

Towards the end of the chemotherapy, she asked me if she could take Tibetan medicine as per the advice of His Holiness Dalai Lama's physicians who visited her. I told her that she could, provided she did not discontinue the allopathic treatment. She then started on the dual treatment. Frankly, I do not know what worked but Mitadi did beat all the odds—and by a mile! She lived for 26 years after the diagnosis of cardiac amyloidosis. I say lived, not merely survived, because it was a full life.

After some years of a professional and personal association that I have cherished, Mitadi's care shifted to the Gangaram Hospital, which Samiran joined after an early retirement from AIIMS. I, too, left AIIMS in 2006 to lead a public health organization but saw Mitadi on different occasions at different venues, lunching with her family or at a condolence meeting for a mutual friend or on a visit to her home. She was still vibrant, with a luminous smile that always lit up

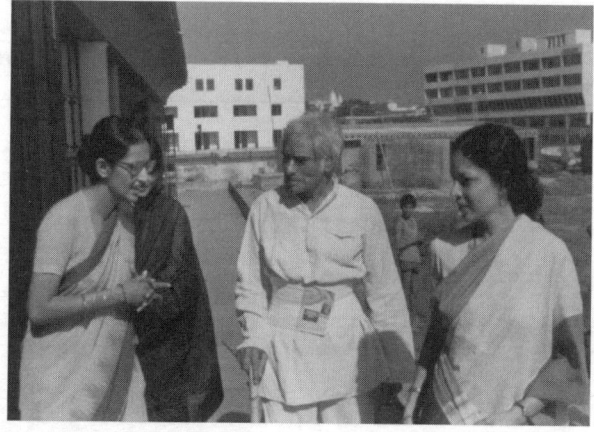

my heart. She gave up her leadership of SSI after suffering a stroke some years ago but continued to inspire her successors with her vision. Even her recovery from the stroke was remarkable and the way she overcame the challenges of the residual disability made me marvel at her will power.

Indeed, it is that indomitable will power that I credit for the medical miracle that was Mitadi's life in the last 26 years. She has not been recorded in the scientific literature as a case of astounding survival. Despite being the dispassionate scientist that he is, Samiran would not have attempted it. I would not only respect confidentiality during her life time but also would not know how to describe the vital ingredient of her therapy—her own unbending spirit that refused to accept the limits that medical science arrogantly sought to set on her life.

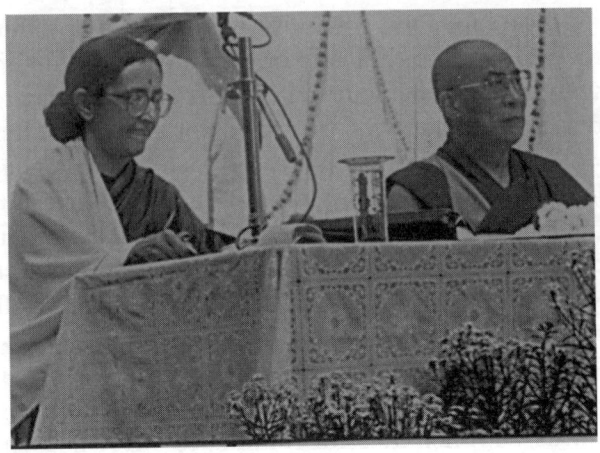

I write this now, a month after her passing, not only to pay a personal tribute to Mitadi's memory but also to thank her for giving me the most valuable lesson as a doctor. Not to take anything for granted. I am still a great believer in science but now I also recognize and respect the tremendous power of the human spirit that extends the power of healing beyond known medical treatments. I have also seen, in Mitadi's face, that the glow of goodness can dispel the gloom of illness. Her life provided proof that love for others can be a more powerful elixir than potent drugs. She will remain forever the inspirational memory of an exceptional human being—truly a woman of silk and steel.

—*K. Srinath Reddy,*
President, Public Health Foundation of India

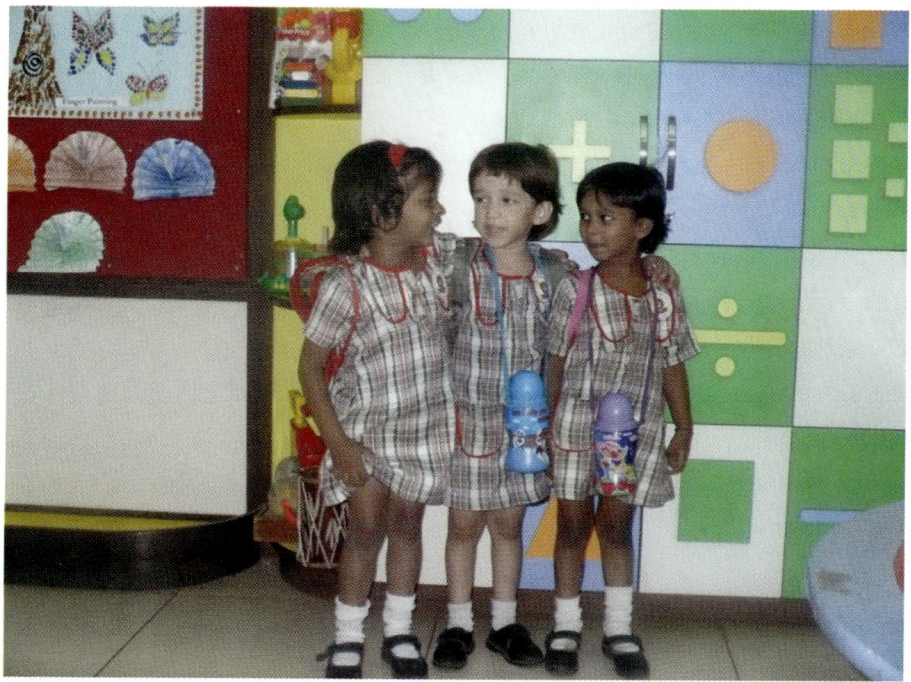

1. School is fun

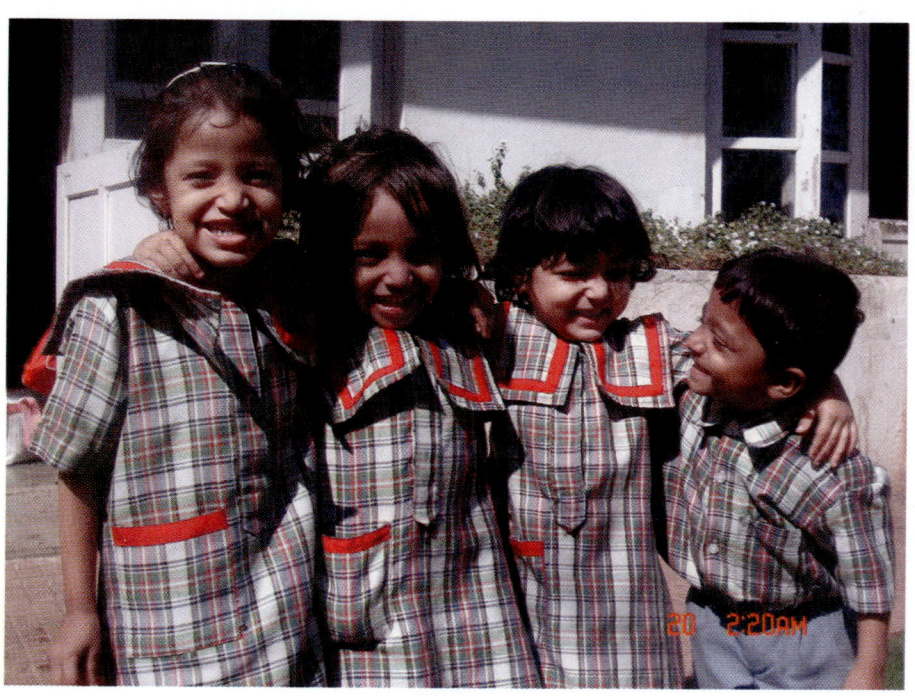

2. We love school

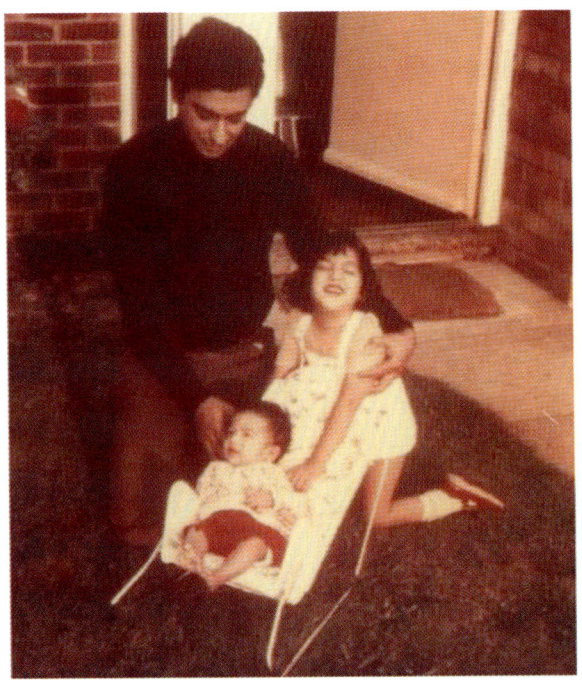

3. Mr Ranjit Chib, father of Nikhil and Malini, at their residence in Richmond, London

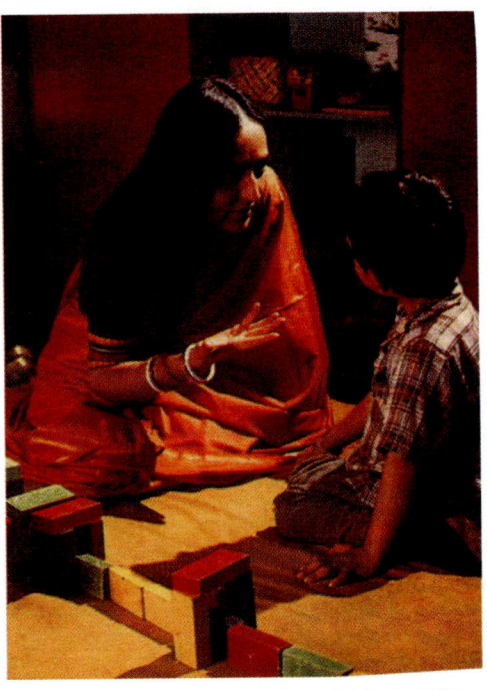

4. A Typical Assessment of a child by Dr Mithu Alur, six years later in Mumbai

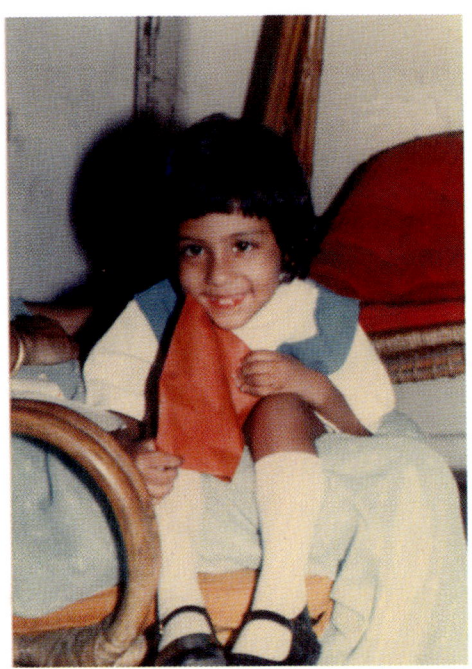

5. Annanya Chatterjee, one of the earlier students, went onto become a lawyer in the UK and was honoured by Her Majesty the Queen

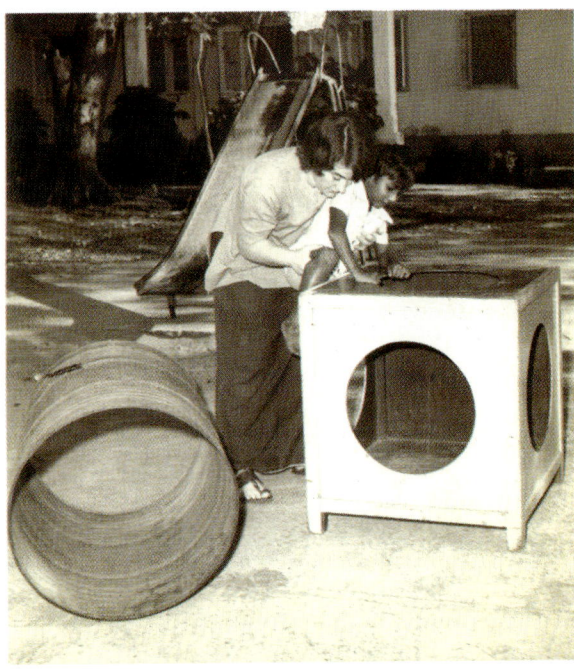

6. Dr Pam Stretch, who set up the Physio Therapy Unit, with a child in the playground

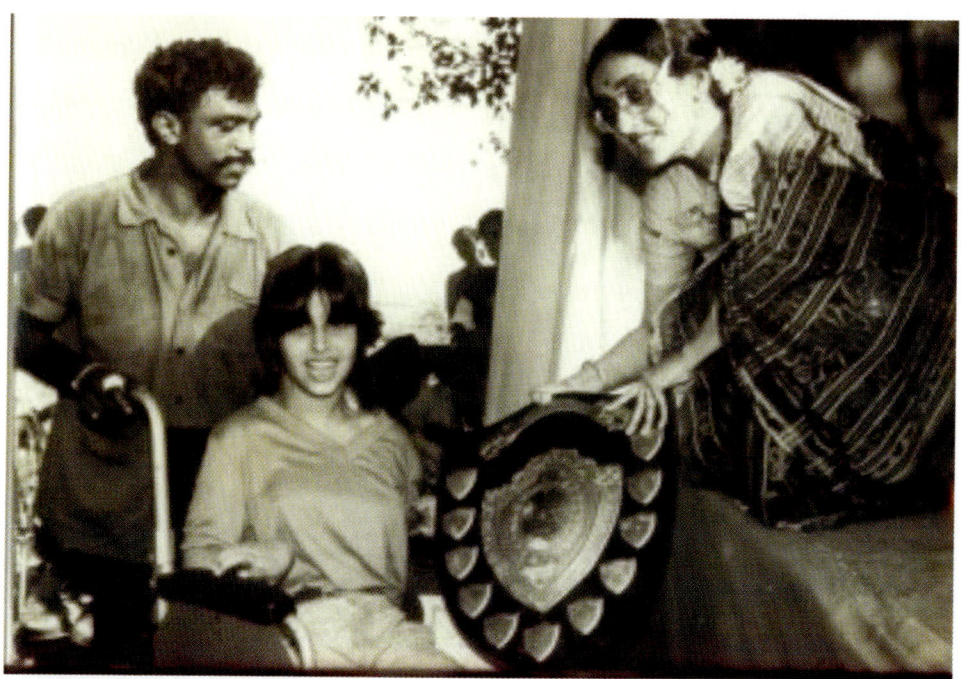

7. Mrs Mita Nundy, Co-Founder of the Delhi Spastics Society, presents Vipasha Mehta with the Shield for Academics. Later she became the first student with cerebral palsy from The Spastics Society of India to have done a PhD; her dissertation was on Foucault and Derrida

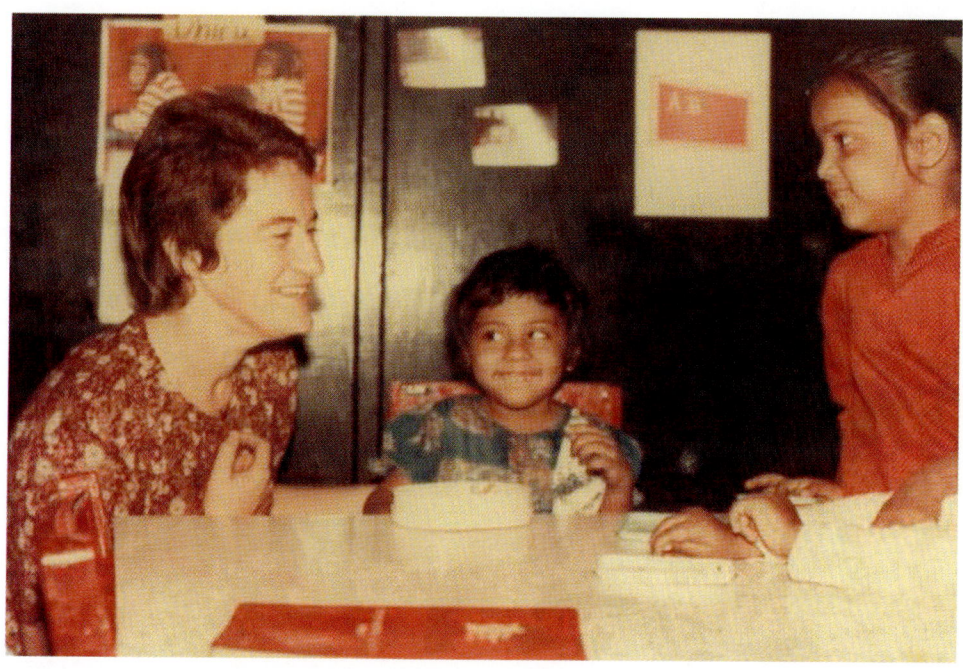

8. Dr Pam Stretch supervising a feeding session in the classroom

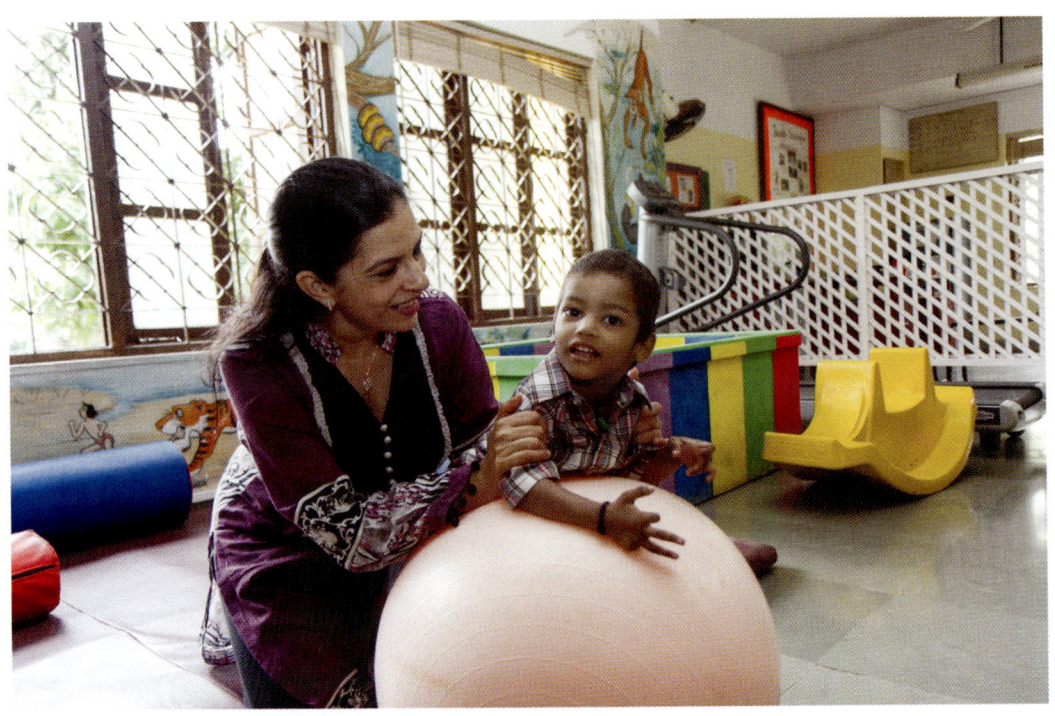

9. Therapy and Treatment can be fun: Dr Shabnam Rangwala enjoys her interaction

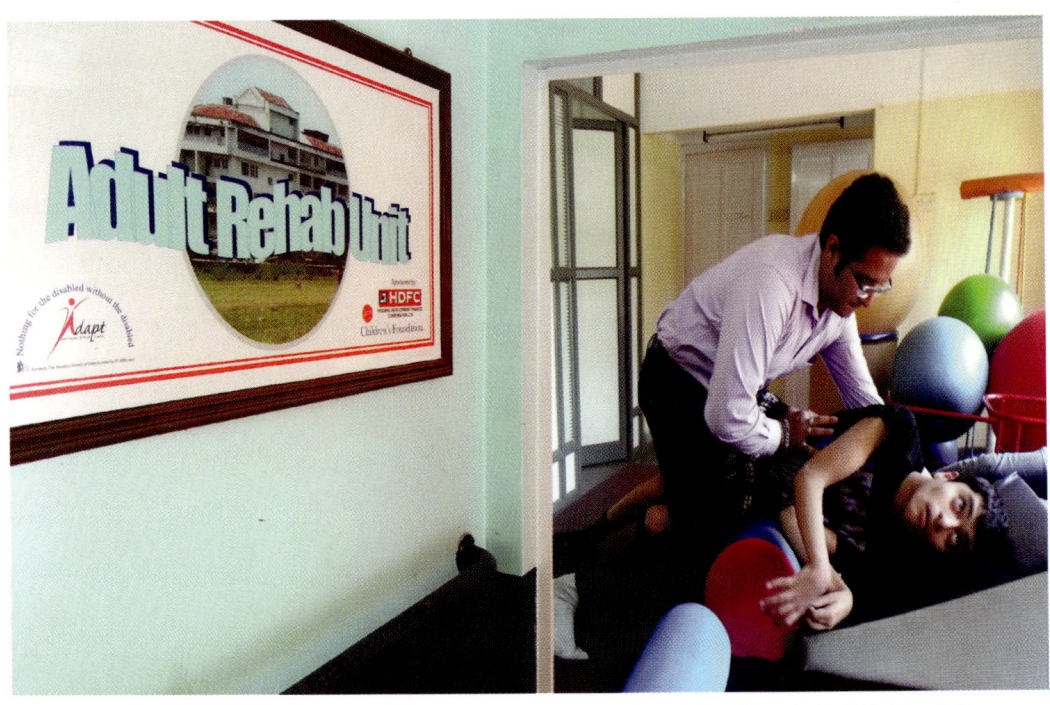

10. Dr Ashutosh Sonawane provides therapy to adults through The Adult Rehabilitation Unit

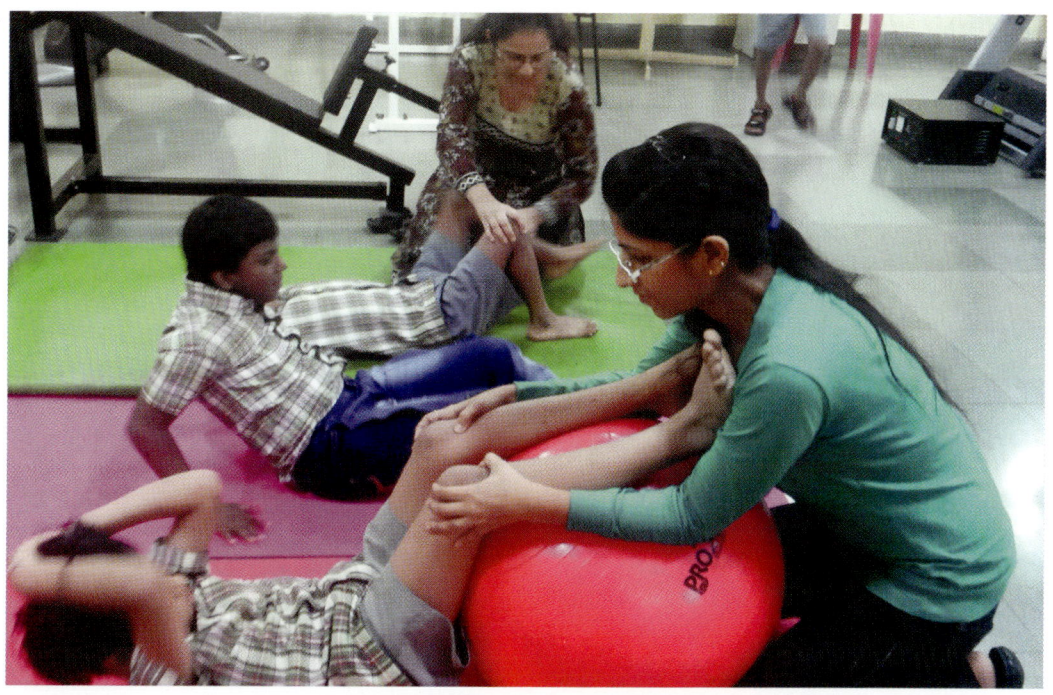

11. *Mothers in Partnership, learning treatment to manage at home*

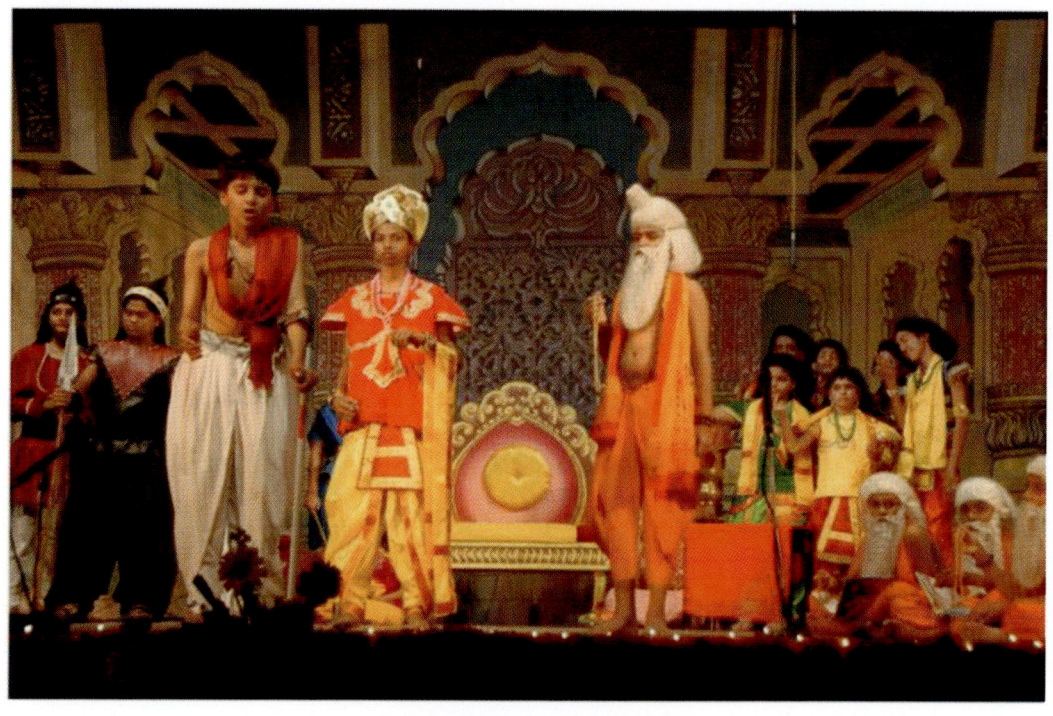

12. *'Ashtavakra' drama in action*

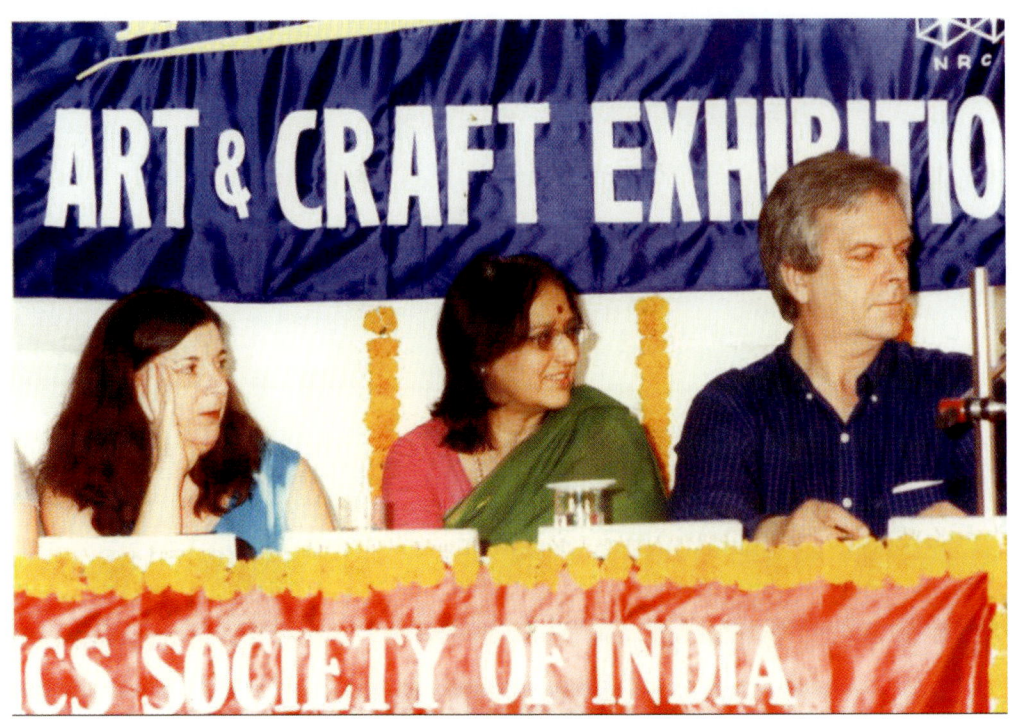

13. Dr Mithu Alur with our Canadian partners Mr Cam Crawford and Dr Vianne Timmons at the Organization's Annual Art & Craft Exhibition

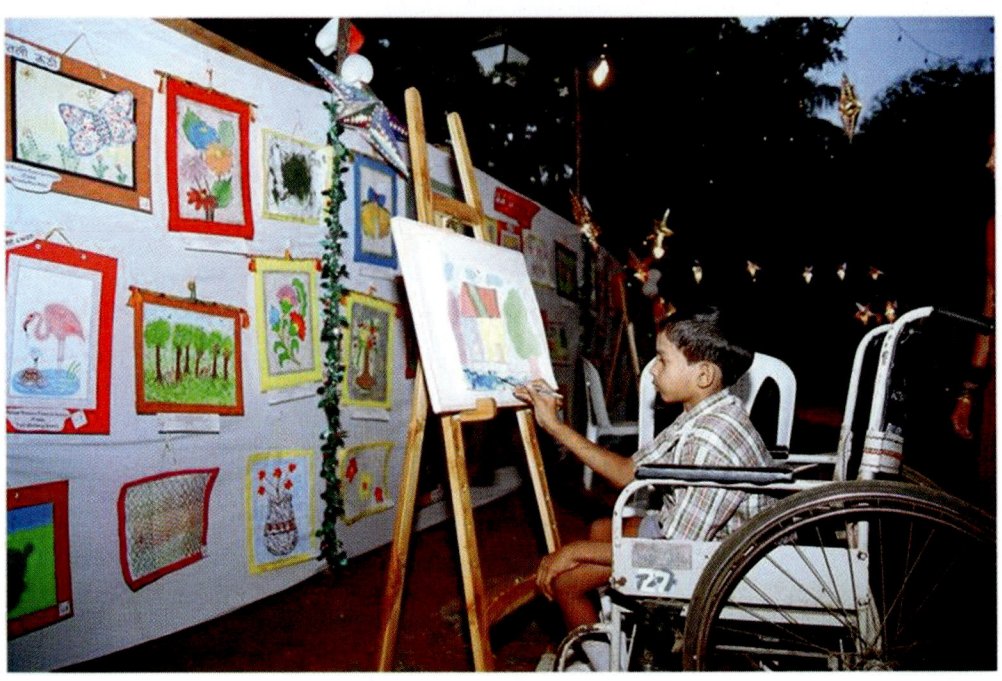

14. A young artist at work

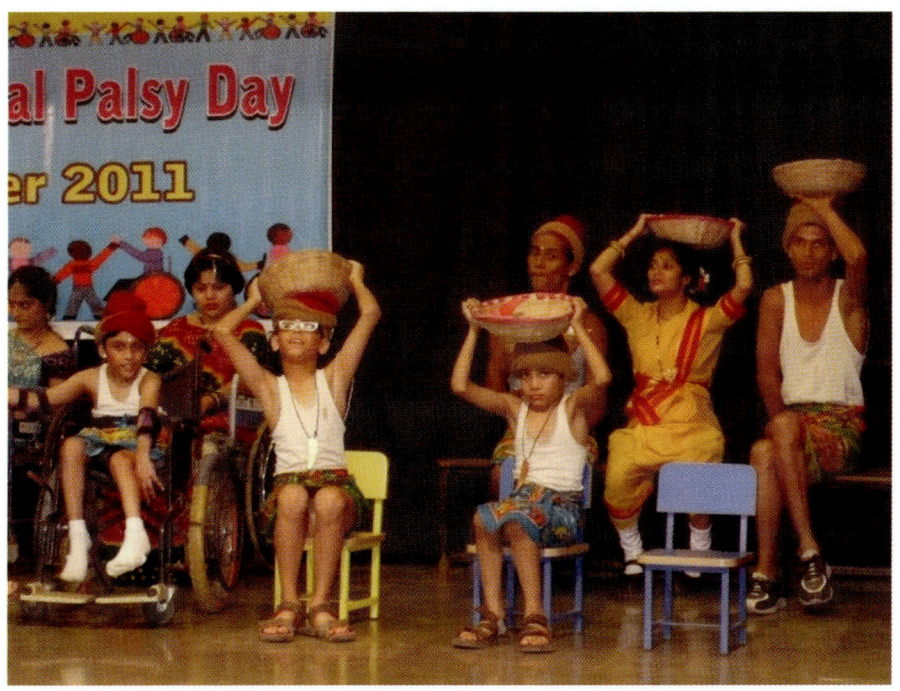
15. Children performing on the World Cerebral Palsy Day

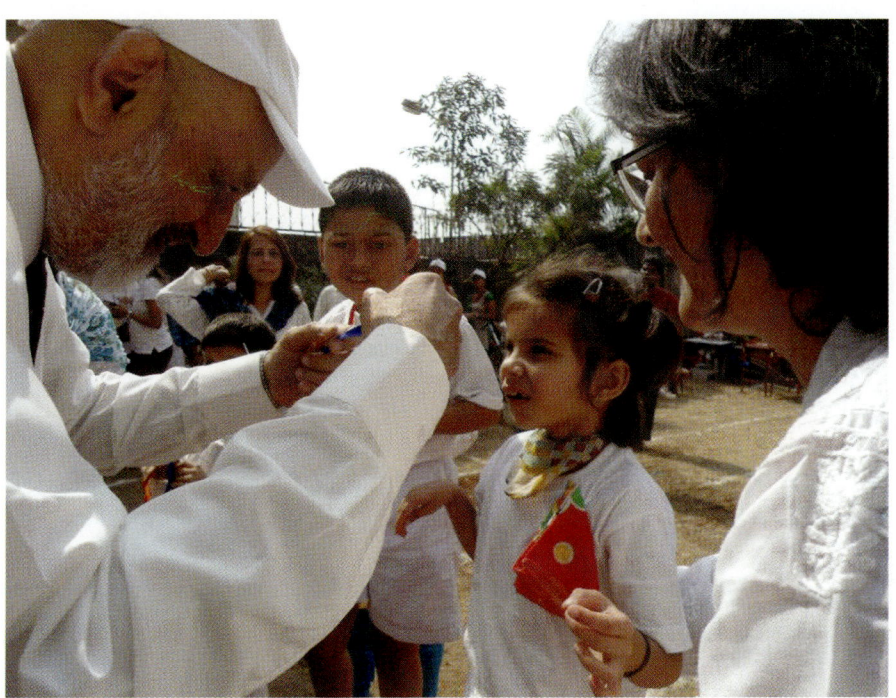
16. Swami Mounananda awards medals to the children at our Annual Sports Day

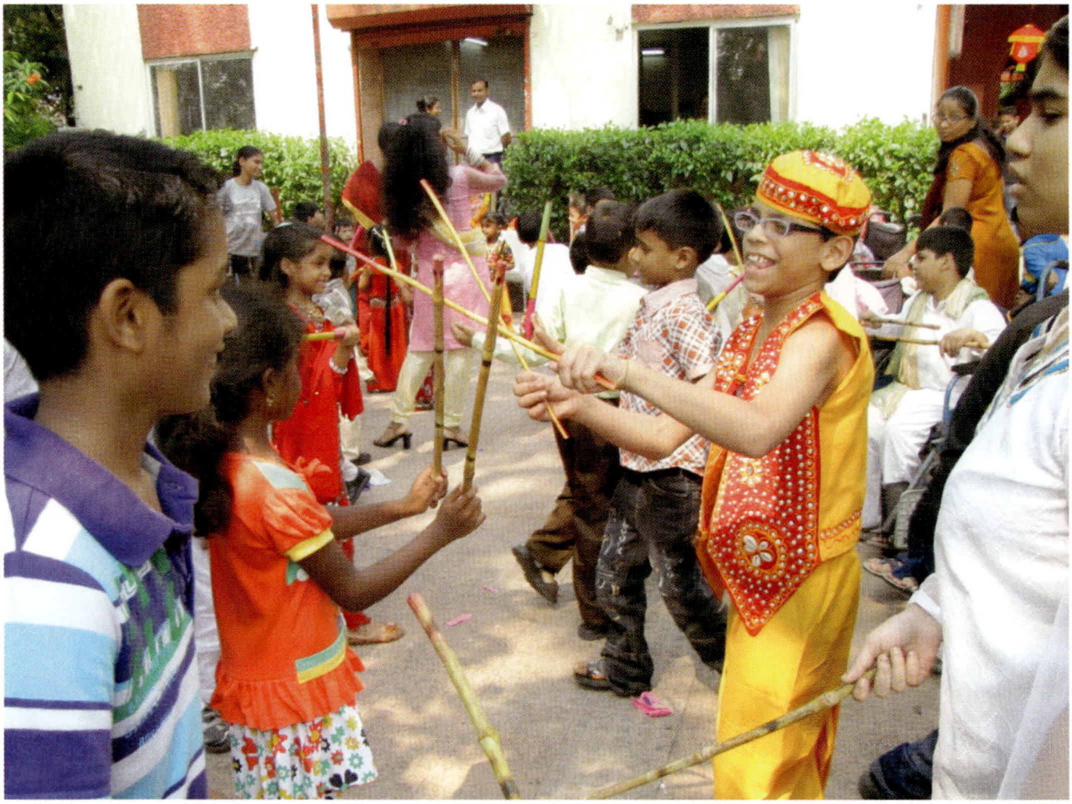

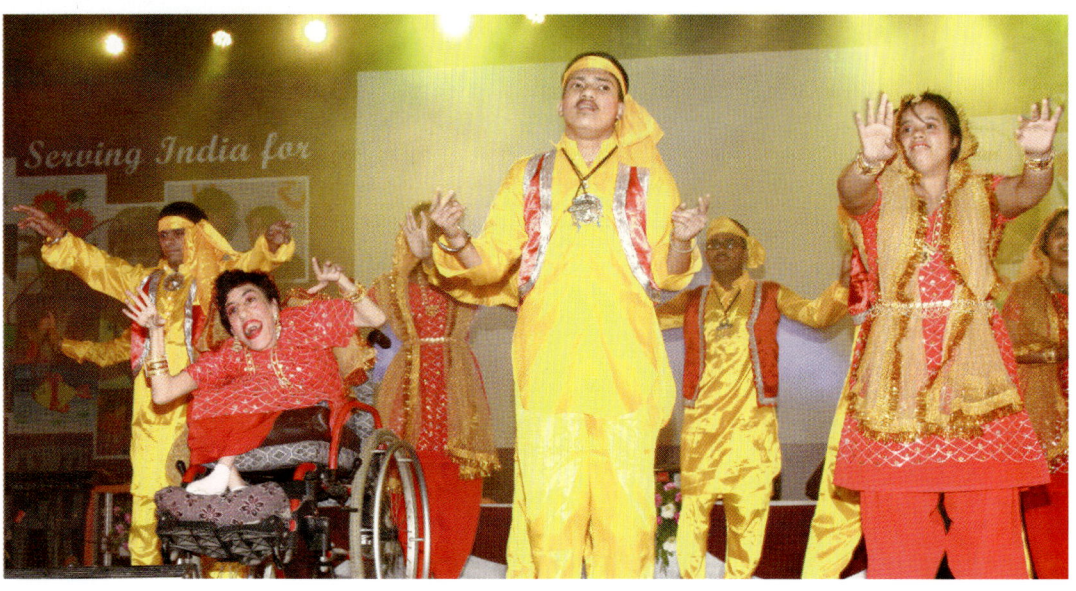

17. We celebrate all the festivals: children dancing during Navratri

18. Children performing at our Annual Concert

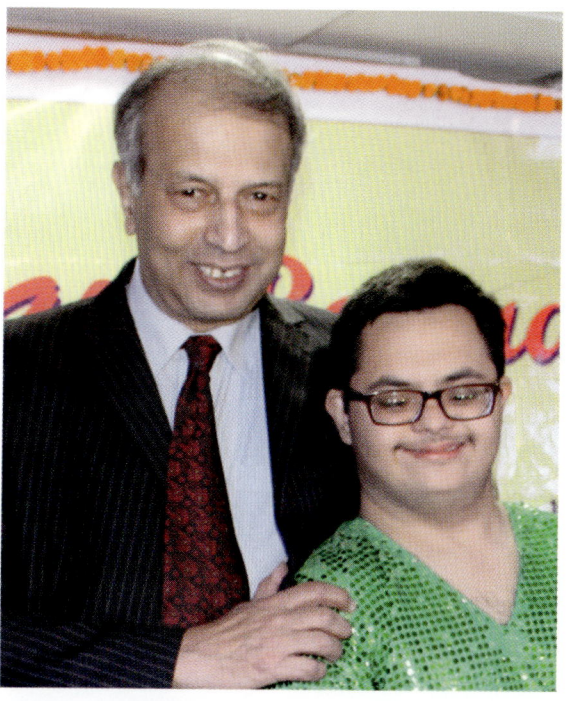

19. Dr Samiran Nundy, Chairperson, Institutional Review Board, congratulates Harsh on his dance performance

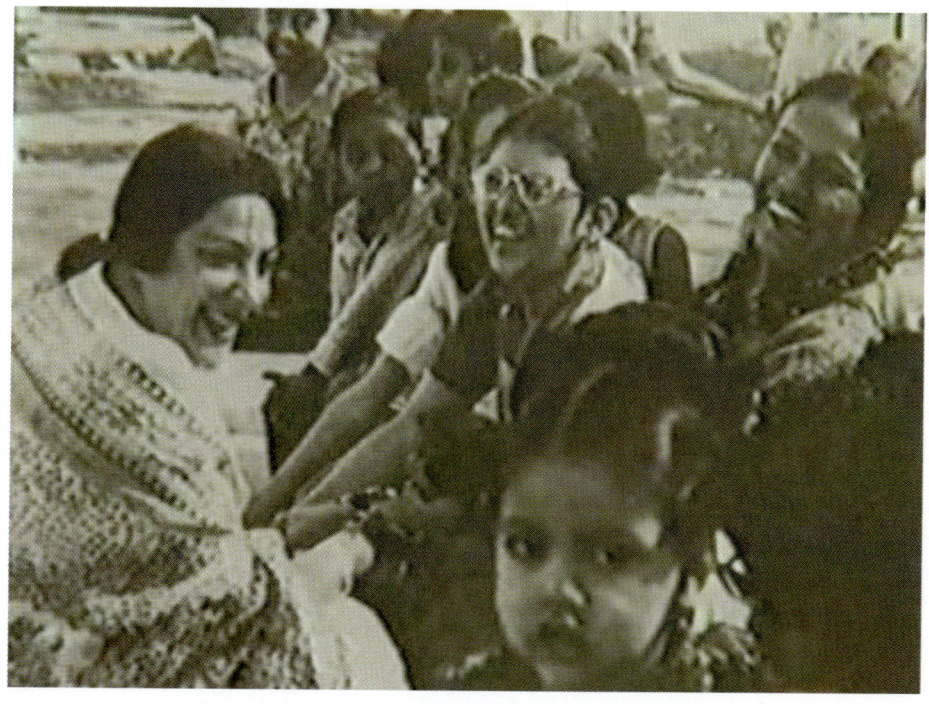

20. Our first Patron Mrs Nargis Dutt with the students

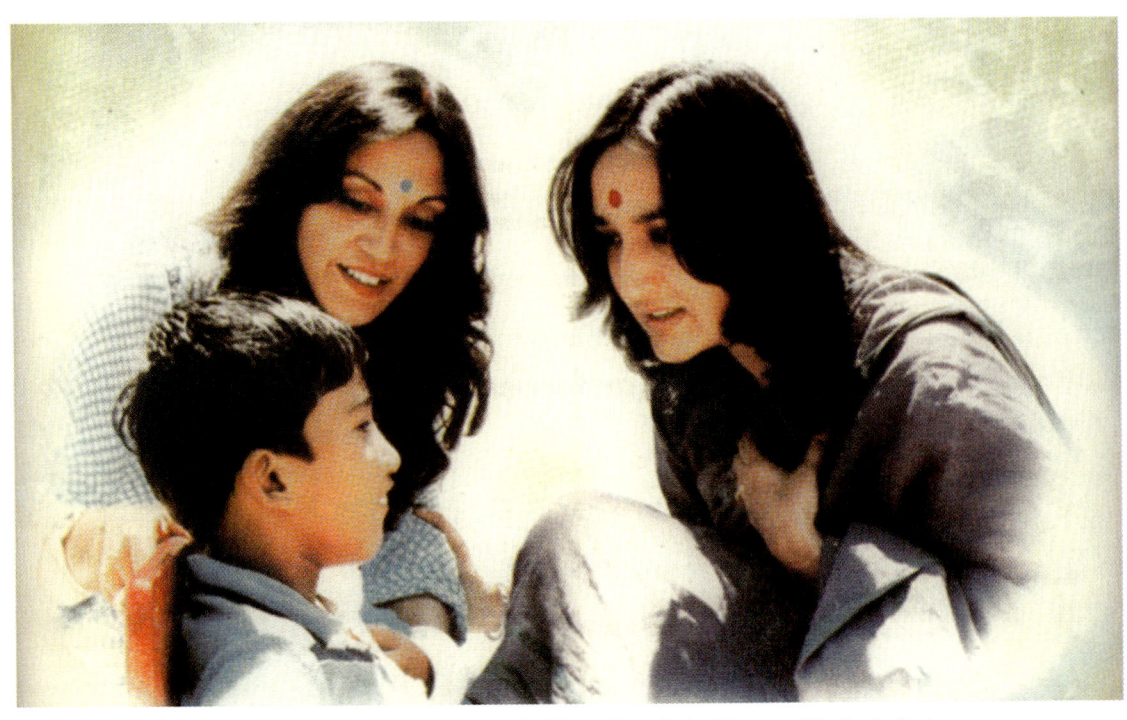

21. *The late Mrs Junie Bose and Dr Mithu Alur chat with one of their students*

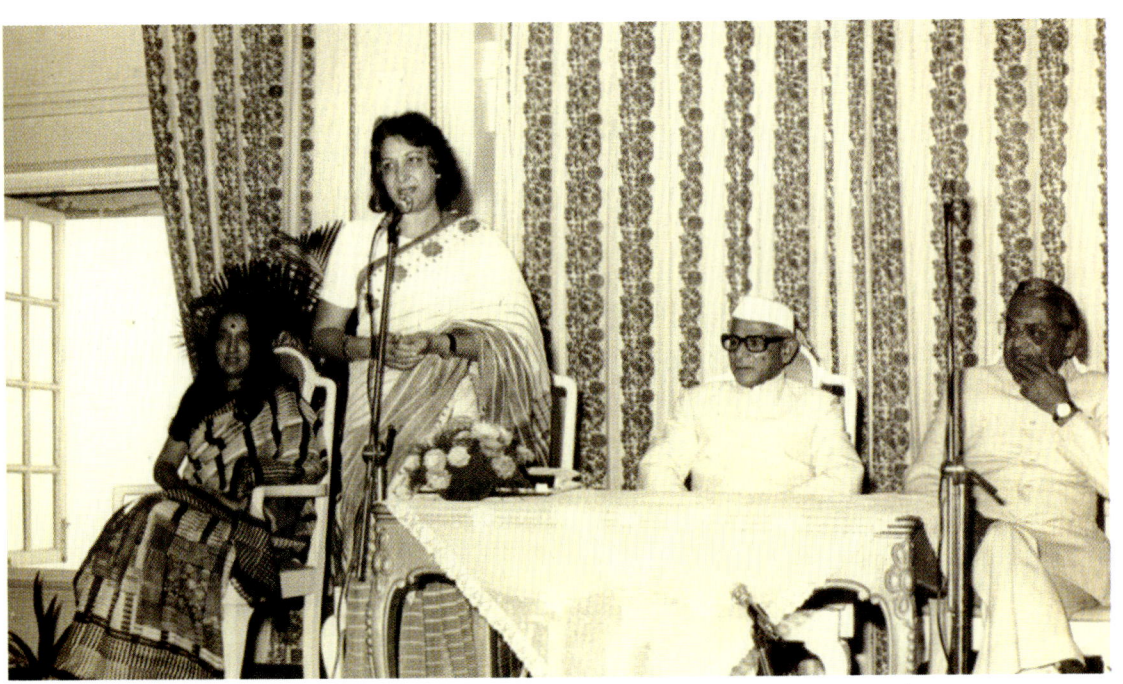

22. *Mrs Nargis Dutt and Dr Mithu Alur with Shri Sadiq Ali, His Excellency the Governor of Maharashtra and Mr Harish Mahindra, President, SSI at a public function*

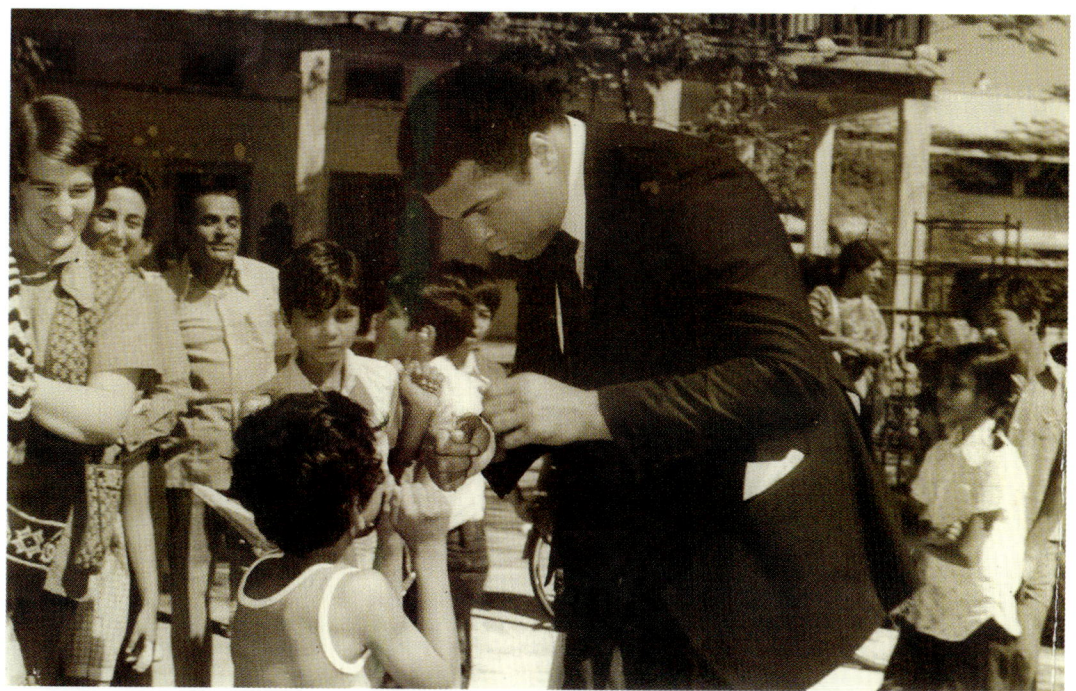

23. *Dr Pam Stretch, Ms Edwina Baher, Mr K.C. Chakraverty, all pioneers look on as Heavyweight Champion Muhammed Ali interacts with the children*

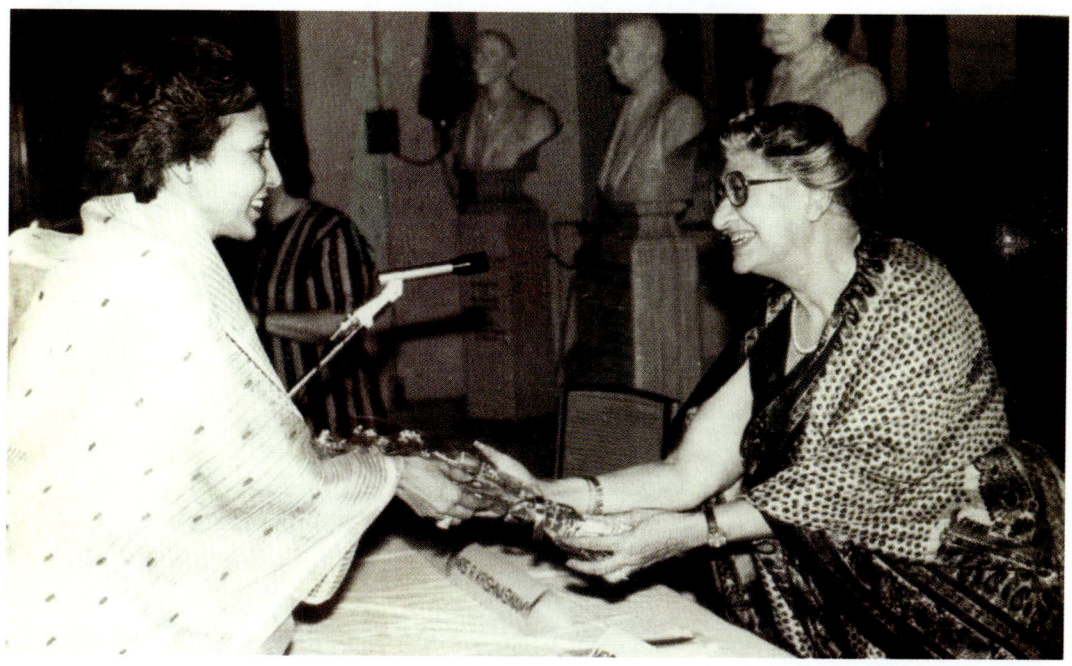

24. *Mrs Uma Bannerjee, Education Consultant, being felicitated by Mrs Kaumudi Kumari who began services in Jaipur with Mrs Deepak Kalra, at the graduation ceremony of the Teacher Training Course*

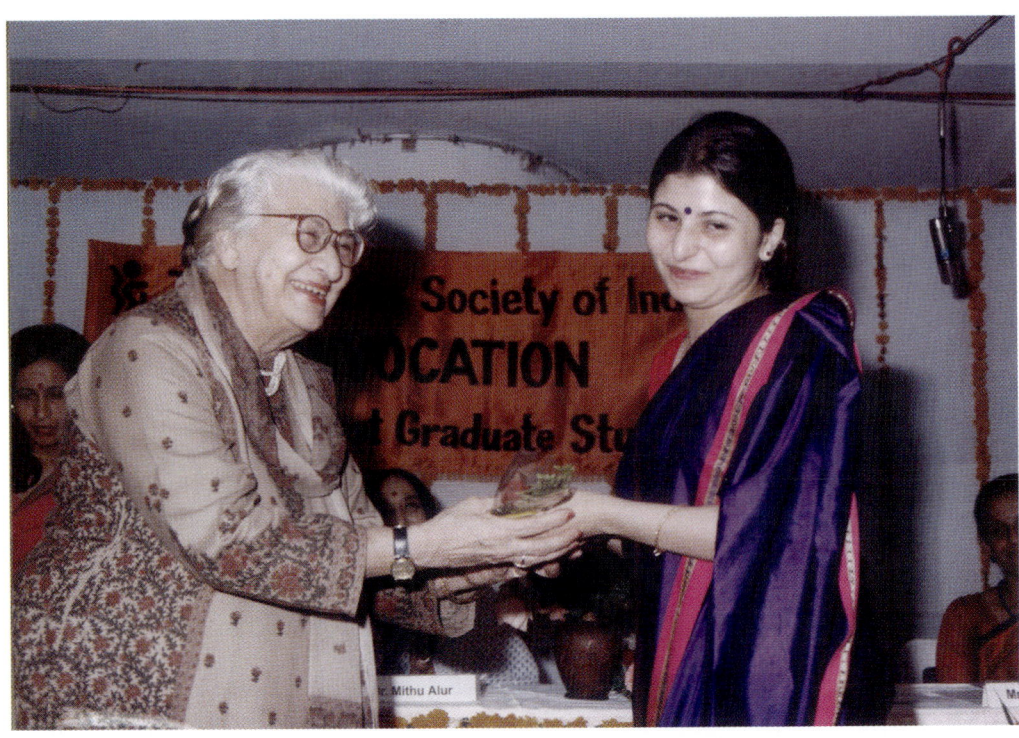

25. *Education Consultant, Mrs Uma Bannerjee, congratulates Mrs Chandreka Maheshwari, a graduate of the Teacher Training Course*

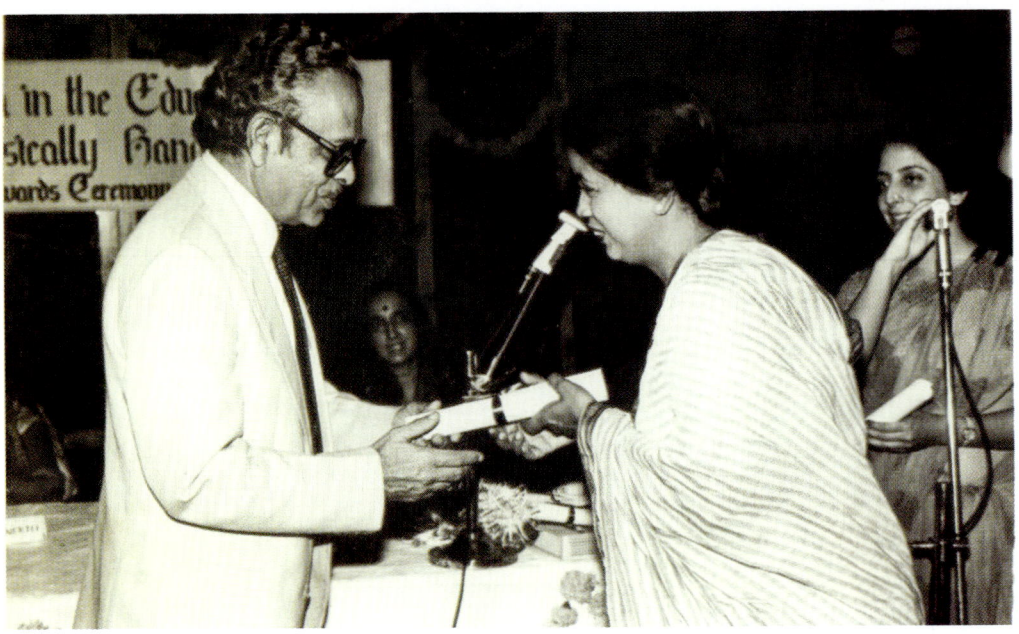

26. *Shri Nana Chudasama awards Mrs Ama Bose, who helped with services in Kolkata, her diploma. Mrs Deepak Kalra, the first Director of Teacher Training looks on*

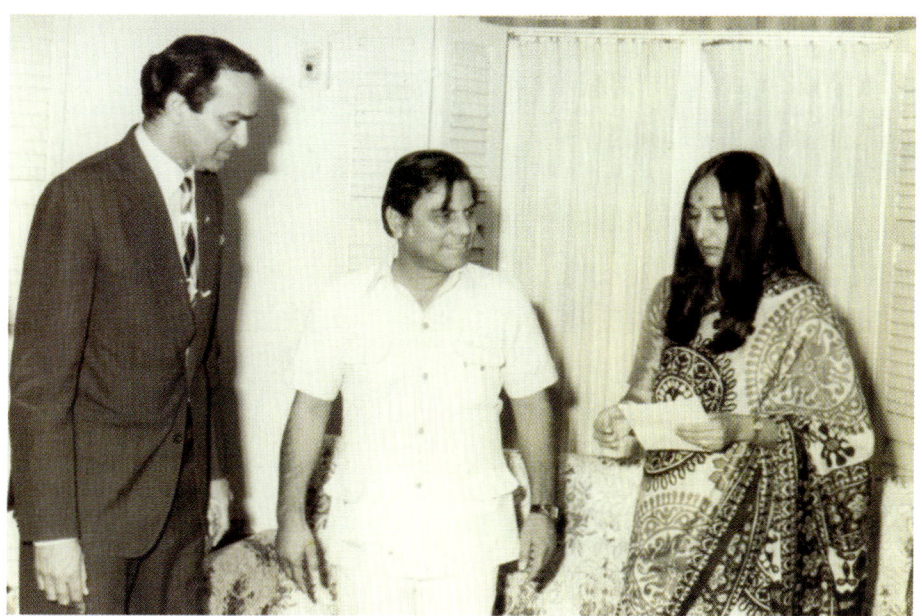

27. Member of Governing Body, Mr H. Kizilbash and Dr Mithu Alur with Shri A.R. Antulay

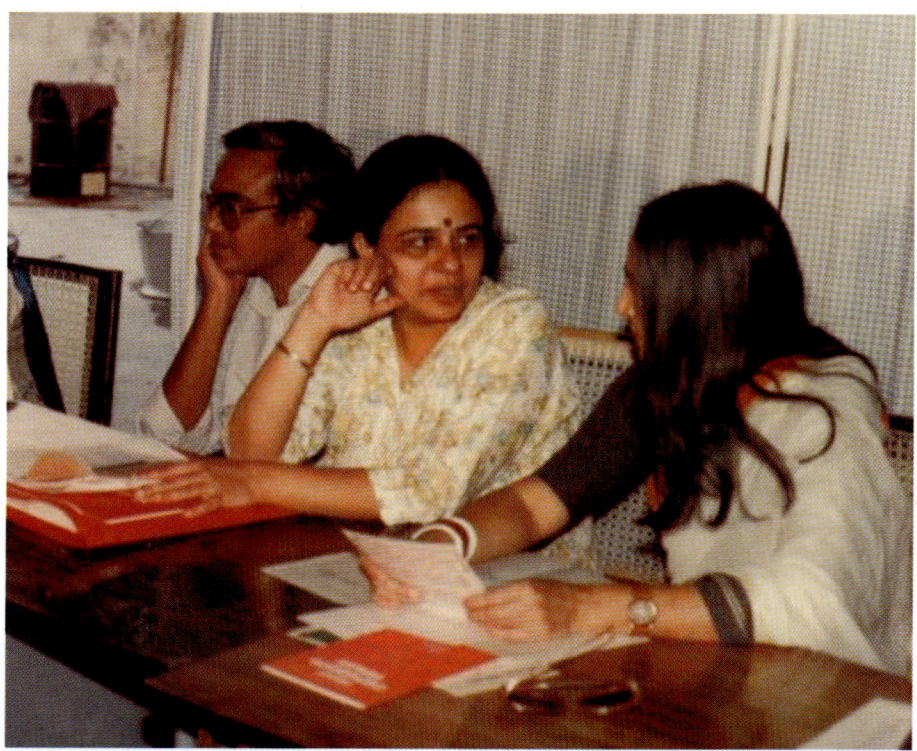

28. Mr G. Natarajan, Trustee, Honorary Secretary and Treasurer of the Spastics Society, Mumbai, Mrs Poonam Natarajan, Founder Chairperson and Director of the Chennai branch of SSI, discuss future plans with Dr Mithu Alur

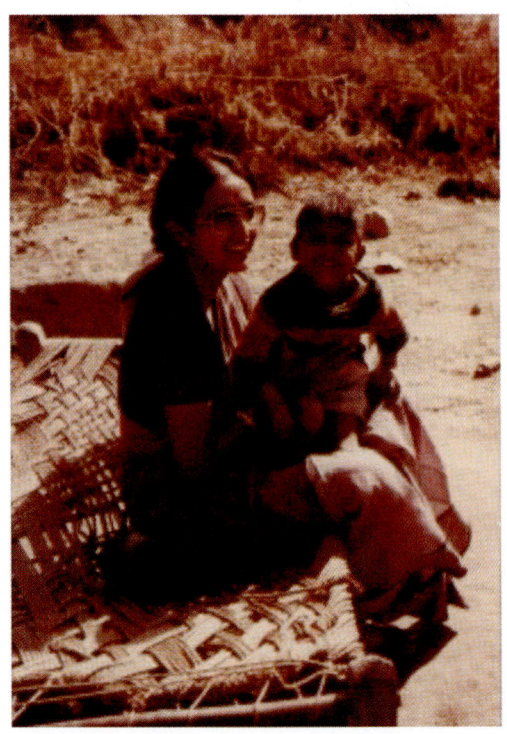

29. Mrs Mita Nundy with a beneficiary under the rural project in Dayalpur, Delhi

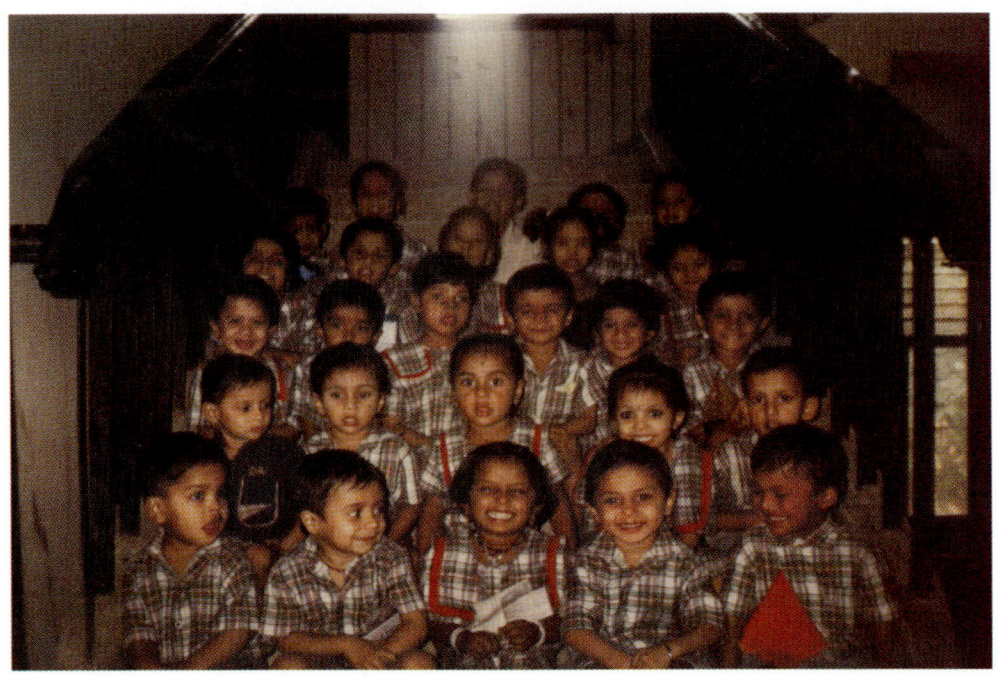

30. Inclusive Education: children with and without disabilities enjoying together: An inclusive nursery

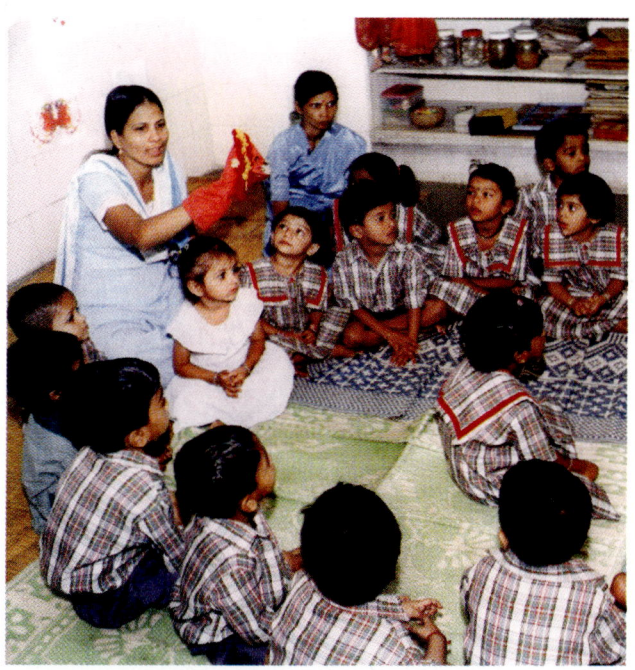

31. Learning is fun: Mrs Gulab Sayyed teaches students in an inclusive nursery in Dharavi

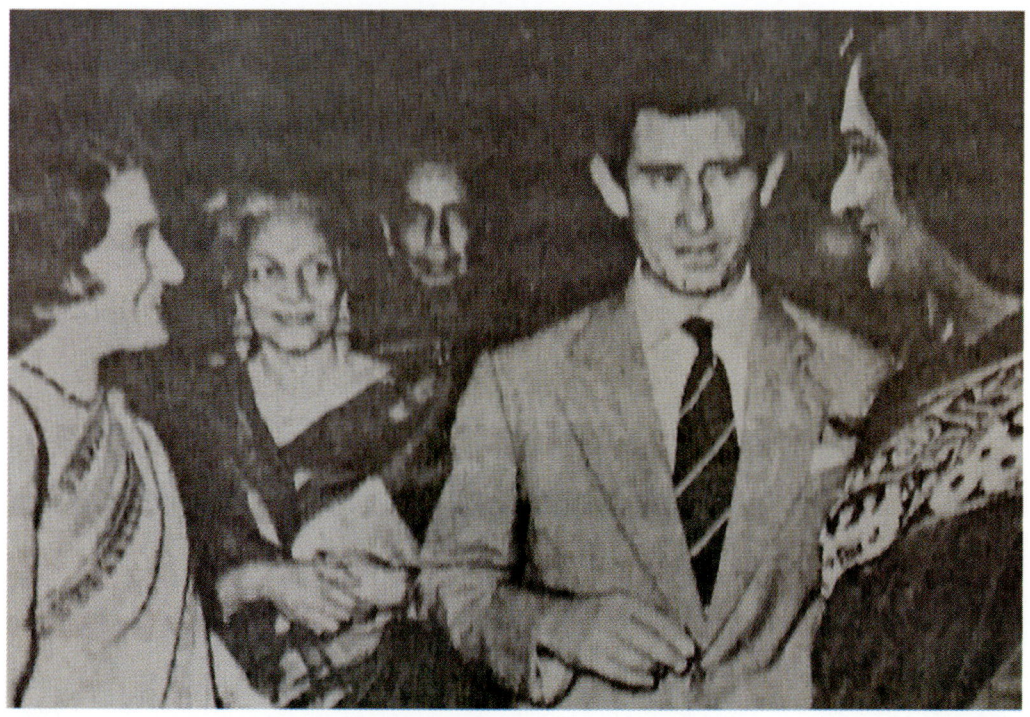

32. His Royal Highness, Prince Charles meets Dr Mithu Alur and Dr Pam Stretch at the Raj Bhavan, Mumbai, when he gifted three Landrovers to the Organization

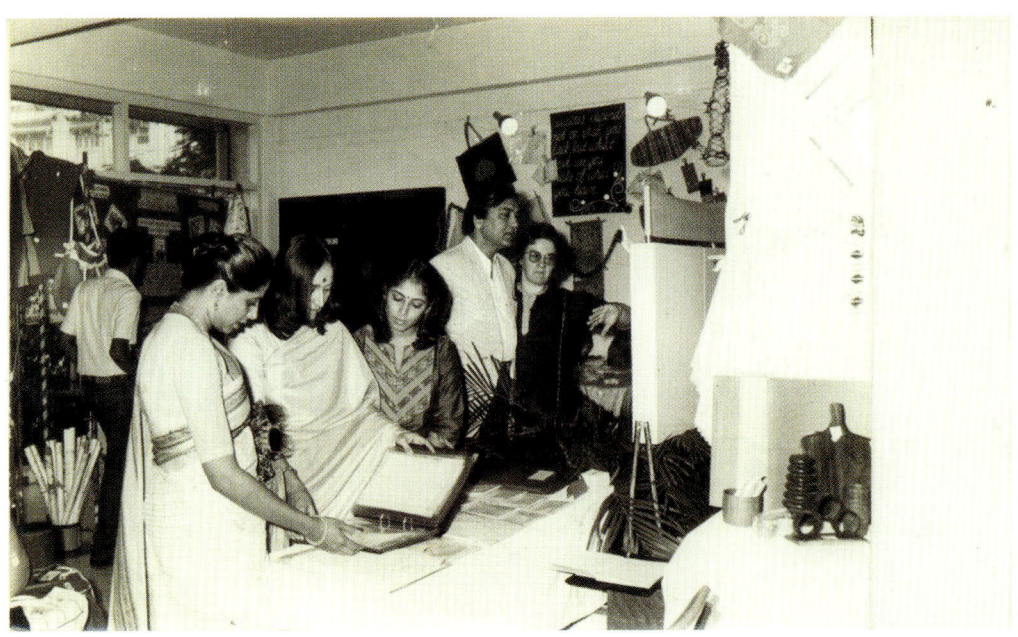

33. Chief Guest the late Mrs Smita Patil inaugurating the I Can Bazaar with Dr Mithu Alur with Mrs Charmaine Lobo, Shri Sunil Dutt and Dr Pam Stretch admiring the articles made by the students

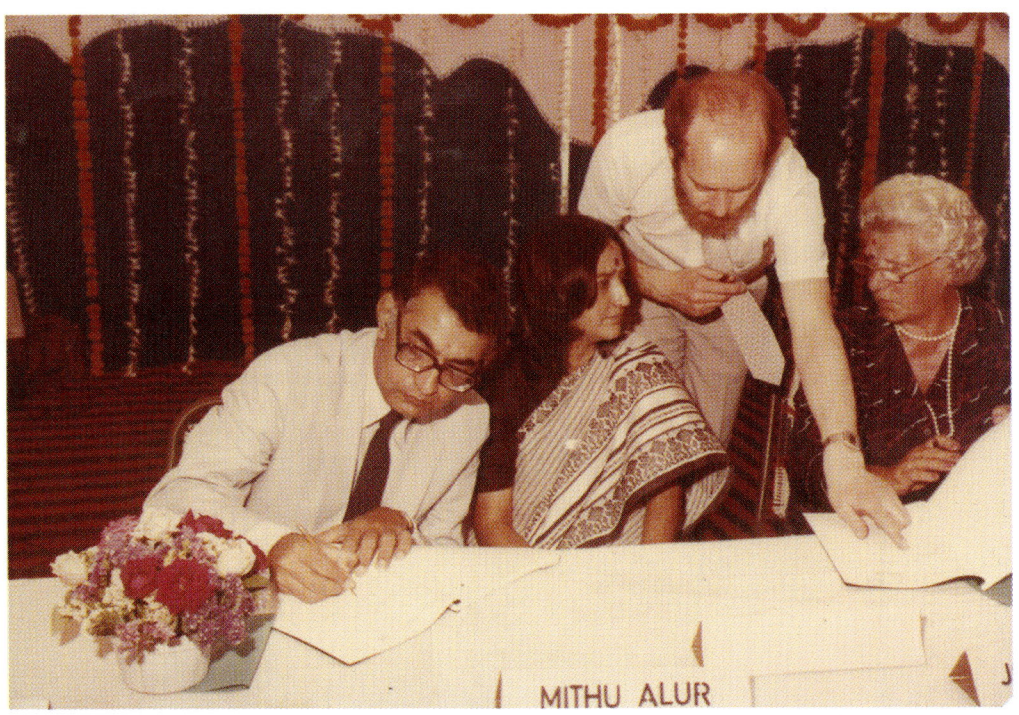

34. Mr Yezdi Malegam, Dr Mithu Alur, Mrs Joyce Smith with Mr Barry Hassell sign the MOU for the Job Development Centre

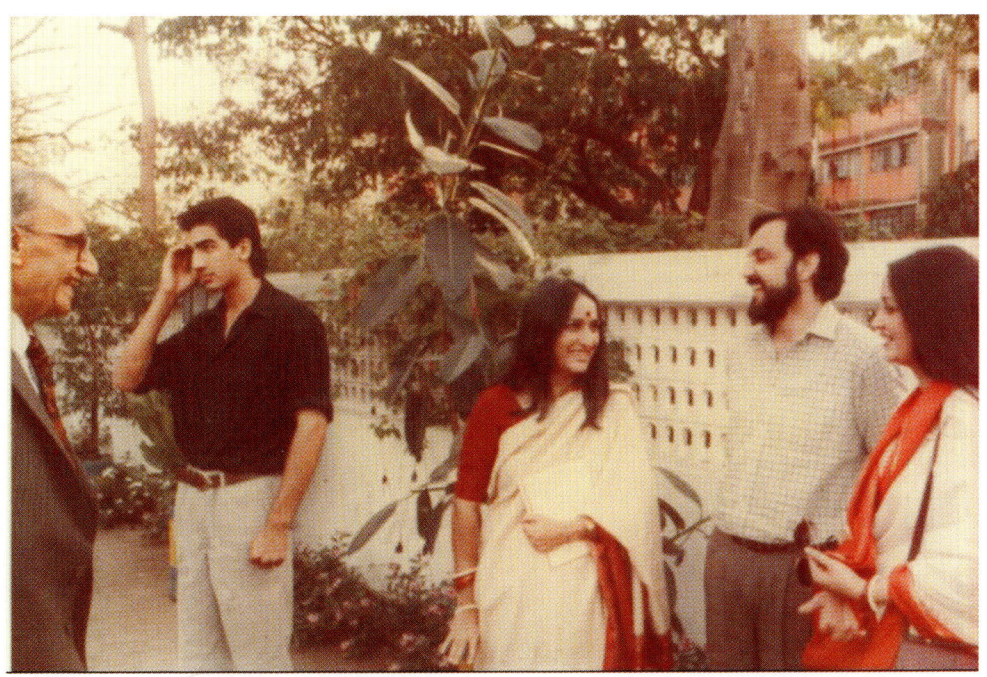

35. Mr Sauransu Bose, Mr Nikhil Chib, Dr Mithu Alur, Dr Prannoy Roy and Mrs Radhika Roy at the inauguration of the National Job Development Centre

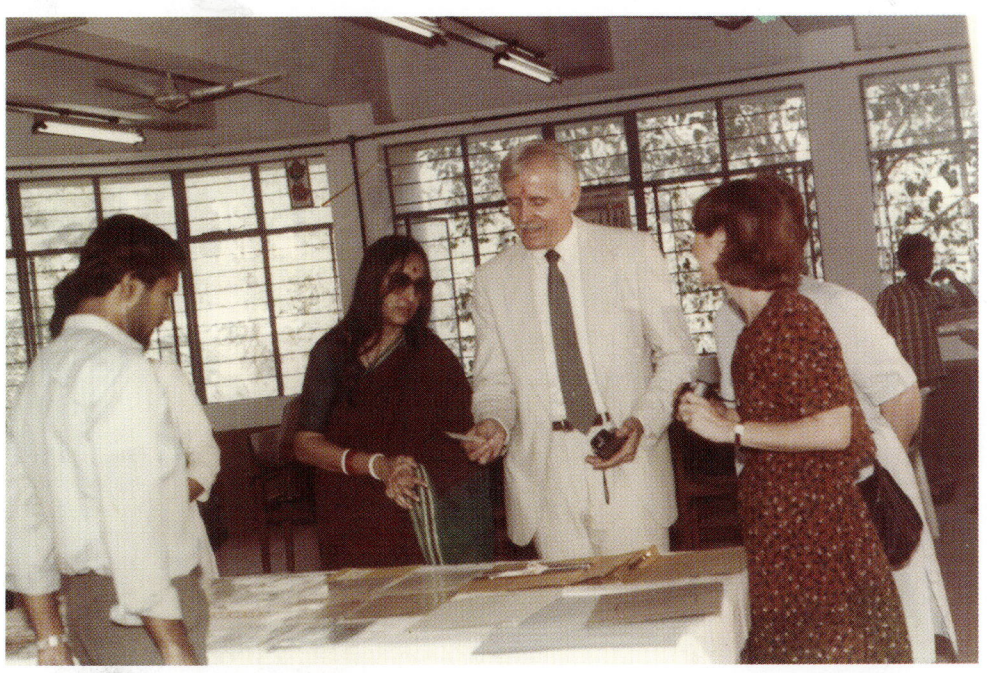

36. Mr Paul Ackerman from the National Institute on Disability and Rehabilitation Research (NIDRR) Washington, visits the Job Development Centre with Dr Mithu Alur

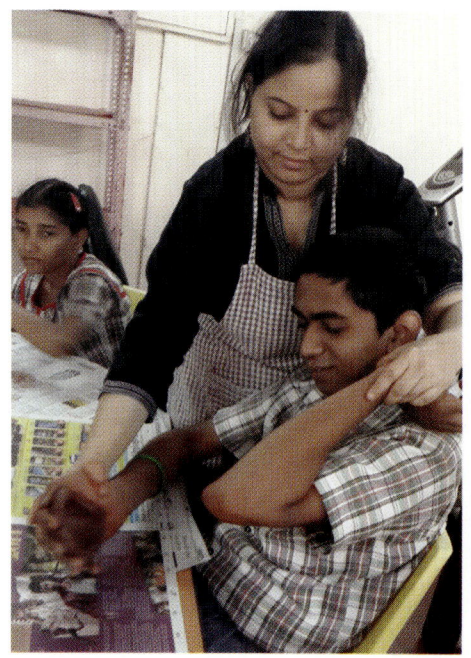

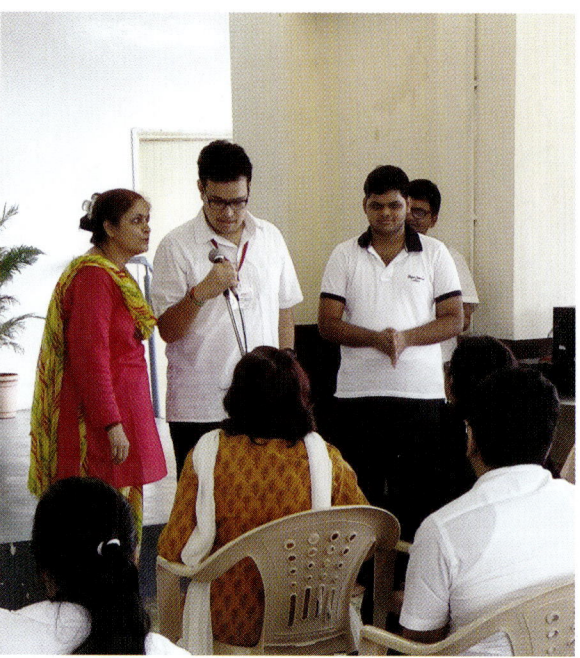

37. Head of Ceramics, Mrs Mamata Mukherjee helps Imran shape a clay bowl with his elbow

38. Deputy Director of Skills Development Centre, Mrs Malka Tandon teaches a young trainee public speaking

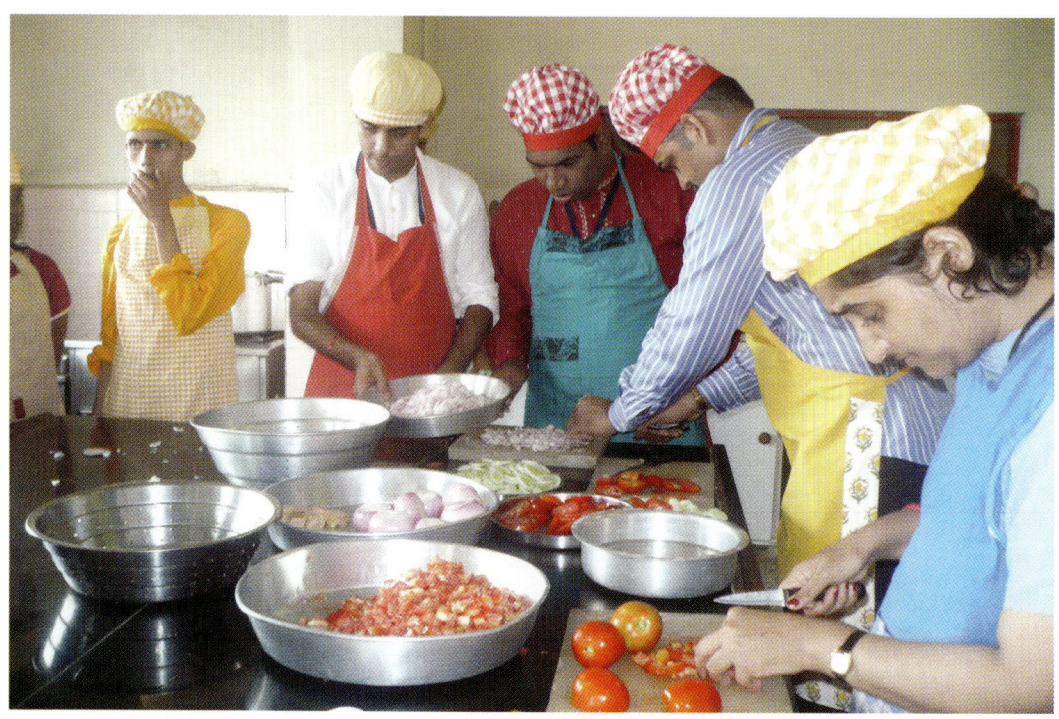

39. Young trainees learning the art of cooking at our Skills Development Centre

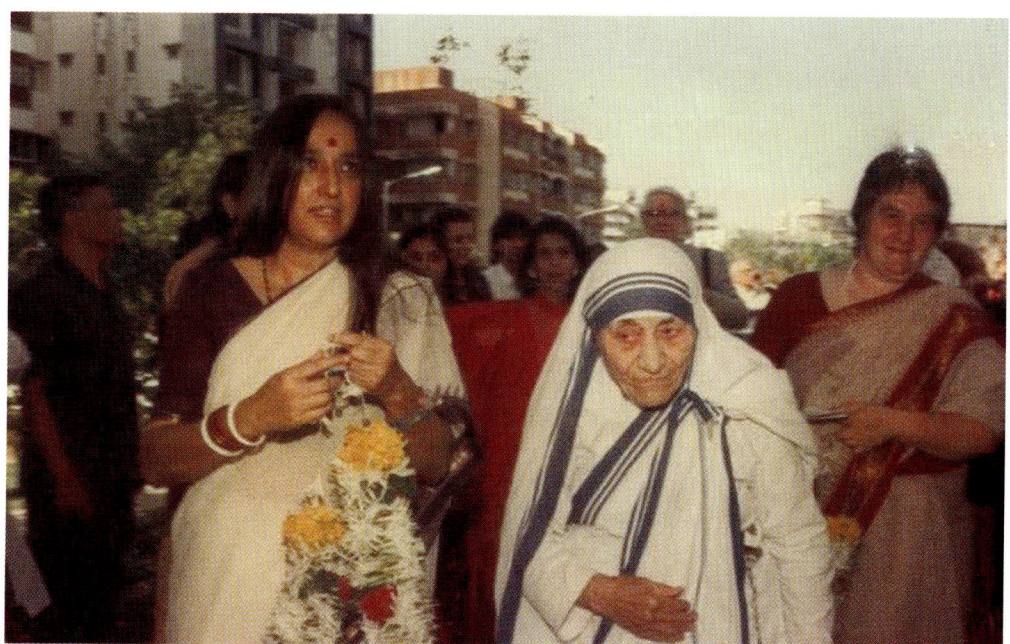

40. Mother Teresa at the inauguration of the National Resource Centre for Inclusion in Bandra with Dr Mithu Alur and Dr Pam Stretch

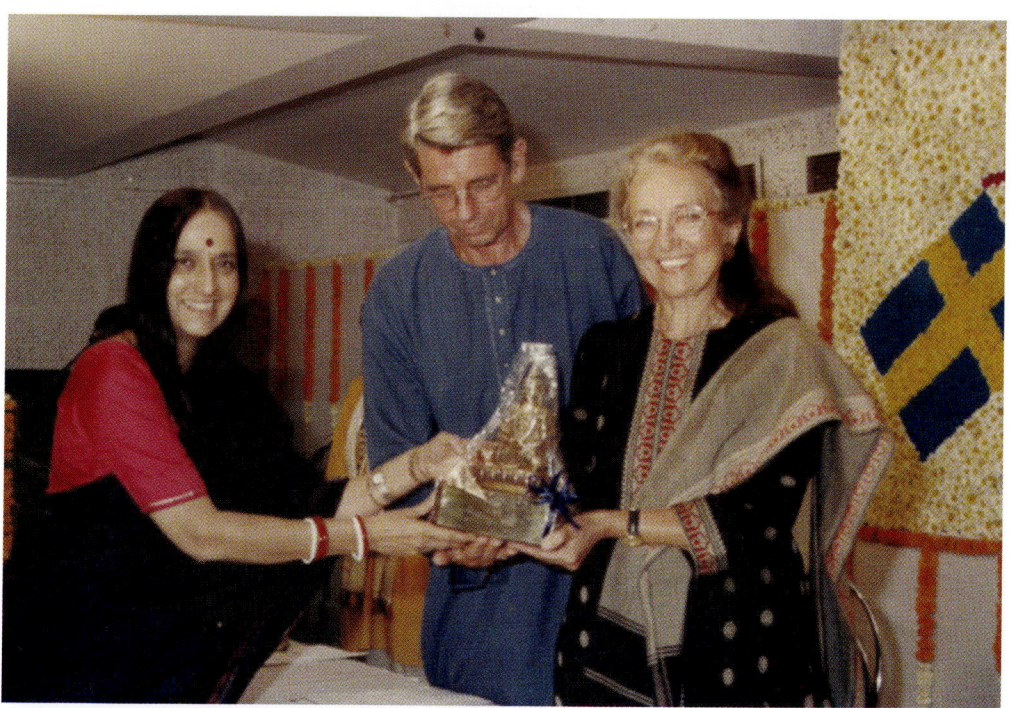

41. Mrs Margaretha Ringstrom, Director of Church of Sweden Aid, Lutherhjalpen, and her husband, Mr Bjorn Ringstrom being felicitated by Dr Mithu Alur, for support in building the National Resource Centre for Inclusion

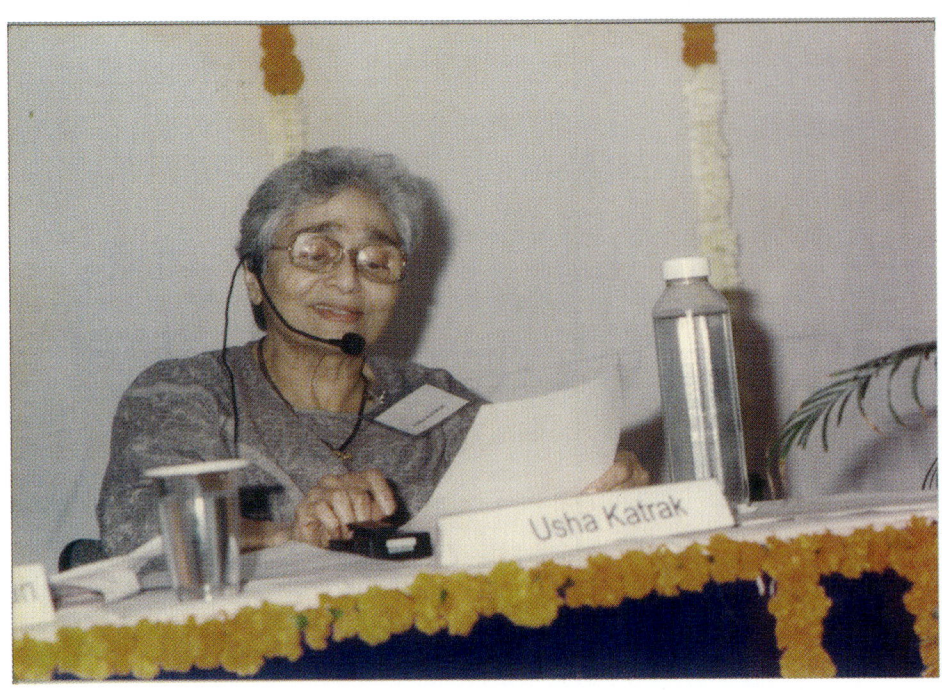

42. *The Best Volunteer Award went always to the late Mrs Usha Katrak, here she is speaking on the marginalization of senior citizens at the Citizenship and Barriers Conference, Mumbai*

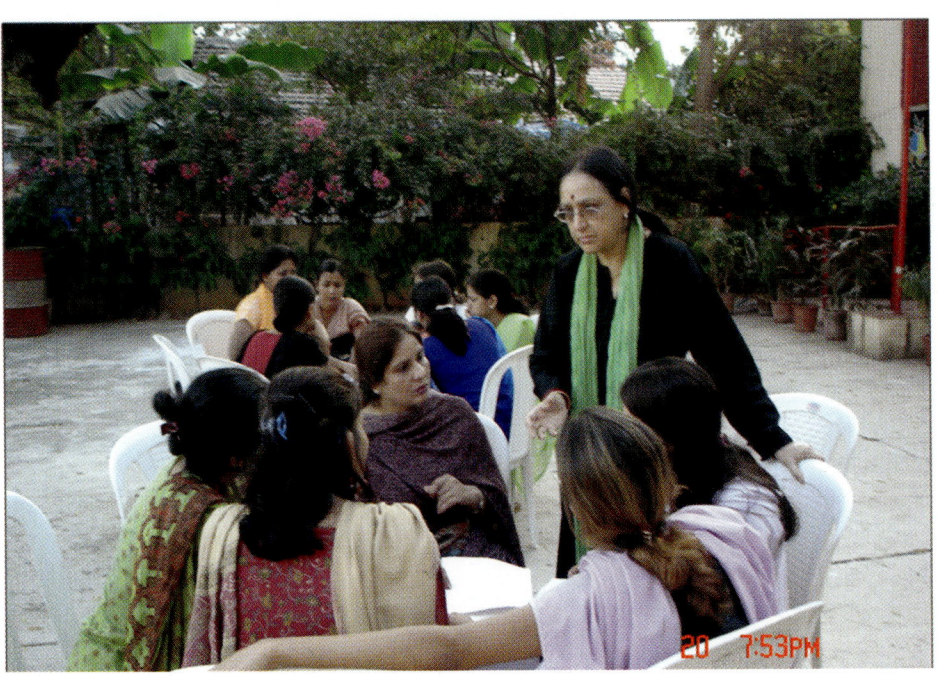

43. *Dr. Mithu Alur introducing the module on Policy to the students of the Asia Pacific Community Initiatives in Inclusion (CII) Course*

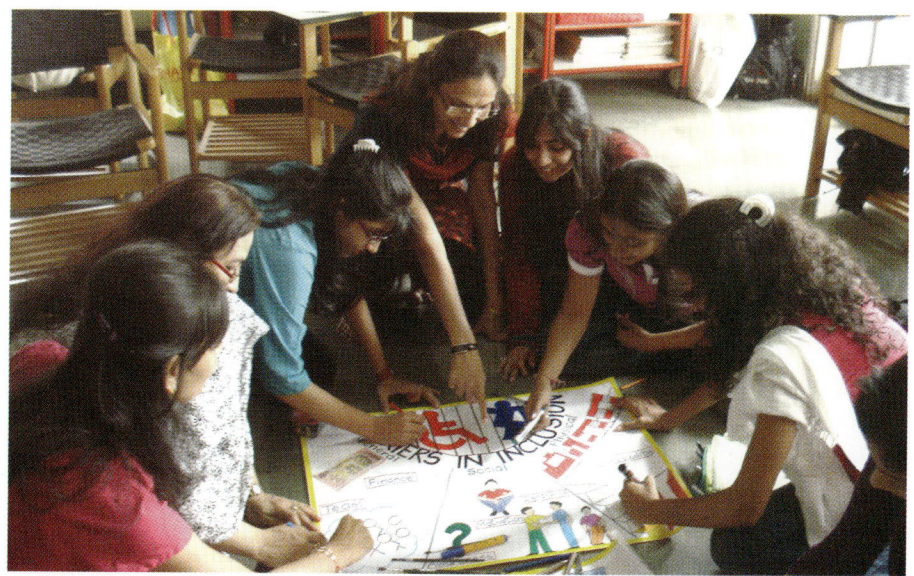

44. *Participants of the Community Initiatives in Inclusion Course preparing their own models of inclusion with Dr. Sharmila Donde*

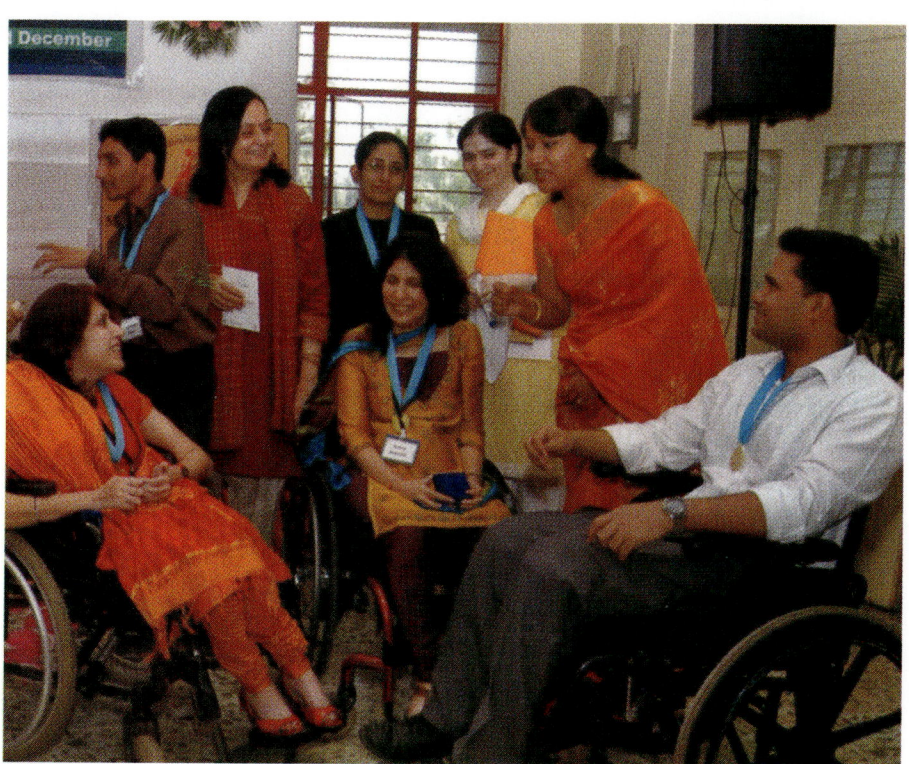

45. *Dr Anita Prabhu, Co-Chair ADAPT Rights Group with Mrs Sumita Sen, Ms Neenu Kewlani and Ms Sunita Sancheti celebrating International Day of the Disabled at the Skills Development Centre*

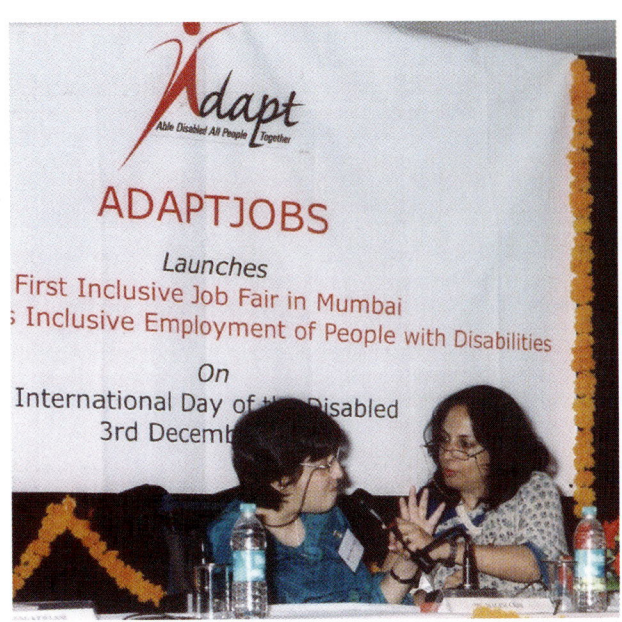

46. Ms Malini Chib speaking on the importance of employment with Mrs Varsha Hooja

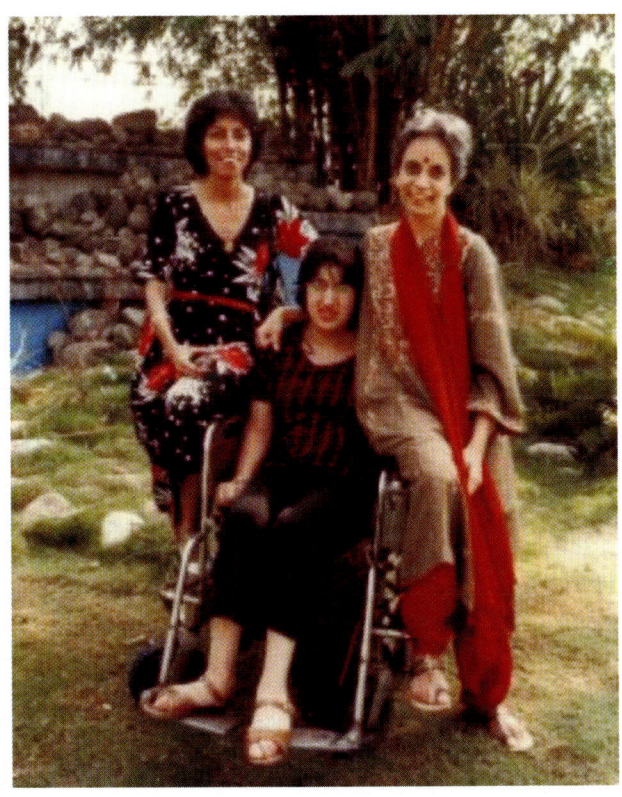

47. A friendship that has survived over the years: Ms Theresa D' Costa, Ms Malini Chib and Ms Amena Latif

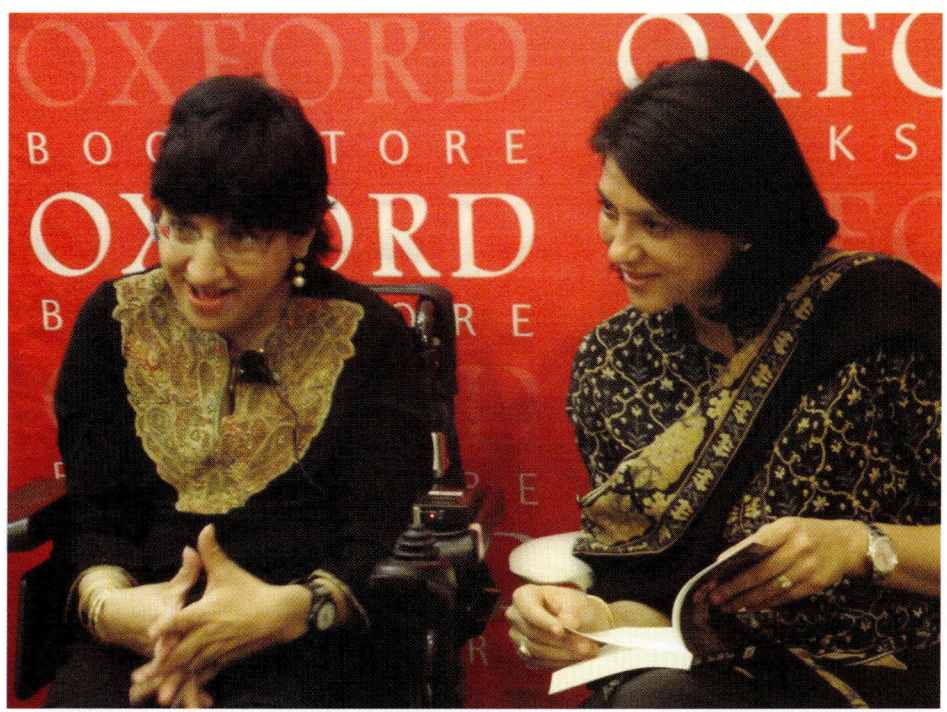

48. Mrs Priya Dutt Roncon and Ms Malini Chib *at the book launch of* One Little Finger *published by* **SAGE Publications in Mumbai**

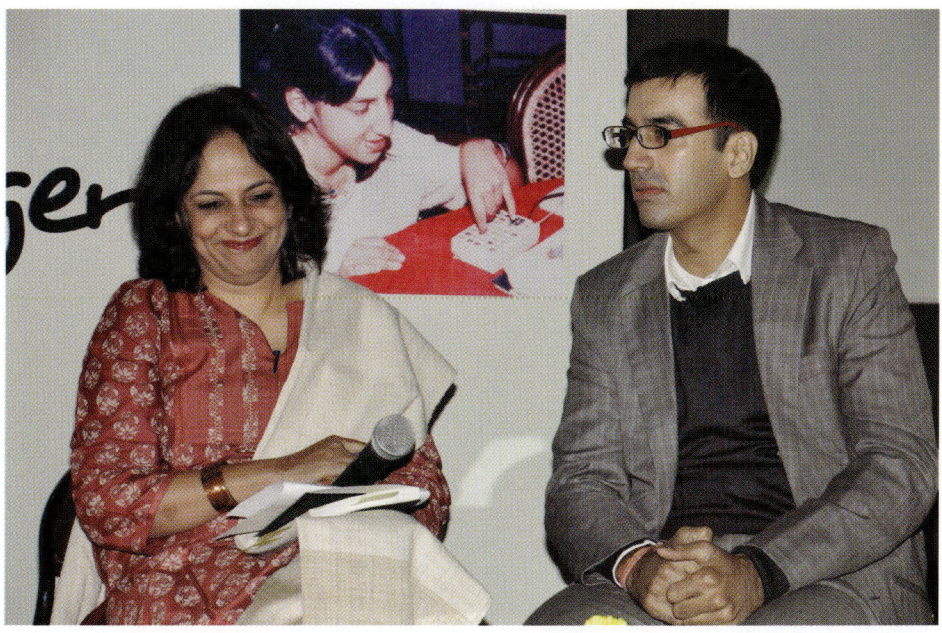

49. Mrs Varsha Hooja and Mr Nikhil Chib *read excerpts of Ms Malini Chib's* One Little Finger *at the launch of the book in Delhi*

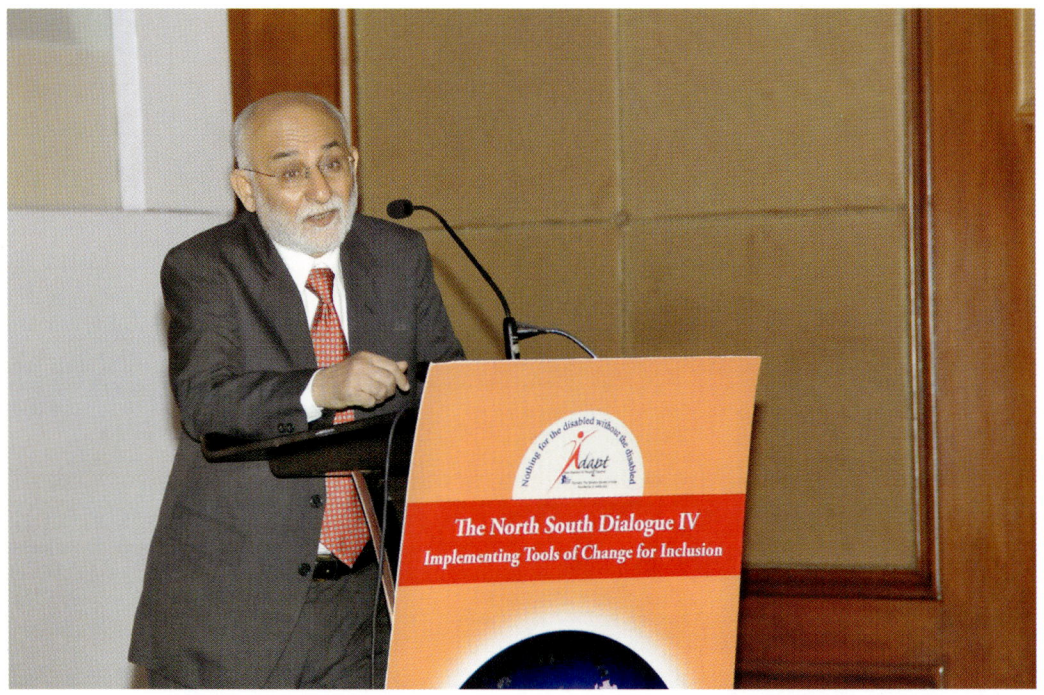

50. Mr Kamal Bakshi, Vice Chairperson, addresses the North South Dialogue IV in Goa

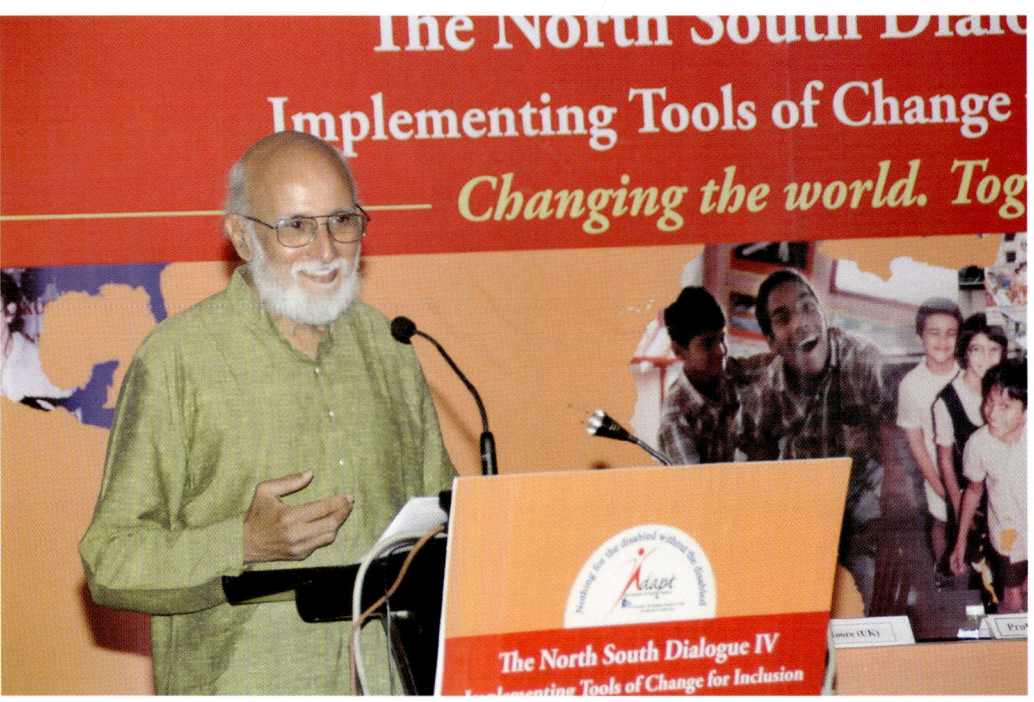

51. Trustee and parent Professor Sitanshu Mehta speaks of his experiences at the North South Dialogue IV in Goa

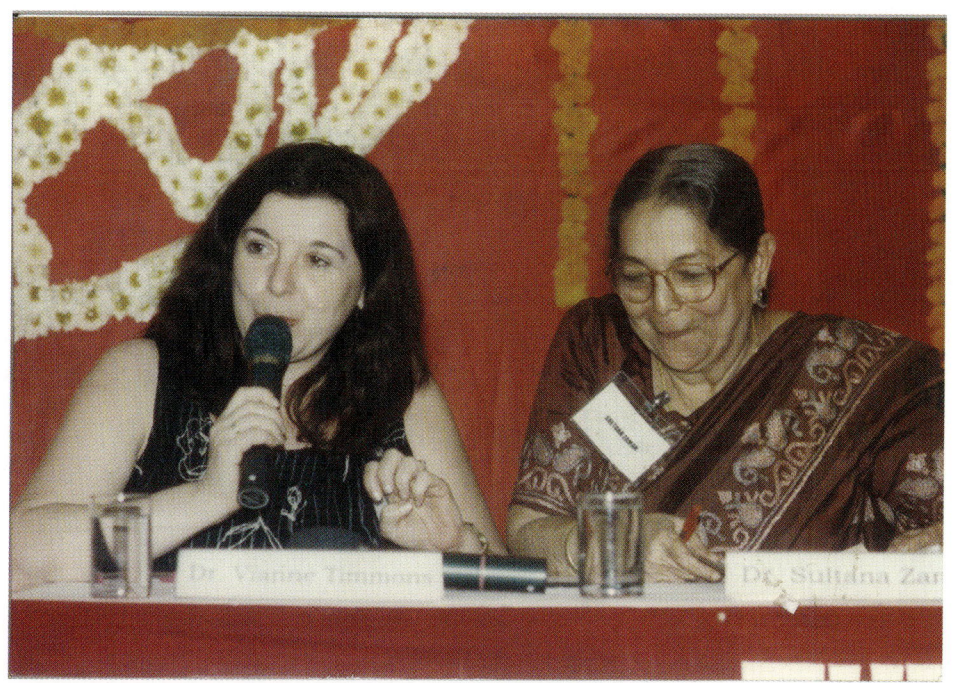

52. Two pioneers, Dr Vianne Timmons pioneer from Prince Edward Island Canada, Dr Sultana Zaman pioneer from Bangladesh, at the North South Dialogue I in Mumbai

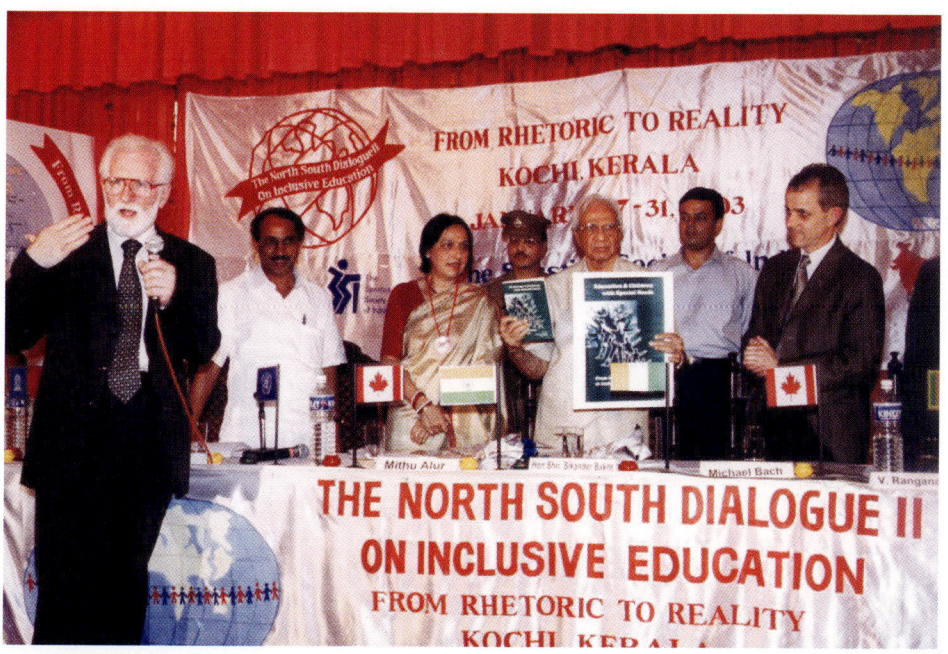

53. Launch of SAGE published book Education & Children with Special Needs—From Segregation to Inclusion edited by Mr Seamus Hegarty and Dr Mithu Alur, by the Governor of Kerala and Dr Michael Bach representing Canada

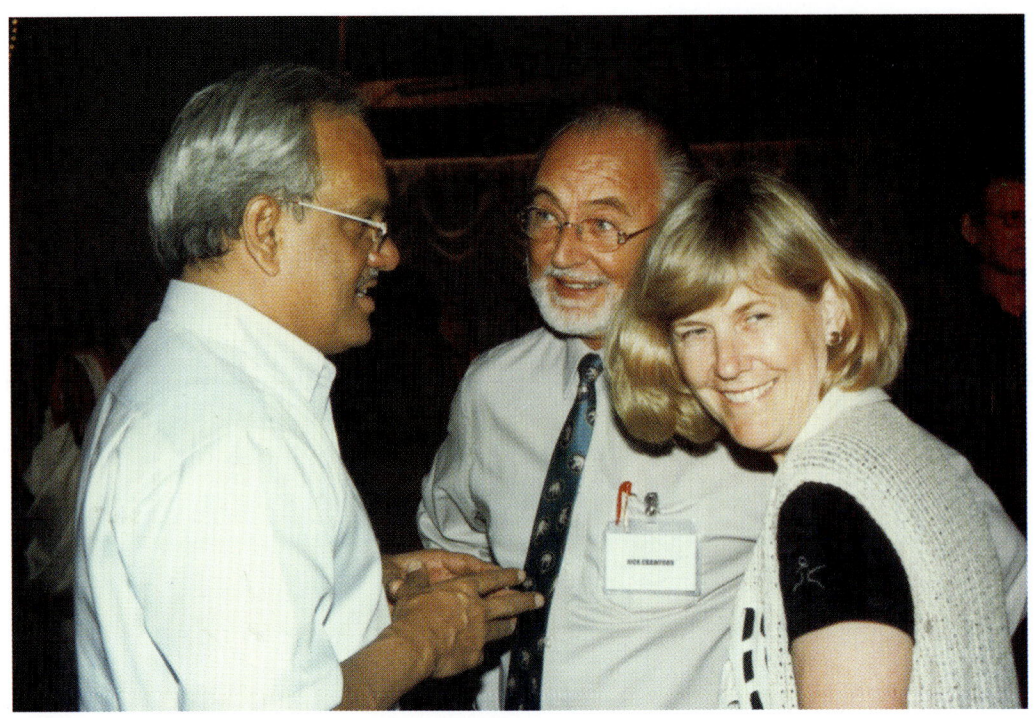

54. Mr Sathi Alur with Dr Marcia Rioux and Mr Nick Crawford at the North South Dialogue I in Mumbai

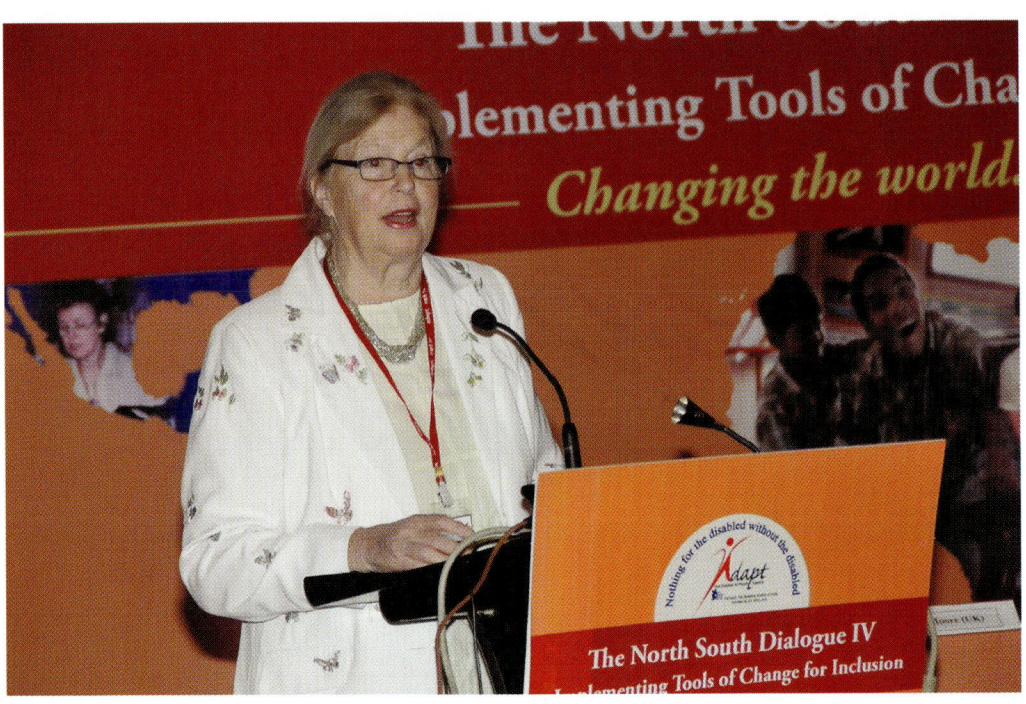

55. Dr Frances Moore, Advisor, Women's Council, UK at the North South Dialogue IV in Goa

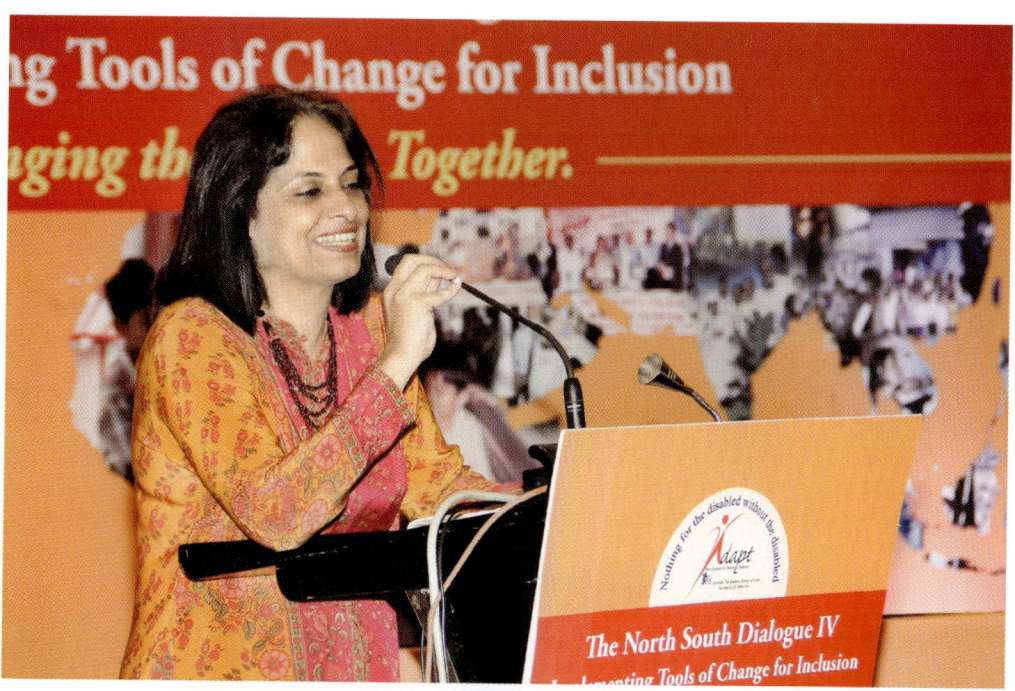

56. Mrs Varsha Hooja presents at the International Conference the North South Dialogue IV in Goa

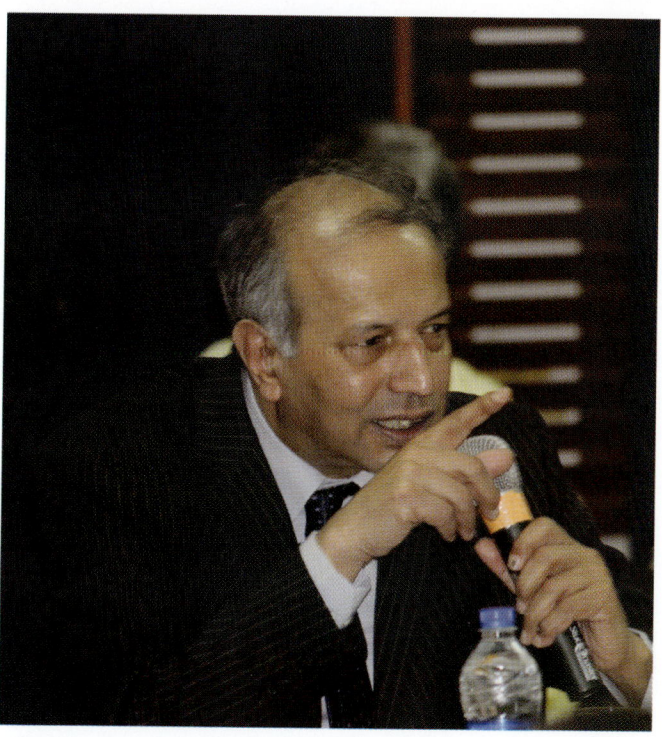

57. The Way Forward: Dr Samiran Nundy addresses the Institutional Review Board

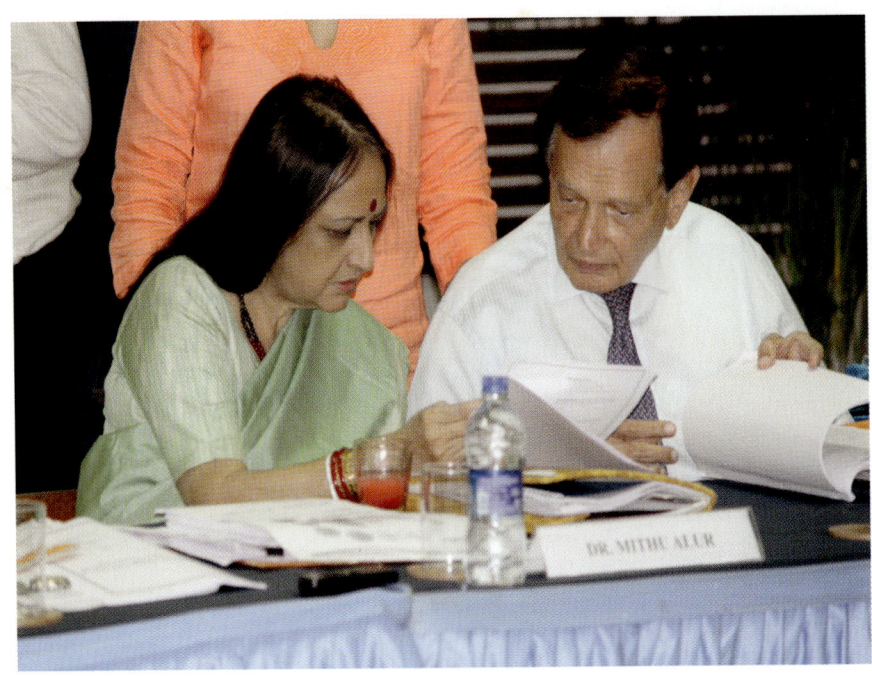

58. *Dr Mithu Alur and Dr Farokh Udwadia discussing the publication of the book* A Birth That Changed a Nation

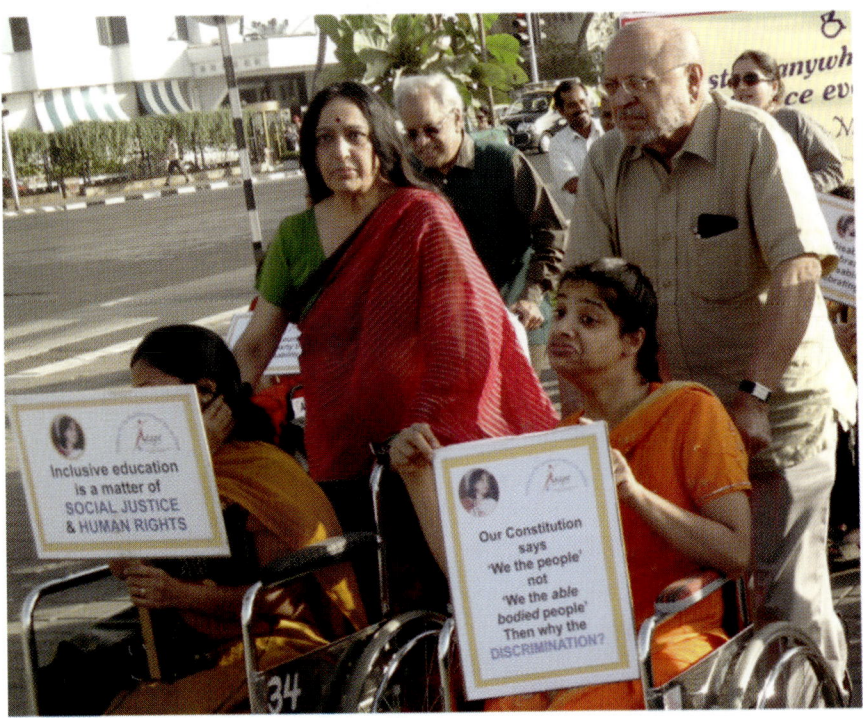

59. *Dr Mithu Alur, Mr Shyam Benegal and Mr Sathi Alur join the demonstration for inclusion*

Domain X

Results and Outcome and the Way Forward

a. The Impact: Overcoming Adversity—Some Stories

The services had a tremendous impact. Innumerable stories emerged of people who had received help and who began contributing in some small way. The director of the National Job Development Centre (NJDC) Vandana Garware, herself a senior social worker, writes about some of them:

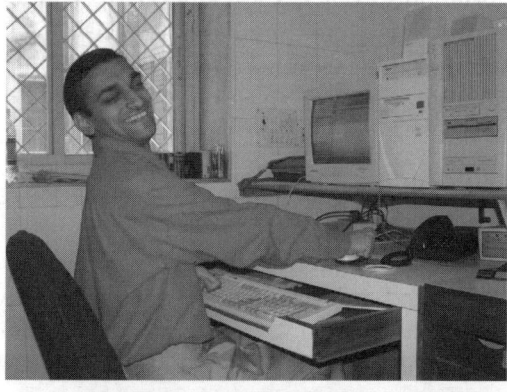

Chetan Mehta: Having worked for over a decade, Chetan is the most senior official in a firm of chartered accountants, Pritesha and Co., in Sion and manages it entirely on his own. Accurate to a fault, his cerebral palsy (CP) and resultant lack of speed has never been a deterrent to him when it comes to getting the job done. Having successfully secured employment after completing his BCom degree, he chose to begin a family of his own! Chetan got married and has settled down to lead an active and happy life.

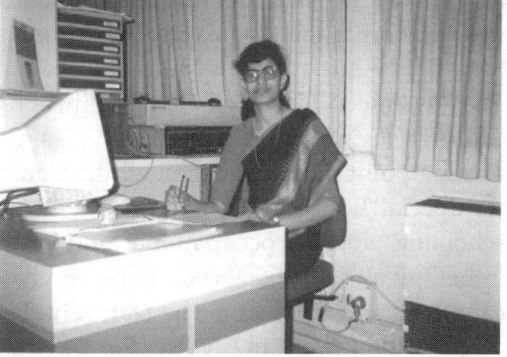

Sunita Thomas: Bright and smiling, Sunita—who has profound speech and hearing impairment since birth—has used her excellent academic records at school (passing out from Std. X) and her training at NJDC to her advantage in acquiring a coveted position in the Confederation of Indian Industry's regional office at Mumbai as a junior executive. In love with her work, the camaraderie she has built up with her colleagues is exemplary.

Arzin Avasia: An enthusiastic and hard-working young lady who has CP, Arzin works as an assistant in the Ratan Tata Institute at Gamdevi. She enjoys her work just as much as she enjoys socializing and travelling during her leisure time.

Ganesh Bhagwat: Ganesh, who has CP, has been working as an accountant-cum-office assistant at the MBA Foundation for quite some time now. Travelling by public transport every day from Dombivili to Chembur, Ganesh's adherence to a strict code of conduct is exemplary. In addition to dealing with outdoor contacts, he handles most of the office work on his own.

Ravikant Redkar: Ravikant, with a disarming smile, formidable courage and indomitable spirit, has battled the odds of CP, economic hardship, access and transportation problems to emerge a winner. Supported by his mother, the NJDC team and the Liliane Fonds Foundation, he owns a communications stall close to his residence.

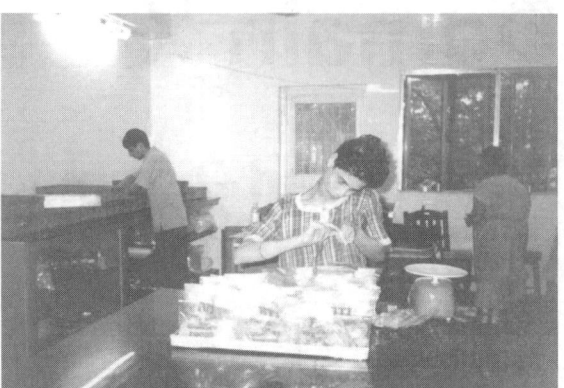

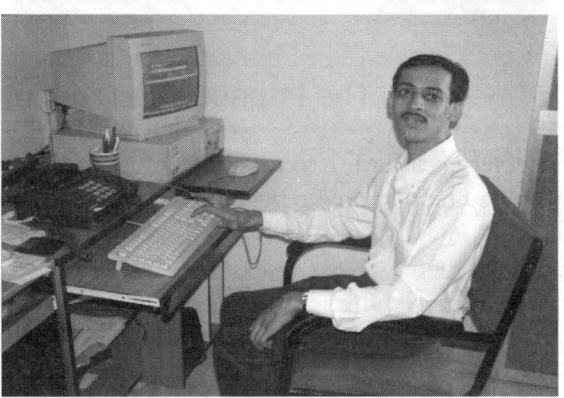

Some Personal Testimony

Ruma Kirtikar writes of her own life journey: 'I had a desire to go to school like my elder sister, but no schools would give me admission because of my disability. My sister's tuition teacher was requested to teach me and she taught me at home, up to the Std. III. My quest for education had begun. The day I met Mithu Mashi and Malini at the Children's Orthopaedic Hospital was the turning point in my life. I joined the Centre for Special Education where I received my schooling, speech, occupational and physiotherapy all under one roof. I also received

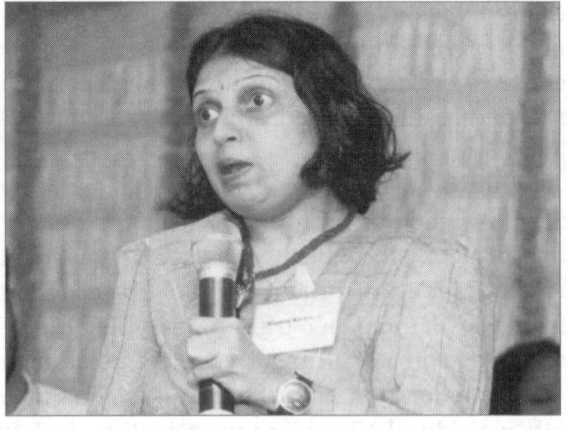

care, love and trust from the staff. The Secondary School Certificate (SSC) examination was an important event in my life. For the first time, I was tested with able-bodied students and came out with flying colours. College life offered newer vistas and put me in contact with a world bigger than my school. Travelling independently by trains and buses were barriers I broke, something I had never dreamt about earlier. My stint at the Nirmala Niketan College for a six-month course furthered my ambition to develop my talents and I decided to take up other courses at NJDC. I did a course in library science. There have been limitations due to CP...Travelling is still difficult. Then people don't understand my speech, so they pass me by, though there are good strangers who will stand and help. The attitudes of family members, neighbours and the general public are a barrier—sometimes overprotective, sometimes insensitive and sometimes inquisitive and probing. Our female role is also put to the test, especially in the Indian context, where girls are supposed to be looked after by either their parents or their husbands. Marriage may not always be an option for us. But we are not allowed to stay on our own, being a woman. I am very grateful that despite all these I have been able to achieve much, that I have worked as the assistant librarian at The Spastics Society of India (SSI). This would not have been possible without the support of all my teachers and particularly Mrs Alur. She showered support, special care and love on me at the right time and this has enriched my life and made it meaningful.

Bharat Shah joined the Children's Orthopaedic Hospital at Haji Ali where he remained till Std. III. He then moved to SSI at Colaba where he was among the first batch of students to pass out from the school, and received the award for best student (academics). He spoke of Dr Mithu Alur with gratitude, saying, 'She is a fantastic person and I am indebted to her.'

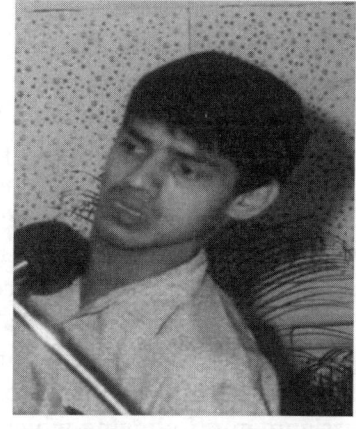

College was a totally different experience because earlier he had always been amongst people who were more or less like him physically. When he decided to pursue a degree in commerce at the Ruparel College, the principal was a little apprehensive that Bharat would feel uncomfortable among the normal students. He hadn't counted on Bharat's determination! Bharat soon became a favourite among both staff and students, participating in extra-curricular activities without compromising on his academics. Bharat gave his exams with the help of a writer and eventually passed out with a higher second class. When it came to employment, his family's business of grocery or powder coating was not what he wanted. He opted for a DTP course at NJDC, where he later trained other students. Subsequently, he started a business in offset screen printing which proved to be successful. He also studied law but did not wish to pursue it professionally. Bharat is fiercely independent, something that his family understands and is supportive of. He, in turn, doesn't grudge them for their concern. When he wanted to get married, they supported him staunchly and he married Anjana, a BSc graduate from Jamnagar who has polio. They have a son. Bharat has received the Jaycees 'Outstanding Young Person' award for distinguished services rendered to the nation. At present, Bharat runs a firm named 'Allied Systems' which deals with DTP, designing and printing.

Utpal Shah was referred to the Centre for Special Education by the Children's Orthopaedic Hospital (COH), where he had been receiving treatment and education services. At the centre, he was eager to learn. Utpal's family was advised to encourage him by giving him simple responsibilities. He was given speech therapy focusing on self-monitoring to listen to, critically evaluate and correct speech. His family was advised to make him read aloud short passages sitting in a stable and relaxed position. Utpal stayed on with the centre till he passed SSC and Higher Secondary Certificate (HSC) with the help of an amanuensis (a writer who could follow his speech) provided by the centre. He joined Podar College

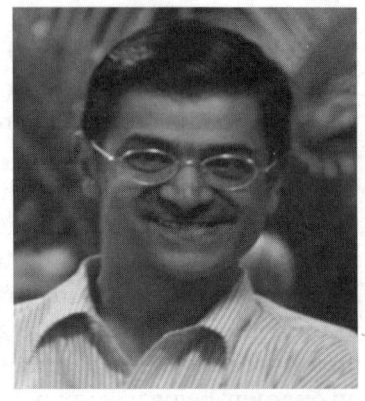

of Commerce and graduated with a BCom in 1992 and MCom in 1994. He then joined NJDC for a computer course. In 1994 he was employed at NJDC as an Assistant Accountant and worked there for 10 years. After that he was with a pharmaceutical company for another 10 years and has recently rejoined ADAPT (Able Disabled All People Together) as the accounts manager. During the course of all this, he got married and has a daughter who passed her SSC with 96 per cent. He says, 'At this juncture, I thank all my family members, teachers and staff at both COH and SSI, especially Dr Mullaferoze and Dr Alur for all their advice and for bringing me to what I am today.' Today Utpal has joined his alma mater, SSI, as a senior accountant in the Finance Department.

Lucas Baretto, who has polio, has been with ADAPT for 22 years. He first joined the NJDC and was on their faculty, where he provided training in computer technology to the centre's trainees as well as to corporates. Thereafter, he joined SSI in Bandra as Dr Alur's assistant, contributing to many projects at the national and international levels. The National Resource Centre for Inclusion (NRCI) was among his first assignments, following which he assisted Dr Alur with computer-related work during conferences held across India. In 2012, he received an award from ADAPT at the international North–South Dialogues (NSD-IV) in Goa. Lucas credits the divine as well as Dr Alur with providing him with the requisite guidance, support and encouragement throughout his

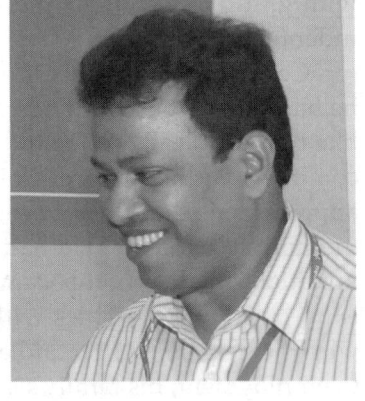

journey. Along the path, he met his life partner and is today blessed with two young children! A proud member of the ADAPT workforce, today he is IT officer heading the department. When asked about the organization, he promptly declares, 'I will always treasure the wonderful memories of the years gone by with the society.'

Rahul Bajaj tells of his experience in joining a regular mainstream school.

'SSI for me was like my world. It was like a fantasy. They all love and care for all their students and never make anyone feel that they are disabled, they always encouraged us to march ahead. They made us play cricket and all other games. Then when I was 12 and

in Std. VII, I had gone to a normal school. I was slightly
lonely in the beginning and Sudha aunty (Nair) used to
come and visit me to make me feel happy. I slowly started
playing with my new friends and I was also in the inter-
house cricket team.

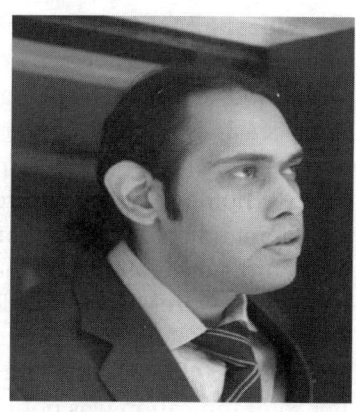

Disability does not start with the person who is disabled.
When parents treat you differently, then you become disabled.
I was lucky and my parents treated me like any other child,
so when I went to a normal school I told them matter of fact
that I had CP and so they never showed any pity and my new
friends always cared for me and no student ever made me feel
out of place. They helped me by writing or sharing their notes
with me. The principal was like my mom to me, she always
pushed me ahead. My teachers helped and encouraged me to go ahead and always taught me
to stand on my own feet. It was an eye-opener when I had to do things independently in a regular
school. I was exposed to an entirely different world and a different perspective of the world. In
retrospect, I was mollycoddled at SSI. My years at SSI, however, had given me a base, a tremendous confidence in myself, the courage to explore and a sense of being which helped me adjust in
every way. Had I gone straight into a normal school, I would have fallen like a fried egg on a pan.
I have a degree in family-managed business (FMB) and am now able and capable of looking after
my family hospitality business and I am grateful to all my teachers and mentors (Mithu aunty,
Pam aunty, Varsha aunty, Shobha aunty, Professor Deshpande and Mr Mahesh Kandpal). I have
learnt that it will be tough but one must never lose hope, must always go on and never forget the
motto of SSI: 'I Can!'

Anup Chakravorty was a bright young boy who studied till Std. X at SSI. Following his
schooling, he was admitted to the prestigious St. Xavier's College in south Mumbai, where he
made many friends and was treated like any other student, albeit with sensitivity, impressing
his teachers and carving a place for himself in the annals of Xaviers' history. He was employed
at the General Post Office in Colaba. A dedicated public servant, satisfied with his work, Anup
is a shining beacon of what is possible if only one puts one's mind to it. We are happy to report
that today, Anup is completely independent and is happily married, with plans underway to
purchase his next car!

Dhawal Chotai: My association with Dr Mithu Alur began in the year 1986 when she inter-
viewed me before admission to Std. I of SSI (now ADAPT) at their Colaba centre. Over the next
10 years, I observed and tried to absorb every value that it stands for. Whatever qualities that
form part of my personality, be it grit, resilience, or the positive and 'never say die' attitude to
life, everything has helped me become successful in life.

Even post schooling, various initiatives taken up by ADAPT such as organizing employment fairs, inclusion initiatives and dialogue with various government authorities have directly
or indirectly benefited me immensely.

Dr Alur is no less than an inspiration and a guiding light to all the disabled in India and
their parents.

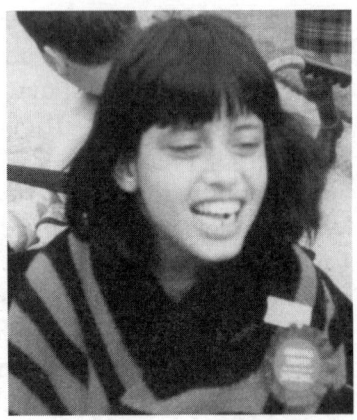

Vipasha Mehta was a unique student. She was one of my first students with whom I experimented with an idea that with good, effective teaching (sometimes one gets this with home teaching) you can cover several classes in a short period. She was terribly bright, sharp, intelligent and scored high in her psychological tests. I decided to teach her.

I remember for the first time, I used a very broad expanded keyboard which she could handle. The idea was she should be able to express herself independently. She soon picked up what I wanted and we covered ground in leaps and bounds. She finished the syllabi of three standards in 2 years. Initially her communication was poor, but soon she began to assert her newly found independence. Vipasha had earlier been taught in her mother tongue Gujarati. However, it did not take her long to master the English language and within a year she was writing poems in English!

She scored very high in her examinations. Vipasha is the only person with CP who has done her PhD and lives independently in Berkeley, California. Her sharp intellect is also manifested in several books of poetry she wrote and I quote below an excerpt!

A poem by Vipasha Mehta

A dense black darkness
Was wandering around
In the sky
Wandering, It spotted a well.
Where
It saw a dense black darkness.
It got really scared.
And collapsed near the well.

Alone sat the mind,
Besides the upset body,
To give birth to faceless demons.
Sits carding faces of people,
to appease,
the displeased
body.

My head is broken
From its remains, rise other heads,
I can't quiet see, what all the heads are doing
Because my head is broken.
places

with warm and dull
colors.

Various
pieces of mind
Live
filled inside
corners
of the…

Farhan—Looking up to Life as a Challenge!

Farhan Contractor operated the computer using a pointer held between his toes. It gave us an insight into the relentless spirit and determination of this young man 'trapped in a disobedient body'. This discerning youngster completed his SSC with a first class. The transition from school to college was not all that smooth and Farhan was initially disillusioned by college—his inarticulate speech seemed to be a drawback in his interaction with normal peers. However, despite all odds he completed his graduation in history and psychology from St. Andrew's College, Bombay. Forging ahead, he is now receiving training in computer programming at the NJDC. His proficiency in typing with the toe proved advantageous to him in operating computers with ease.

Apart from being a vociferous reader, his favourite pastime also includes watching cricket and listening to both English and Hindi music. You attempt to ask him, 'What about Classical Music?' 'Oh no!' comes the reply, emphatically. And before you wind up, you ask him about his immediate desire to which he replies, 'I don't want to depend on others'.

Some Stories from Our Workers and Beneficiaries

What of the People Behind Their Success? Who Were Some of Them? What Did They Say and Do?

A senior speech pathologist Anaheeta Nariman writes about her early experiences:

'Earlier, I used to get very irritated with people who thought I was being charitable by working in the job I do. Now, however, I explain that I am a qualified professional who finds her work rewarding and I get paid for it.' Miss Varsha Uttamsingh, a teacher, says 'There hasn't been a dull moment in the past five years that I have worked here. Each day has been filled with new experiences. One is always on the move, both teaching and learning and quite often, the latter outweighs the former.' Miss Amena Latif, teacher and special assistant to director, writes 'I was in school when I first decided that I wanted to get involved. And when I came here, I felt: This is it! I enjoy my work and find every day is a new day.' Mrs Mangala Dhingra, senior occupational therapist, describes her work 'I don't know what it is about working here, but I can't think of leaving. It's an attachment. Maybe it's the family-like atmosphere or the easy relationship with my superiors. I have lived at various places in Bombay—some quite far out of town—but that never hindered me from getting here.' Miss Nirmala Chhugani, physiotherapist, said 'When I was working at a hospital, CP was considered a dangerous area! No one wanted to get involved with CP children. But when I started working here, I realized I was learning something new every day. I would never opt for another job even though I have a problem getting here. I stay at Ulhasnagar and have to travel two hours each way. But my ties with the children are close and this is the most fulfilling aspect of my work. If a child is absent for a day, I wonder what's happened.' Mr A.G. D'Mello, manager—personnel and administration, wrote 'I am deriving greater satisfaction from the realization that I am contributing my might in doing virtually God's work on earth, caring for the handicapped spastics who would, otherwise, have been left high and dry in this world, as it were, bereft of opportunity.' Miss Zomrote Irani, teacher, said 'Oh what a noble thing you're doing!' is what people say when they learn that I'm working at SSI. And my reaction is 'No! It's not noble. I'm as selfish as anybody else and I'm doing my job for my own selfish reasons. Because it gives me tremendous satisfaction.' Mrs Maya Muddaiyya, teacher, said 'Working here has been very rewarding. I have learnt a lot of good things, especially patience and hard work.' P.K. Basu, finance manager, said:

> After working 33 years in the corporate sector, I decided to work for a charitable institution. That is how I came to join The Spastics Society. Having never seen so many handicapped children my initial reaction was of shock and a feeling of despondency. Slowly that feeling started fading as I could realize how valiantly the handicapped children were trying as well as how the teachers and therapists were helping them in the rehabilitation process, and then a feeling of joy and fulfillment replaced the despondency in me.

Anand Singh, establishment officer, who has been in the organization for 35 years says 'I have grown up here and it has been like my home. Over the years I have learnt many values.' Shasti Biswas, peon, says 'I know I could have worked somewhere else, but I won't do it as I love our children very much. When they leave the school I feel so bad I can't tell you. They are a part of my life and I am very happy to be a part of theirs.' Mrs Mahrukh Kapadia, manager—appeals and public relations, says 'It is a symbiotic relationship where the take on my part is far greater than the give on the children's part. SSI has given me the opportunity to work for spastics, which has given me a sense of inner fulfilment and satisfaction. It has made me a more sensitive, patient and caring person.' Mrs Ruma Sikka, senior superintendent—work training unit, says 'Government reservation of jobs for the handicapped is a myth. We train them and find that no one wants to take them in. So, three years ago I had a talk with my boys and girls and told them that if they wanted they could work harder, produce more and get more pay. (The government pays only ₹100 per trainee.) They agreed to this and today we get more orders from companies and are in a position to pay more than what other vocational training centres for the handicapped are paying.'

Charmaine Lobo Suri, Special Educationist of Primary Section, said 'I was fortunate to have been associated with the Centre for Special Education from 1983 to 1991. Its warm, cheerful, family-like atmosphere appealed to me immediately and I started working here as a teacher with the reception class after I completed my Teacher Training Course (TTC). We had limited space—rooms were partitioned to form classrooms. Funds were limited, too but, the staff were steely in their resolve to do the best for the children in their care. When one walked into the centre, you heard chatter, noise that told you that here's a bunch of people that mean business.

We put together an annual week-long fundraiser exhibition and sale at the Max Mueller Bhavan called 'I CAN'. This exhibition showcased the work of the students over the year and was always a huge success. Beautiful pieces of pottery, embroidery, craft work and greeting cards were quickly snapped up by our patrons and the delicious food cooked by our catering department was a sure-shot hit.

We had mentors like Mrs Alur, Ms Pam Stretch and Mrs Uma Banerjee, who had fire and inspired passion despite the dismally low salaries. Those were great years!'

Uma Banerjee, head, primary section. 'After 29 years of teaching in various types of normal schools in Calcutta and Bombay, it was with a certain amount of trepidation that seven years ago, I offered my services to the spastic child. I was prepared for anything, but nothing prepared me for the cheerfulness and loving care which I encountered in that school. The children, with multiple handicaps, smiled, laughed and with a persistent doggedness and determination tackled each task given to them to the best of their ability. Their patience and good humour was motivating and I learnt so much from them with regard to nature—human nature.'

Writes a volunteer and a mother of a boy with disabilities about her experiences of working as a volunteer:

'Life is sometimes filed with hardships
But rainy and cloudy days, too, are followed by sunshine
That's when you appreciate
The dauntless spirit of flowers of the field.'

'All mothers of special children will probably agree with these beautiful lines as we all sail in the same boat. My son Yash was on the Glenn Domans Program in the USA. The programme required Yash to be at home and hence school was not possible, but after two years of rigorous training I, as a mother, felt the need to send Yash to school. I thought of Manju Chatterjee because I knew her from my therapy days. She was enthusiastic and encouraging and helped with the formalities of enrolling Yash as a part of resource support for students. Yash used to look forward to meeting his friends and teachers and always talked about them. Though there was no formal education at this point of time, there was immense satisfaction that my child was a part of such a wonderful organization. The school would take children for picnics, they participated in *melas*, fun fairs, there were educational field trips organized to the aquarium, and children–teacher participation in the Kala Ghoda Festival. Children were taken to nearby gardens and shown plants and flowers as a part of education as well as recreation.'

'Every now and then we would hear of some well-known person from the corporate world coming to the school to meet and spend time with our children. Also students from other schools came to play, interact and encourage our children with special needs. All this and the celebration of festivals like Diwali, Holi, Christmas and so on at school would in their own little way bring so much happiness into Yash's life and our life. All this support emotionally helped us and brightened my son and my life in many special ways. As a parent I am very grateful and thankful to ADAPT for accepting my child as part of their organization.'

(Source: Annual Report 2008–09)

Isabella Onslow, international volunteer: 'I come from England and am working as a volunteer in the Bandra centre for 3 months. I arrived here in January and since then have learnt and experienced a huge variety of things that I never thought I would end up doing! My main task is to prepare for the annual show, which celebrates inclusion and differences and which takes place on 30th of March. My job involves teaching a group of the students a variety of songs which are all in English and providing an accompaniment on either the piano or guitar. From teaching this group I have learnt patience. And optimism, which I have discovered, is also hugely important; if one goes into a lesson thinking that what you are about to try and do is impossible then nothing will ever happen; your pessimism projects onto the students and they will start to think that they can't, for example, learn a new song. If, however, one goes into a lesson with the attitude that anything is achievable, then you are not only able to teach with more enthusiasm and energy, but are also able to tell your students convincingly that they can do it. I have learnt that the attitude with which you approach something is more important than the task itself. Working at ADAPT has completely changed my perception of disabled people. Before arriving here, I was of the view that disabled people are made of glass and that one has to be very careful when working with them. Now, thanks to ADAPT, I have come to see that they are just the same as anybody else; just because someone may not be able to walk or talk doesn't mean that one can't have the same expectations of them as one would of any other person. In fact, as I observed while I was at ADAPT, the achievements of people with disabilities are often much higher than those of an able person. After my time at ADAPT, I will go back to England with an experience of a completely different culture, new friends and a changed perspective' *(Source: Annual Report 2008–09)*.

Sangita Vaswani, volunteer Std. II (2008–09), said 'First I would like to tell you how I have become a volunteer at the ADAPT school. One day I came to school to meet Mrs Manju Chatterjee and to give some snacks to the children. I found her very friendly and she appreciated my gesture. She asked me to give my time to these special children. I agreed with her and I started coming to school. Now I have got so attached to the school that I eagerly wait for the three days that I come here to spend time with the children. I wish more people would come forward and give their time to these special children. I wish the school all the best for the good work that each and every one is doing.' Tristan S. Kaufman, international volunteer from New York (2010–11), says 'I came from New York in 2010 and during my time working with disabled students at your fine institute, my life has changed dramatically. I am honoured to have participated in an organization where people dedicate themselves to helping and educating those in need. I have developed strong bonds with each and every one of the children in the class. I grew attached to them. I will never forget these children that I have come to know and loved.'

Deepak Kalra, parent and founder of Umang, Rajasthan, says

I've got used to people staring at me and my son wherever we go. In the first year however, I used to re-act very differently. I avoided going out altogether. Now, I myself am so much more confident and realize that if I get onto a train with my son, some amount of time will have to be spent satisfying curiosity. Now I answer people's questions or intercept them if they are talking among themselves about my son, and give them the correct picture. And in answering their questions, I am using the most basic tool for increasing public awareness—word of mouth.

Some awards were given at that time. They were for exceptional and outstanding service to the disabled in India. The Nargis Dutt Memorial Award was given to Pam Stretch for her pioneering services in the area of treatment. Pam made an exceptional contribution in virgin territory in India. The work, which was of a pioneering nature, has often been arduous, physically and mentally, but her courage and her boundless missionary zeal overcame everything that came in her way. She was very well-respected and loved by Mrs Nargis Dutt, our late patron, and was most deserving of the first Nargis Dutt Memorial Award, instituted by SSI, for her meritorious service. Besides her passion for CP, she was very interested in 'natural' systems of medicine and therapy. Through and because of her work with SSI, she was trying to develop a new therapy called 'Intrinsic Development'.

'I consider myself very fortunate to be working in such an exciting, pioneering field and with so inspirational a person as Mithu. This is why I have stayed on here in India for 15 years,' writes Pam.

The Radhakrishna Award was given to the late Mrs Uma Banerjee for innovative and exceptional work for the disabled in the field of education. She had worked in the field of education for 40 years and specialized in infant and junior levels. From 1950 to 1964, she taught in Calcutta after which she became headmistress of the junior department of Bombay International School. In 1967, she became headmistress of the Infant Department of the Cathedral and John Connon School, Malabar Hill. After her retirement in 1982, she joined SSI as an educational consultant at the Centre for Special Education and also as a senior lecturer on normal education for the society's postgraduate TTC (affiliated to Bombay University). She was an English consultant at the J.B. Petit School and her specialties were remedial reading and developing the English language. She published four infant arithmetic books entitled *Counting in Easy Steps*. Mrs Uma Banerjee made a significant contribution in setting up the primary section at SSI. Her interventions in the educational field of disabled children were innovative and creative. In SSI, she laid the foundations for formal study for the brighter, intelligent disabled child preparing for public examination, thus making a pioneering critical contribution to special education. During her eight years with SSI, her work was highly creative and innovative. She helped to build up a fine cadre of teachers through TTC. For her exemplary contributions to education, it was most befitting that she received the first Radhakrishna Award for education instituted by SSI.

The Junie Sethi Award was given to Shanti Nundy from Kolkata where Junie had worked for many years with her. It was for exceptional and selfless services rendered to disabled children in India. Mrs Shanti Nundy had been teaching for over 30 years, both in India and overseas. She had worked with culturally disadvantaged children in Malaya, normal children in Calcutta and physically disabled children in the British Honduras. Mrs Nundy qualified as a Special Educator from Brandon University, Canada. From 1976, she was associated with the Spastics Society of Eastern India (SSEI), where she was a senior teacher in the Extended Education Department at the Centre for Special Education in Kolkata. Mrs Nundy's selfless dedication to disabled children is quietly reflected in her work. Her affection for the students and staff, her ability to see that everyone was given equal attention and her determination to fight for the cause made her one of the strongest pillars at SSEI. She worked closely with Mrs Junie Bose Sethi. Her modesty, her compassion, her warmth for all who worked with her and her love for the children made her a very suitable candidate to receive the second Junie Bose Sethi Award from SSI which had been instituted after Junie's demise.

For selfless and devoted service for disabled children, Maya Muddaiya received The Swami Vivekanand Award. Mrs Maya Muddaiya was deputy principal of the Centre for special education, Colaba. Her earlier teaching experience was in Vishakhapatnam and New Delhi. During her six years of work, Maya worked indefatigably. Her commitment to her work and her conscientiousness and her warmth and affection for children and staff made her a rare individual. Her exceptional selfless dedication made her an excellent candidate for the first Vivekananda Award being given by SSI.

The Lillian D'Souza Award was given to Theresa D'Costa for exceptional and meritorious service rendered for the disabled for 35 years. As the chairman's secretary, she had played a valuable role and wore multiple hats! She is virtually a historical encyclopaedia and has played a key role for every single event and function. Armed with a degree in psychology and with very good public relations skills, she was able to interact with colleagues as well as the public with ease. Above all, being thoroughly conscientious and sincere, she put her heart and soul into her work, giving of herself generously and making a deep impact with the way she sustained the pace. Having graduated with an honours degree in psychology from K.C. College, Bombay, she joined SSI in November 1977 and claims there has never been a dull moment for her since! She feels she is working in a family where 'give and take' exists. She says 'I have drawn great inspiration from Mrs Alur and have always loved social work. I look forward to a long and continuing association with the cause of the disabled who are still a low priority in our country.' Theresa wove into her service, of over 35 years, a spirit of dedication and commitment with a religious fervour. In the pioneering stages, there were numerous and multiple jobs that needed to be done. She did this quietly with patience and with indefatigable zeal.

In recognition of dedicated service as a volunteer at the Centre for Special Education for over seven years, the late Mrs Pam Advani received the Appreciation Award. A regular and contributing member of the team, Pam writes, 'I was inspired by all the work Mrs Nargis Dutt had done with SSI and thought I, too, would like to contribute by becoming a volunteer. I have learnt so much from working with the children and have found that it is I who need them not they who need me.'

What of Malini?

Malini has a Double Masters' from the University of London. The first Masters' was in Women's Studies from the Institute of Education (IOE) under the guidance of eminent academic, Professor Diana Leonard. The second Masters' was from The Metropolitan College, University of London, in Information Management and Technology, which made her a fully qualified Librarian. On her return she expanded the library at SSI into a Library and Media Resource Centre (LMRC). Moving the Society's service delivery mould from Charity to Rights she together with others formed the ADAPT Rights Group (ARG), a unique inclusive group that brought together persons with and without disability battling for their rights.

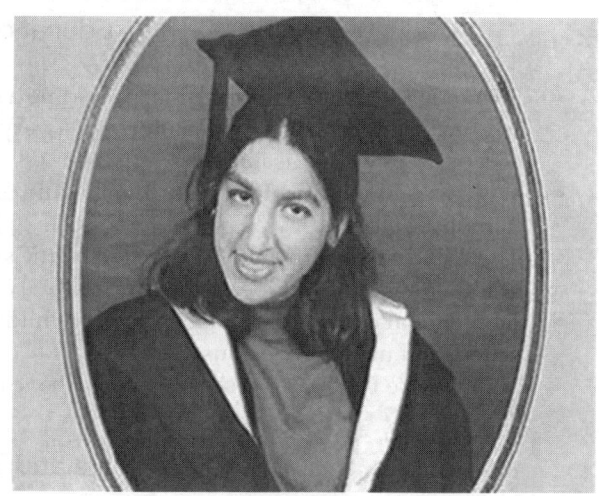

Ms Malini Chib

Trustee and Honorary Secretary, ADAPT Founder Chairperson, ADAPT Rights Group (ARG)

Believing in the larger issues of marginalization she expanded the Rights Group to include concerns such as women's rights and LGBT issues. Malini is a member of the Research Action Committee of the IRB and one of the Trustees of the Governing Body of the Spastics Society.

Malini's greatest contribution has been the sharing of herself ... of having the courage to put out in the public domain her sorrows, her thoughts ... of constantly reminding everyone that persons with disability need to be a part of the mainstream and not apart from them ... of reiterating the international thinking of *'Nothing About the Disabled Without the Disabled'*.

An author, researcher and academic activist she expresses an inner world with graceful candidness through the pen rather than demonstrations. Malini's debut autobiographical work was a book called *One Little Finger*, published by SAGE, which contributed tremendously to awareness about disability and in recognition of this, she was honoured with the National Award by the Ministry of Social Justice Empowerment (MOSJE) Government of India, for being a role model in spreading awareness for persons with disability.

Today, Malini is working with Tata Consultancy Services (TCS) London as Diversity Consultant for Women and Disabled people in London.

She has been the inspiration behind the film *Margarita with a Straw*, directed by her cousin Shonali Bose with Kalki Koechlin in the lead role, and which won numerous international and national awards.

Malini is one of the many disabled pioneers who paved the way for others to come in the following years. Given the modifications, the care and professional support, combined with their own grit and determination, they proved that adversity could be defeated. Certainly they demonstrated that individuals with CP reap the benefits of education and proper management, just as much as other young people.

b. Results and Outcome

Education

- SSI made a technical contribution, providing a holistic programme combining education and treatment under one roof. This formed a very strong base for children and youth with CP and other physical disabilities.
- With a slight modification in the curriculum and with skilled trained teachers, the students demonstrated that it was perfectly possible to be educated.
- The schools were officially recognized by the state board. Students appeared for the SSC, the National Institute of Open Schooling (NIOS) and went onto universities.
- Educational reforms took place allowing children to have writers and get extra time for their school and university exams.
- Today more than 3,000 cases of children have been educated through the first centre.

Healthcare and Treatment

- Early infant clinics, where high-risk babies were assessed, helped to create awareness that children must have early detection and management. Screening, identification and assessment of newborn and high-risk babies along with neonatal support and care is now available at the centres. Intervention focusing on better health for the child and mother is an integral part of the services provided.
- More than 5,000 babies, children and young people have come for assessment and remedial programmes over the last 40 years (Alur 2009).

Treatment and Rehabilitation

- New concepts previously unknown in the country such as Bobath, Vojta and Peto, Conductive education and individual therapy concepts were introduced. The importance of the use of the 'eclectic approach' was established.
- A large number of children came from different parts of the country to avail of the services offered comprehensively under one roof.
- The 'Management of cerebral palsy and other physical disabilities' course established the much needed therapy training in the country. Therapists came from various parts of the country including Baroda, Bhuj, Cuttack, Bangalore and Mumbai and some also came from neighbouring countries like Pakistan and Bangladesh. Through the training of therapists, the organization was indirectly impacting the lives of large numbers of parents and children with CP throughout the country.
- A new Interdisciplinary Team Approach was successfully created. for cerebral palsy. Here doctors and paramedicals consisting of physiotherapists, occupational therapists and speech therapists, psychologists, social workers and special educators worked together under a special school setting rather than a medical one, conforming to a current social rather than a medical model (Ibid 2009).
- Professionalism combined with care was introduced.

Pedagogy

- First training courses for teachers set up in India decentralized services, allowing knowledge to spread was introduced. A change of attitude and perception, teamwork and the strengthening of the knowledge base became the mainstay of the courses. These became recognized by the University of Bombay and the Rehabilitation Council of India (RCI).
- On the macro level, there was now an attempt to influence pedagogic changes in the curriculum of the general teacher education by National Council of Educational Research and Training (NCERT), National University of Educational Planning and Administration (NEUPA) and National Council for Teacher Education (NCTE), creating a cadre of educators who believe in the abilities of 'all' children and in their right to study side by side, learning from the strengths of each other.

Engagement with Parents and Disabled Activists

- Parents and families of the children got trained at the various training programmes of SSI resulting in SSI model being replicated in various cities like Delhi, Chennai, Bangalore, Kolkata and Jaipur by parents and family members.
- Empowered parents and families set up services around the country. The various SSIs provided help from their own bases under a special school setting.

Engaging with Government Has Resulted in the Following

- CP, which had previously not been recognized amongst the government's classifications is now recognized as one of the 11 official classifications accepted by the Government of India's ministry of social justice and empowerment.

Replication and Spread of the First Model

Towards the end of the 1970s, SSI nurtured the expansion of services across the country as part of its growth plan.

The organizations that emerged were largely initiated by parents, family members and close friends.[1] The result of this was the incubation and development of services in virgin territories

---

[1] To name a few in Kolkata it was begun by Mrs Junie Bose, Mr Abhijit Bose, Mrs Sudha Kaul and Mr Om Kaul, Mrs Perin Aibara, Mrs Shanti Talukdar, Mr Ahmed and Mrs Uma Ahmed, Mr Sen and Mrs Reena Sen, Mrs Indrani Mazumdar, Jayobrotho and Mrs Subhra Chatterjee amongst others; in Delhi, late Mrs Mita Nundy and Dr Samiran Nundy, Mrs Anita Showrie and Mr Arun Showrie, Dr Lotika Sarkar, Mrs Minu Jalan, Mrs Manju Dubey, Mrs Radhika Roy, Miss Gloria Burrett, Ms Shyamala Gidugu, Ms Vandan Bedi amongst others; in Bombay, Mr Ranjit Chib, Mr and Mrs Vishesh Bhatia, Ms Lillian Khare, Ms Pamela Stretch, Mr Kamal Bakshi, Mrs Nergish Pakhivala, Mr Sathi Alur, Professor Sitanshu Mehta and Mr Natatarajan; in Madras, Mr Natarajan, Mrs Poonam Natarajan, Rajul Padmanabhan, Usha Ramakrishna and many more who were touched by the fever and thirst to serve the country; in Bangalore, Mrs Rukmini Krishnaswamy and Mr Adhip Chowdhury; in Jaipur, Mrs Deepak Kalra, Bina Kak and team.

in Delhi, Madras, Bangalore, Calcutta and Jaipur among other states. The organizations were initially named after the parent body as The Spastics Society of India, Delhi, Madras, Bangalore and so on; later when they moved away they changed their names. Central government grants-in-aid and matching funding, and applications for land, organized and released through SSI for several years until the organizations were developed to take over as independent and autonomous organizations.

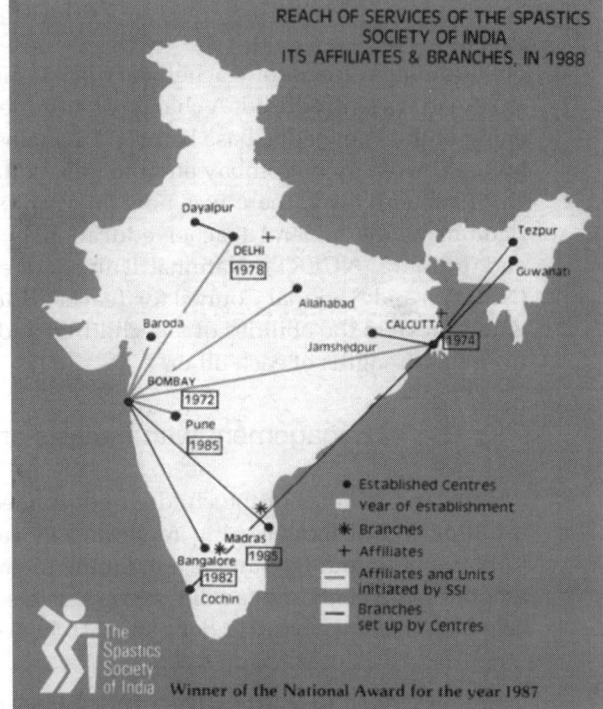

This figure is not to scale. It does not represent any authentic national or international boundaries and is used for illustrative purposes only.

Research

- Research paved the way to showing how children could be educated in special schools as well as ordinary schools. Research also showed the way to how mapping, identification and assessment and screening of babies could be done.
- Research developed a code of practice and the best practices were recorded under the CAPP I, II, III as instructional resource material to propagate inclusive education.

Community

- Deinstitutionalization, and demystification, took place. A whole community approach was developed involving the slum and rural folks and district officials.

Policy

Reformative action took place. The Right To Education (RTE), today, makes it legally mandatory to include all children with disability, giving them the constitutional right to education.

On the legislative front, a landmark legislation in India has been passed beginning with the Persons with Disability Act in 1995.

- This was followed by the 86th Amendment of the Education Bill. When people talk about education for all, the all does not include children with disabilities. The amendment of the education bill has made a positive statement. The clause states that 'all' means children with disabilities as well.
- A question on disability has now been included in the census.

- The Persons with Disability Act was passed in 1995. It went under a review process by the NGO sector together with government officials so that it incorporated the internationally recognized convention of the UNCPRD. The amendments have now been done through many consultations. However, it still remains a Bill and not an Act as it has not been passed by Parliament yet.
- A new ministry of women and child was constituted. This was a major focus which would help the 4 million children under the age of five who had been left out of the government preschool programme.
- Government reconstructed a body, which is the highest authority today in education, called the Central Advisory Board of Education (CABE) committee which had been started by the British. This has as its members all education ministers of the different regions of India as well as eminent civil society people, where I was among those invited.
- In conclusion, we had certainly made progress on a macro level, initiating change all over the country. Disability issues, which were earlier ignored within the policy framework in India, are now being addressed in all major policy documents.

The Meta Theories and Key Lessons That Emerge

- *Micro efforts* of civil society are valuable in being catalysts in *generating macro outcomes.* Micro efforts have a ripple multiplying effect which can spearhead governments into action before state initiatives can take effect. As we have seen, in a country like India where universal education has not yet happened and where there is a lack of cohesive policy leaving millions of children out of the educational circuit, *faulty systems* need to be addressed.
- *Demonstration of inclusion* was important. *Identification of an issue* in the policy agenda is the first step towards policy formulation. Non-identification of issues leads to neglect. The `How' of inclusion within government's existing programmes has been demonstrated; however, operationalizing and implementing the policies into action on a national level have not been done. *What is now needed is to scale it out.*
- The entitlements regime, targeting all citizens, is unlikely to happen in the current lifetime of most people in a developing country. Therefore it is critical to ensure that some basic services are available and for this it is necessary to identify *key resources* to achieve this. The one way this is possible is through *community and family participation.* The cornerstone of my inclusive policy is *cost neutral.* The cost neutral philosophy requires key elements to be resourced such as empowering disabled people and their parents to lobby for their rights. *In the area of practice… inclusive practices within the child's community and neighbourhood need to be adopted quickly and efficiently.*
- Inclusion is a process, it is evolutionary and it needs preparation. In countries where systems and policies are still not in place (and working with countries in the Far East), I can safely argue we will continue to need *a dual system.* I am not a radical. Unfortunately, inclusion cannot be accomplished overnight. We cannot throw the baby out with the bathwater and choke the baby! While I strongly believe that children with disability should be given equal opportunities, *the truth is that special schools would be needed for a while for children with more severe difficulties until the whole system has evolved.* Recently, I have had distressed members of Parliament telling me about parents who have been asked to leave special schools and thrown out to go to regular schools. This is not the process of change I believe in.

- Given the problem of numbers, integrating all disabled children immediately may not be the right paradigm for India. Yet, in areas where there is no option, like in the villages and slums, the common school must admit all children including children with disability. I believe in the dual system as well as advocate common schooling in the villages.
- The cost of exclusion is staggering. On the other hand, inclusion is cost-effective. The cost of inclusion is manageable. My experience shows that inclusion can take place within existing resources, regardless of however poor the country is. The experiences related showed that it can be done amongst the poorest communities in a cost-effective manner with relatively little investment. In fact, wealthier nations have arguably created greater, more insurmountable obstacles to inclusion because of their relatively vast material resources. In the South, by contrast, the rehabilitation and special needs industry is much smaller and less powerful and human resources can be harnessed to bring about inclusion. Here, implementation of inclusive education may simply involve the positive reinforcement of a well-established community, based on inclusive attitudes and practices. Tapping existing resources such as the efforts of civil society and working with the community are valuable resources for advancing one's beliefs.
- Inclusive education is not just a recipe for the rich affluent countries of the Northern hemisphere. Inclusion is not about funds… it's about ideology, it's changing one's own mind-sets, it's about evolution and a process of change in attitude and lack of funding should not mean certain children are segregated.

The Way Forward

There has been undoubtedly a quantum leap. The educational needs of children with CP and other disabilities have been noted. Inclusive education has taken centre stage.

The RTE has been a landmark legislation. It is imperative to ensure it does not remain another piece of legislation gathering dust, but is put into action. However, the challenges are huge, when we think of an approximate figure of 51 per cent of children with disabilities (CWDs) being illiterate, with no schools to go to. If the RTE is to be operationalized and not merely remain a document collecting dust, clearly reforms are urgently needed.

Given below are some recommendations for the way forward.

Mapping

Robust data about the whereabouts of children with special needs is still not available; there is a startling discrepancy between existing data and ground-level findings. There is a need for *disaggregated data of CWDs* in order to facilitate micro planning for educational and health supports for CWDs in their jurisdictions. This will determine what needs to be contained within local resource support organizations and it is only through this process that CWD can be supported for their identified needs.

Identifying children with disabilities using survey and screening instruments is not an easy task. Some previous efforts in developing countries have had some measure of success. Building on that knowledge United Nations Children's Fund (UNICEF) and the UN Statistical Commission's Group on Disability Statistics have developed a new approach. The new tool for identifying and screening of childhood disability is the international standard for monitoring childhood disability. This is now being called by UNICEF Multiple Indicator Cluster Survey (MICS). It should be adopted as it has been tested in 15 countries.[2]

Intervention

SSI's Shiksha Sankalp model of mapping could be incorporated as a best practice model with its various activities on the district level through the setting up of a Hub framework that flows from district level down to the block, cluster and school levels to the class where the child is located. The Inclusive Education District Hub (IEDH), known as the Hub, will maintain information, identify the needs of the children and connect them to existing schools. As per the rules of the RTE, it will synergise the different agencies. Setting up of such a Hub has been included in the guidelines for implementation of RTE. Sarva Shiksha Abhiyan (SSA) has agreed that their existing block and district resource centres (BRCs and DRCs) need to be upgraded to IEDH.

The Cluster Resource Centres (CRCs) and DRCS exist only on paper for the multiply disabled population as they are at distances that are impossible for parents of physically disabled children or adults to walk to. The *needs of the child with disability are not identified. Only the* children with the most obvious disability are being identified.

Teacher Preparation

Education for all cannot happen without inclusive education. The training of regular teachers is imperative. By understanding that changes in teaching methods can make the curriculum accessible to all children, including those with disabilities, a teacher or principal is well on the way to improving the overall quality of their school.

The government's teacher training courses also need to be upgraded. All schools, private and government need to make the RTE operational and synthesize it with the existing government programme of SSA and NCTE as well as programmes being run by NCERT, University Grants Commission (UGC), Indira Gandhi National Open University (IGNOU) and the central universities to make RTE a reality.

The need of the hour is preparing teachers, transformation of schools, changing role of teachers, redesigning syllabi. Without this RTE would fail to bring justice to children who have suffered exclusion and neglect for years (Alur 2012).

Health Services

The health system, too, needs to be improved. Health and educational services need to be synchronized. Medical and paramedical courses still do not provide the necessary training on how to deal with CP. Special modules and courses for doctors need to be added to the syllabi.

---

[2] A report on a study on this by Dan Mont and Sathi Alur has been accepted as part of best recommended practices of UNICEF, New York, in the World Bank. It has also been included in the Q Bank of the National Centre for Health Statistics, US government.

Monitoring and Evaluation

It is critical to ensure that rigorous monitoring and evaluation of projects are done to ensure the targeted beneficiaries are able to access good quality basic education.

Women and Child Development Schemes

The ministry of women and child development runs the largest preschool programme, the Integrated Child Development Scheme (ICDS), but still excludes children with disability by not specifically including them in its definitions of target groups. The ICDS needs to fall in line with what is now law in the country and their training programmes of *anganwadi* workers need to include modules about identifying and teaching special needs children.

Interdepartmental and Interministerial Convergence

There is a need to dovetail the activities of various ministries, departments and the Centre and states so as to achieve uniformity across the country and reduce duplication of effort that would result in greater efficiencies and achieve better results. Figure 10.1, below, represents the interministerial convergence for inclusive education.

The procedure for transformation has begun but an Interministerial Convergence of the Ministries is recommended with a regular evaluation of whether this is being implemented or not.

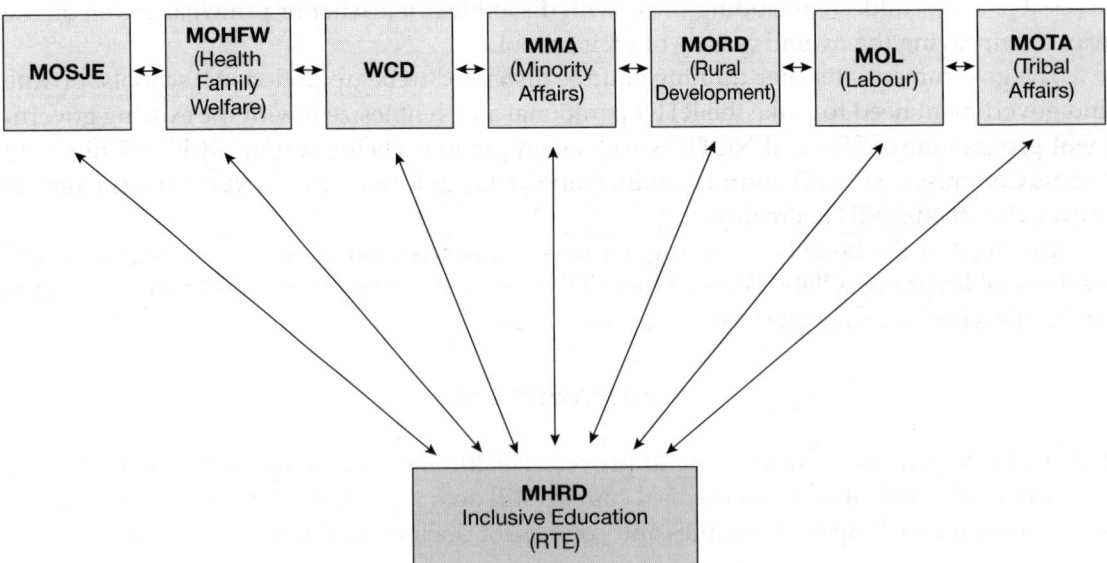

Figure 10.1. Interministerial Convergence for Inclusive Education

Source: Author.

c. Reflections, Discussion and the Way Forward

Among the most important and unique achievements was moving a chronic disability like CP away from dreary hospitals to a special school model and providing a social setting where the children received social, emotional, therapeutic and academic support. We were able to humanize a group of people who were earlier neglected or patronized or sometimes treated as morons and idiots. Certainly, they were grossly misunderstood. Through our models of intervention, we showed that they are individuals with potential and ability. Today, they have passed out and become computer analysts, accountants, authors and lawyers; some have done their PhDs. They now have the dignity they deserve, despite being different.

When SSI started in 1972, physiotherapy, occupational therapy or speech therapy was a specialization known only to these experts. Children were more of a 'diagnosis' to be discussed amongst colleagues. As reported in this study, a leading doctor in Bombay said 'Parents are patients and you cannot share their file with them—they do not understand.' We changed that and ensured that parents, rich or poor, got the status they deserved! Discussion and conversation with the parents was non-existent. From 1972, a strong focus on parents as an important member of the team was given.

SSI introduced the concept that expertise and specialist knowledge is certainly necessary to achieve the desired progress, but should be provided in a humane and compassionate manner. The interdisciplinary team kept in mind that in the early days, our patient who is an infant is not aware of what has happened to him or her. It is the parents who are caught in a quagmire of trauma. Their grief, their bewilderment and confusion about what is going to happen to their child, became their primary concern. The concept of explaining to the parent why a certain exercise or activity was being done, or what was the purpose of doing it, gave them the knowledge they needed to get empowered. In addition to managing their children at home appropriately, parents were encouraged to become professionals and help as teachers, therapists, sometimes becoming principals of schools and occupying management positions. Our close work with the families kept the work on the ground level with a bottom-up approach.

The methods used for preparation of parents paved the way for another new model for empowered parents to take up the cause of their own children in regular schools. No middle person was needed to speak for them. Parents took over the ownership of ensuring that their child settled into a regular school and directly worked with principals and teachers in regular schools. *A cost-effective model of inclusion* emerged which has been documented as a good code of practice for successful inclusion to happen in developing countries. This new cost-effective method has been applauded by colleagues internationally. To create that empowered and confident parent took 40 years!

'Segregation dehumanizes' writes Chib (excerpt from speech given in 2009).

With the RTE happening, we have been able to demolish a few myths; the myth that only special schools are appropriate for children with disability, the myth that it needs vast resources for inclusion to happen and that there are vast numbers of disabled children hidden out there waiting to consume all the resources. The truth is that inclusion is not about money but ideology. Inclusion is the challenge of addressing differences and diversity. Mindsets and attitudes need to be more inclusive.

What we were able to do has been well expressed by a Nobel Laureate of India, Rabindranath Tagore, who said,

> 'the problem is not how to wipe out the differences but how to unite with the differences intact.'

Demonstrating special educational practice, inclusive education on the ground level gave all the practical infrastructural knowledge that needs to be done for services to spread and the special child's needs to be understood.

To conclude I would say simply *what worked* is that policies and *practices needed to have a bottom-up, top-down approach*. Fortunately, now, there are legislations and constitutional instruments in place. *Engaging with government at top levels was important.*

Inclusion has to be context- and culture-specific. The ideology of inclusion and the methods to achieve it is differs with each situation and each country. It is not necessary to transfer Northern paradigms and take them out of context as we have done during the colonial and the postcolonial period... *inclusive education clearly needs to be context- and culture-specific to each country.*

What the children taught us through all their struggles, was about their courage, their grit their determination to succeed, given little modifications and the important question ... who is disabled? *Is it them who may see, walk, think, move differently ... or is it us who cannot understand differences, who cannot see or hear them?* (Alur 2009)

d. Ideology and Philosophy

Gandhiji said: 'A small body of determined spirits fired by an unquenchable faith in their mission can alter the course of history.'

This the organization endeavoured to do, during 45 years, by creating a civil society movement built on the bedrock of social justice and human rights.

It may be years before India's disabled are fully accepted as citizens with their own rights and needs. However, we have brought the handicapped out of institutions, hospitals, bedrooms and slums and humanized them, shown them as people...people who can think, laugh, cry, who feel sorrow, pain and above all joy—just like you and me (an excerpt from Dr Alur's speech in 1976).

An important lesson, in our philosophy of service and professionalism, is that it is crucial to make the disabled person, however rich or poor, feel emotionally and socially strong. They will always need determination, grit and moral stamina, to face up to the lifelong battle of having a handicap, a lifelong suffering. Human suffering needs a large dose of nurturing through love and care to build up self-confidence and to rise up to the struggle for better understanding. Emotion is essential in the rehabilitation process and, most important, is a humane contact between patient and specialist.

Our journey has been not for money, not for personal power, not for personal prestige, but purely for the spirit of service... and a belief in what all scriptures say that *the right is to work only and not to the fruits.* As a sage has said, 'all religion is only true if it is religion in action, real feelings of love are of value, if it is translated into some form of action' and as the great thinker and philosopher Albert Schweitzer has said:

> That everyone shall exert himself in that state of life in which he is placed, to practise true humanity towards his fellowmen, on that depends the future of mankind.

The overall idea has been for us the bigger goal… for building a caring nation…an India that cares for its *needy, the helpless, the poor and the disabled.* Suffering, social injustice has no territorial barriers. To create a*n India that celebrates diversity and includes all excluded and margin-alized people, moving towards equal opportunity and equal participation as Tagore writes in his poem* 'Where the mind is without fear… into that heaven of freedom let my country awake'.

Inclusion challenges our own value systems of tolerance. In a subcontinent as large as India, with so many issues that inundate one, working in an area of darkness in virgin territory, *one needs detachment* and a large dose of tolerance. One also must be ready to walk alone…. 'Ekla Challo Re' as Tagore says: to fall, to bleed but to pick oneself up and walk on. There has to be the grit to survive … to serve beyond personal wealth, personal ambition, personal power … *but for the good of the country* … we hope we can continue to serve in the right spirit (Alur 2010b).

I sincerely hope that this book will be a beacon of hope and have a message for the new pioneers of tomorrow, showing the way, that many more children, who are neglected and even locked away in the far-flung areas of our country, and other countries, will get their needs recognized and be included into our lives and that many more parents will wipe away their tears and be encouraged to have faith and belief that 'all is not lost' when a child with CP is born in their family.

Mithu Alur, 2015

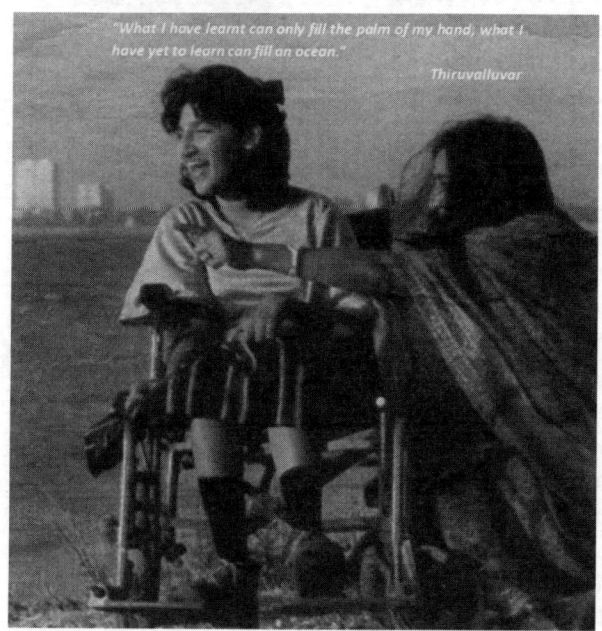

"What I have learnt can only fill the palm of my hand; what I have yet to learn can fill an ocean."

Thiruvalluvar

> A relationship between a normal and a disabled person should be like all other relationships – based upon mutual respect rather than pity. I move away when it is the latter. Life is a challenge – there are many mountains to climb. But for me the most important thing is to climb it with a smile.
>
> —*Malini Chib*

Annexure I

Developing a Code of Practice for Inclusive Education; Culturally Appropriate Policy and Practice (CAPP)

CAPP I (Alur and Bach 2005b) works on a macro level of policy, legislation, formulation and implementation that will work on a state, national and global levels. This is *the whole policy approach*. It is targeted at policymakers and administrators, teachers, educators and civil society, which includes non-governmental organizations (NGOs) working in the field of disability and education, teacher unions and human rights organizations and provides strategies that will aid teacher educators to train teachers implementing inclusive education practices.

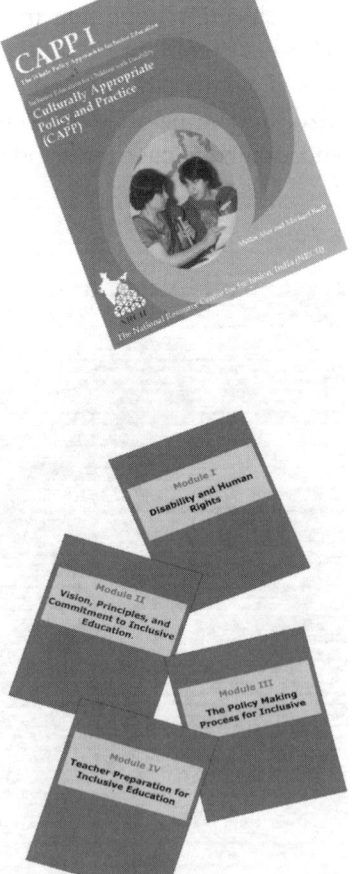

Module 1—Disability and Human Rights. The objectives of this module are to introduce participants to the following concepts and ideas: the global demographics of disability and education; the history of oppression of the disabled and the disability rights movement; the shift from a medical model to a social and human rights model; and international human rights and policy commitments to inclusion.

Module II—Vision, Principles, and Commitment to Inclusive Education. This module introduces participants to a broad framework for understanding inclusive education. It describes the vision, principles and commitments on which public policy, teacher training and civil society activism for quality education for people with disabilities is based.

Module III—Policymaking Process for Inclusive Education. This module is designed for policymakers involved in making decisions that affect the education and educational status of students with disabilities.

Module IV—Teacher Preparation for Inclusive Education. The objective of this module is to reiterate the philosophy, the key principles of inclusion and to introduce the participants to the following units: multiple intelligence, differentiation of needs and curriculum, changing roles of teachers and students and teaching strategies to facilitate inclusion.

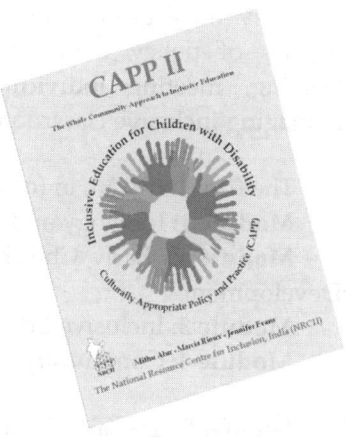

Inclusive education is about commitment—it is about a change of attitudes and it is about excellent teaching. The CAPP hopes to provide ways and means for achieving this. It is the first step towards a just, humane and equal society (Alur and Timmons (2009).

CAPP II (Alur, Rioux and Evans 2005) works on a mezzo level of community, workers, local administrators and bureaucrats. This is *the whole community approach*. It consists of 16 manuals and 4 flip charts targeted at training for teaching at the preschool level. CAPP II was bought by the Ministry of Human Resources Development (MHRD) for their training programmes in various states.

The manuals have been written on four levels.

Level 1 (LI PM) is for policymakers, academics, administrators and non-governmental agencies. They are the people who formulate policies and programmes. They explain the 'why' of inclusion and details about the available guide and manuals.

Level 2 (L2 P) deals with professionals who have a substantial degree of knowledge in areas of disability, health and education, have working experience and are able to train others in their field with the guide and manuals. This resource will also be appropriate for senior health and education officers, and NGOs in the field.

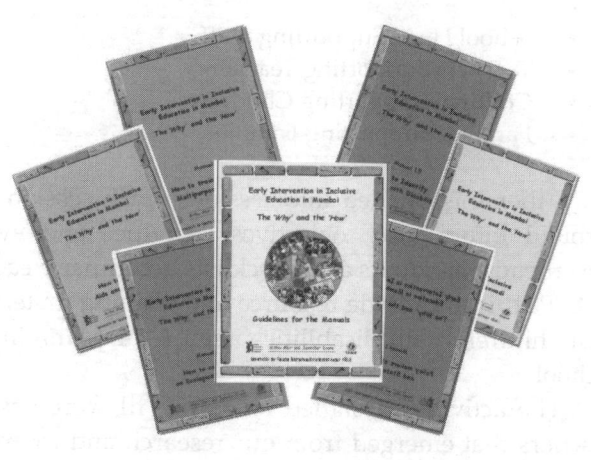

Level 3 (L3 MT) is for master trainers or those who will go into the community to teach *anganwadi* workers, parents and other members of the community how to handle the child with disability.

Level 4 (L4 AMW) is for *anganwadi* multipurpose workers who deal with the capacity training of community *anganwadi* workers who will be actually involved with the day-to-day handling of children with disability.

Source: Alur, M., Rioux, M. and Evans, J. 2005. *Capp II: Culturally Appropriate Policy and Practice II: The Whole Community Approach to Inclusion*. Mumbai: National Resource Centre for Inclusion.

They have been grouped in six basic themes of policy, community, education, training, meeting individual needs and managing inclusive classrooms.

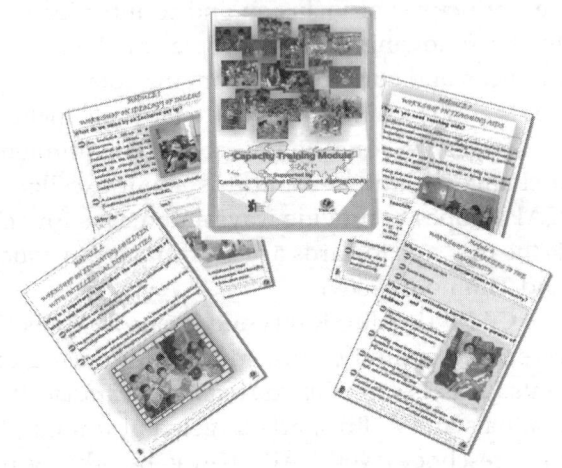

The flip charts are in four modules:
Module 1: Ideology and Philosophy
Module 2: Early Childhood Care and Development
Module 3: Inclusive Educational Inputs
Module 4: Community

Jennifer Evans said, 'Include parents and the community members, because it's only if parents and the community members and professionals work together that they can have a truly holistic service, which will then support the inclusion of all children within an inclusive school' (Alur and Bach 2005).

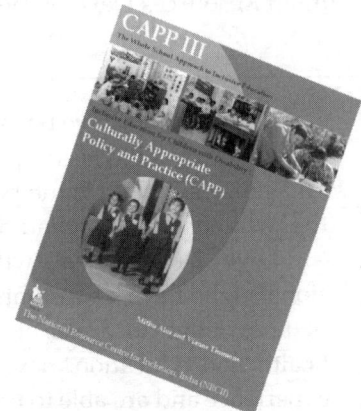

CAPP III (Alur and Timmons 2005) works on a micro level of classroom and school values and culture/policies/ practice. This is *the whole school approach*.

It has four major units:

- School Head Supporting Staff
- Teachers Supporting Teacher
- Children Supporting Children
- Families Supporting Families

Each theme is divided into sessions. Each session has background information, objectives, activities and evaluations. Overheads, handouts and checklists accompany each section. CAPP III is to provide resource and training material to help put children, with disabilities aged 6–14 years, into regular school.

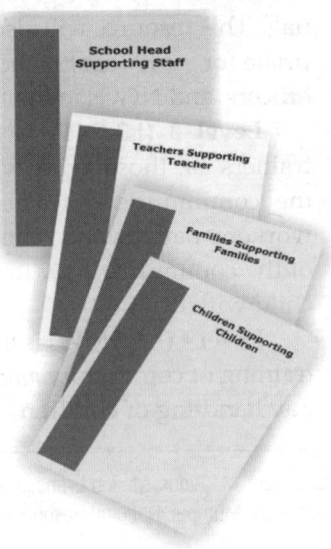

The activities designed for CAPP III were based on the barriers that emerged from our research and examination of key factors. They are designed to enable the stakeholders to create their own solutions through brainstorming and sharing of successful stories of inclusion and were based on actual situations that the researchers identified and for which, as an Inclusive Education Coordinating Committee (IECC) team, they helped develop proactive responses.

We found it was key to get principals, as school heads and as primary stakeholders, to take leadership in effecting changes in the mainstream school system. The unit on school heads explains what inclusion is and emphasizes the importance of treating children with disabilities as full members of the school, working with families, providing adequate support to teachers, working in a collaborative way and demonstrating by example.

The unit on 'Teachers Supporting Teachers' includes training sessions on understanding inclusive education and creating a child-centred curriculum; welcoming the child and full participation; enabling families and involving parents; working in collaboration with other teachers and professionals; and creating an inclusive environment. Case studies of successful inclusion are shared and give ideas about possible solutions to commonly faced barriers. Common guidelines to be used for teaching various disabilities are also included.

'Children Supporting Children' includes sessions on how to welcome a new classmate and how to work together. This unit includes activities to increase children's understanding of different disabilities in a caring and compassionate way and to promote interactive teaching and learning. Suggestions for encouraging peer support and buddy systems are also presented.

The 'Families Supporting Families' unit includes modules that help explain to parents what inclusion is and to encourage them to express fears and hopes about inclusive education. It provides guides to sessions on introducing inclusive education; involving families and supporting each child; preparing the child; parents as advocates; communicating with the teacher; and forming support groups.

CAPP III concludes with 'Tips for teaching all children' with specific reference to children with hearing impairment, Attention Deficit Hyperactivity Disorder (ADHD), Down Syndrome, autism, visual impairment, reading challenges, learning challenges and cerebral palsy (CP).

This infrastructure has to be in place to begin inclusive education.

It is necessary for school leaders to be informed about the best practices in inclusive education and encourage staff to adopt the principles and practices. Inclusive education needs to be on the school agenda. The culture of the school needs changing. The 're-culturation' of the whole school environment leads to a whole school approach. CAPP III outlines the whole school approach to education and is targeted at the 6–14 years age group (Alur and Timmons 2005).

Annexure II

Organizational Structure: People Behind the Scenes

The Governing Body

The management style of functioning: Board members of the organization always have been grass-roots workers and professionals. Most of the present board members are working trustees and co-opted members who are very closely involved in the planning, implementation and monitoring of the organization on a day-to-day basis. The tradition of the board's close involvement in both the micro level functioning of the organization and macro level planning continues till date. The board of trustees meets as often as required.

Managing trustee and founder chairperson, Mithu Alur; vice chairperson, Kamal Bakshi; trustee, Sitanshu Mehta; joint honorary secretary and acting CEO, Malini Chib; Parliamentarian and trustee, Priya Dutt Roncon; honorary treasurer, Nikhil Chib; trustee and acting CEO, Varsha Hooja; members, governing body, Ami Gumashta, Deepak Kalra, Vishal Bakshi, Aslesha Gowarikar, Nikhil Dhanrajgir and Jayabrato Chatterjee.

The Institutional Review Board (IRB)

There is an Institutional Review Board (IRB) as referred to earlier which serves as an independent representative and competent body to review, evaluate and decide on the scientific and ethical merits of research. The primary purpose of this committee is to protect the rights, safety and well-being of human subjects who participate in a research project. The IRB is entrusted with the initial review of the proposed research protocols, prior to initiation of the projects, and also have a continuing responsibility of regular monitoring of the approved programmes till their completion. The board ensures a critical review of all ethical aspects of the proposals and is free from any bias and influence that could affect objectivity. It also checks the scientific soundness of the proposed research projects and advises researchers on evaluation and technical excellence of the study.

Dr Samiran Nundy, Chairperson; Dr Farokh Udwadia, co-chairperson; Dr Surajit Nundy, Dr Mithu Alur, Dr Armida Fernandez, Dr Anaita Hegde, Professor Zenobia Nadirshaw, Dr Anuradha Sovani, Ms Malini Chib; action research team, Mrs Varsha Hooja, Dr Shabnam Rangwala, Ms Sangeeta Jagtiani, Mrs Deepshikha Mathur, Mrs Shobha Sachdev, and Mrs Gulab Sayyed.

The Board of Advisors

In addition to the board of trustees, governing body and IRB, a board of advisors has been constituted of eminent personalities who lend their presence from time to time throughout the year for public events, conferences and meetings of importance.

Mr Shyam Benegal, Mr V. Ranganathan, Mrs Vera Udwadia, Mr Arup Patnaik, Mr Nagesh Kukunoor, Ms Dia Mirza and Ms Shonali Bose are members of the board.

Reflections and Reminiscences

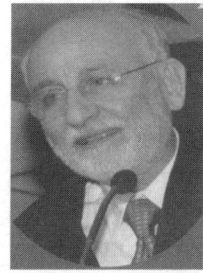

Mr Kamal Bakshi, former Indian ambassador and vice chairperson, governing body, Able Disabled All People Together (ADAPT).

'Reporting on the railway budget on February 27, a national newspaper highlighted some "disabled-friendly" items. Earlier, this paper had prominently published a photograph of differently abled artistes. Forty years ago, could one have seen one such item even once a year? If we were to credit ADAPT with only one achievement after four decades of dedicated work, against all odds, indifference and hostility, it is this: our country has become aware of the existence of our citizens with disability and their rights. ADAPT has achieved this in cooperation with many others; but, more importantly, it has been achieved as our successful struggle to include children with disability within the ambit of the Right to Education (RTE) Act is now heard. We will continue our struggle for a disability friendly India until the country recognizes the contribution that the differently abled can potentially make to our progress, prosperity and peace!'

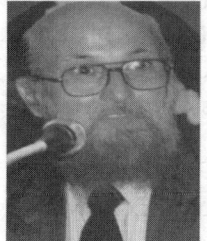

Professor Sitanshu Y. Mehta, poet, critic, Fulbright scholar, recipient of Padma Shri and trustee

'As parents and workers associated with ADAPT for more than three decades, my wife Anjani and I have witnessed, worked for and greatly benefited by the pioneering and peerless work at ADAPT, so ably and insightfully led by Dr Mithu Alur and carried out with such expertise and dedication by her extraordinary team of teachers, therapists, administrators and financial managers. ADAPT enhances not only the cause of the physically challenged but also, in its, unique, idealist-practical way, the entire Indian society and our sense of being human.'

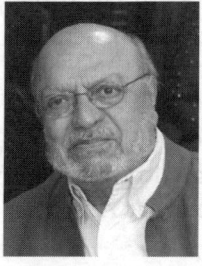

Mr Shyam Benegal, ex-Rajya Sabha member, eminent film director, recipient of national and international awards and recipient of Padma Bhushan and member of the board of advisors

'To make disabled children able to cope, compete, function and excel in the hurly burly of everyday life is perhaps among the most difficult challenge to meet. ADAPT, headed by Dr Mithu Alur and her dedicated team, is fully committed to meet this challenge. Each day, everyday.'

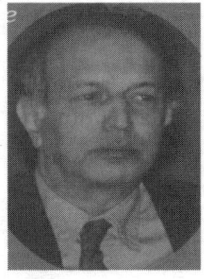

Dr Samiran Nundy, surgeon and Emeritus Professor, Department of Surgical Gastroenterology and Liver Transplantation, Sir Ganga Ram Hospital, recipient of Padma Shri and chairman, IRB

'I am proud to have witnessed the birth, growth and development of such a magnificent institution as ADAPT. The birth was when Malini and her family came to stay with us for a few months in Cambridge where she attended the Roger Ascham School, later moving to Cheyne Walk in London. Mithu then resolved to set up a similar institution in India to not only provide therapy but also a formal education to the physically challenged. Starting from the Colaba school, "Spastics Societies" have now been started all over the country. I, of course, have a major conflicting interest when I write all this laudatory stuff. Not only am I Malini's uncle and Mithu's brother-in-law, my wife started the Spastics Society of Northern India (SSNI) and my mum banged tunelessly on the piano in the mornings for the long suffering students and staff of the Spastics Society of Eastern India (SSEI) in Calcutta. She said those were the happiest years of her life. As the present chairman of the IRB, I now want to see the history of these 40 years properly assembled and chronicled into one large, fat book with plenty of pictures. My colleague on the IRB, Dr Farokh Udwadia and I have promised to help get it published so that the world will know what a fine and worthwhile journey it has been.'

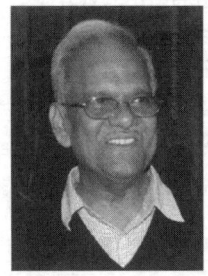

Mr Sathi Alur, is lead consultant on mapping for the World Bank. He has served in an advisory capacity to various UN agencies and international governments as well as The Spastics Society of India (SSI) for many years. As honorary financial advisor to ADAPT, he has guided the budget planning exercises and suggested innovative administrative and financial reforms. In recent years, he has provided valuable inputs to the government in areas of legislation, national policy, economics and health. A visionary, he had the far-sightedness to create the First Five Year Plan. He moved the organization to the idea of sustainability making all financial system transparent and exposed the society to more than five governments on the international front.

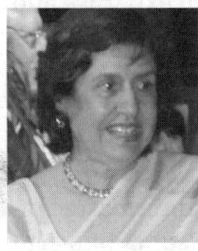 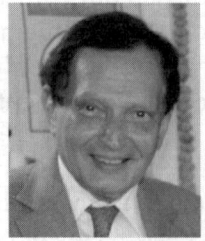

Mrs Vera Udwadia, member of the board of advisors ADAPT and Dr Farokh Udwadia, recipient of the Padma Bhushan, consultant physician, Breach Candy Hospital and member of IRB ethics committee.

'Forty years ago, Dr Mithu Alur had a mission and a dream to start an institute like ADAPT. Today, it has borne fruit and she manages three excellent schools in Mumbai for disabled children. The first thing that strikes a visitor to the ADAPT schools is how dedicated, kind and cheerful all the teachers and therapists are and how affectionate and happy the children look. In fact, these children probably spend the happiest hours of their day at the school where they not only study but play, swim, listen to music, paint and do pottery. One can learn so much from them. Dr Alur and

Malini need to be congratulated for bringing sunshine into the lives of those who are fortunate enough to attend such a happy school. She has also succeeded in making the lives of their anxious parents easier by giving them hope in a country where so much more needs to be done for the handicapped. ADAPT is also to be congratulated for doing and publishing research on the various aspects of disability through workshops and conferences.'

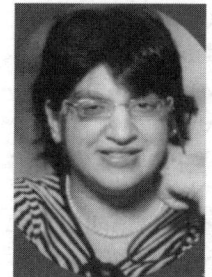

Ms Malini Chib, co-CEO and trustee, ADAPT, founder chairperson, ADAPT Rights Group (ARG) and recipient of many national awards

'Today, I reflect on 40 years of ADAPT. When we came back from England, disabled people were non-entities. We were considered vegetables. Seeing my mother's distress at me not being accepted by India, my father Ranjit Chib urged to set up a small school. I think both my parents didn't imagine the need and demand for services for disabled people. Parents flocked to the centre in Colaba as if it was nectar. The founding of the school has been a landmark in the country. I think the organization could not have grown without the vision of both Sathi, my mother and Pam.... Today, we have done our BAs and MAs and hold jobs and are wage earners. Indeed, we have come a long way from being called "plastics" and recipients of charity. My vision for the next 40 years is to see more disabled people leading "normal lives". I hope we can access transports and pavements. We must fight for our rights as citizens of India.'

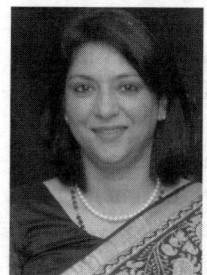

Mrs Priya Dutt Roncon, Honorable Member of Parliament (Lok Sabha). Trustee, ADAPT and Nargis Dutt Foundation for Cancer.

'My sincere appreciation to the children for teaching me more about life, love and laughter. I believe life is a beautiful journey for those who bring about a positive change in the lives of others. As I look back, I can't help but be thankful for all the wonderful memories. For the past 40 years, the organization has been encouraging and empowering children with disabilities to live meaningful lives. Many lives have been made beautiful because of your dedication and passion. Your aim to create an inclusive disability-friendly nation has my full support. My parents, Nargis and Sunil Dutt, were both patrons and I am only humbled to carry their legacy forward. My journey with ADAPT has been a beautiful and meaningful one.'

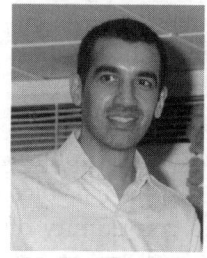

Nikhil Chib, economist and entrepreneur, Honorary Treasurer, ADAPT

'We managed to touch the hearts and lives of many and continue to do so. From the children to the teachers, all I see is happiness, love and commitment. These are necessary ingredients to life and you are an inspiration to the world outside. Well done! The battle is not over. Today, the corporate social responsibilities (CSR) policies of companies do not include disability as one of their issues. We need to move to skills development and employment. The challenge ahead to include all our disabled people is great and we should continue to work hard.'

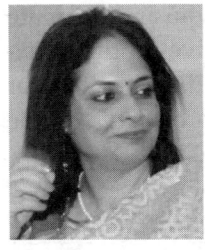

Mrs Varsha Hooja, CEO and trustee, ADAPT

'The Buddha has said, "Thousands of candles can be lighted from a single candle and the life of the candle will not be shortened. Happiness never decreases by being shared." ADAPT has been one such a candle and it has been a privilege and honour to have been a part of this incredibly enriching journey that began with the birth of Malini (who is today a successful author and lecturer and an inspiration for all of us) and led to the setting up of the first ever special school for children with multiple disability; a model that spread services across the nation and led to a movement that is now working tirelessly towards ensuring that every child is able to avail of her/his right to education. Synonymous with ADAPT has been its creator Dr Mithu Alur or Mithudi, as she is known who has had the courage to critique her own highly successful model of special education and then move away to establish another paradigm, that of inclusive education, expanding the concept to include all marginalized groups. History will look back at these 40 years and fondly record how she has transformed the lives of not just persons with disability but also their families, many of whom have found their dignity and self-respect because they have been supported to stand on their own feet and write their own future.'

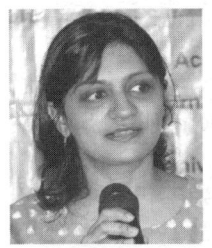

Mrs Ami Gumashta, honorary director, finance and member, governing body, ADAPT

'MEMORIES...MOMENTS...MILESTONES make this journey. A path-breaking journey of 40 years. A journey started by a mother drawing inspiration from her daughter. Today they are both trailblazers in their own right, who have borne the torch strongly with passion and commitment, with sincerity and loyalty and with sensitivity and love. Their spirit is unmatchable, bringing a special light into the lives of many and making a difference to this nation. I am only one of those many whose lives have been touched and it has been a pleasure to be a part of this 40 year journey and to support it. I have grown with Mithudi, Mr Alur and Molly over the last 18 years. The journey has been inspirational, empowering and a learning process. The nurturing has drawn the best out of me, making me a strong individual in my own right. They are my mentors in the true spirit of the word and today as I stand proud with them, I acknowledge with humility that I am honoured with the respect they give me and the trust and faith they have in me. I cherish the energy which flows here, the emotions and the spirituality which makes ALL the difference and makes our lives special.'

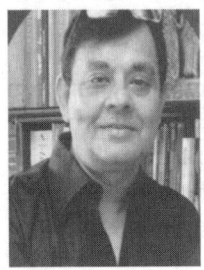

Mr Jayabrato Chatterjee, writer, film-maker, corporate communicator and member, governing body, ADAPT

'Forty years! It has been a long journey indeed; a journey that pioneered the disability movement in India; a journey that was arduous but fought relentlessly by Mithudi and her dedicated team; a journey that gave a voice to the voiceless, to the physically and mentally challenged community of our country, to the poorest of the poor and to the weakest and downtrodden sections of our society. Today, as Mithudi walks on in her sojourn to make inclusive education the right of every child in India, it is time to applaud her selfless work and salute the savant in her. She looks frail but has a will of steel. She seamlessly combines in her the artiste and the administrator. That, perhaps, is the greatest lesson we need to learn from Mithudi and her stupendous work.'

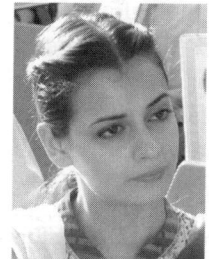

Ms Dia Mirza, celebrated film actress and producer, social activist and member of the board of advisors

'No society can possibly be healthy if it does not believe in being inclusive. This is our chance to celebrate an inclusive society. Give all those that have been forced into the shadows by generations of ignorance a chance to come out and shine! These little stars can and will sparkle. All we need to do is embrace them and their cause of being a *part of us* not *apart from us.*'

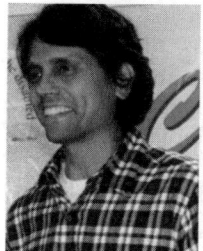

Mr Nagesh Kukunoor, well-known film director and producer, social activist and member of the board of advisors

'ADAPT is my family. Over the years of my association, I've been constantly humbled by their commitment to make India a better place for the disabled. Way to go ADAPT!'

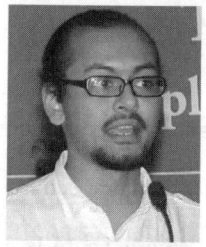

Mr Satyen Bordoloi, writer, journalist, film-maker and social activist

'The beginning 'small step', made with only 3 children in one small house, today has helped millions of children and adults with disability gain services that are available in almost every state of the nation. The time is indeed ripe to go from one small step to many, many giant leaps of inclusion in the next 40 years.'

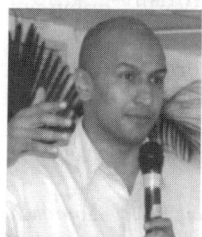

Dr Surajit Nundy, Fellow at the Center of Brain Science at Harvard University and member of IRB ethics committee, ADAPT

'If one said that the only achievements of ADAPT were that it had pioneered over 40 years the creation of services, training programmes, rehabilitation, research and education for the disabled, that would be enough to ensure ADAPT's place as one of the truly remarkable institutions of India. But to say only that would be to ignore, perhaps, ADAPT's greatest achievement—that it has inexorably annihilated our blindness to that integral part of all of us, our disabled citizens, and, thus, made us whole.'

Bibliography

ADAPT (Able Disabled All People Together). 1973–2013. *Annual Reports of the Four Decades*, ADAPT, formerly The Spastics Society of India, Mumbai.

Alur, M. 1978. 'The Multi-disciplinary Approach to Cerebral Palsy'. Paper read at ICPS International Conference, Riyadh, Saudi Arabia.

Alur, M., ed. 1982. *It's Ability That Counts*. Mumbai: The Spastics Society of India.

Alur, M. 1988. 'Comprehensive Services for Cerebral Palsied Children in India, with Bombay as a Model of the First Program Created'. Paper presented at the 16th World Conference on Rehabilitation, Japan.

Alur, M. 1989. 'A Model in Employment and Vocational Rehabilitation Services in India'. A brochure printed by the National Job Development Centre, available in the library.

Alur, M. 1998. *Invisible Children: A Study of Policy Exclusion*. Thesis submitted for the degree of Doctor of Philosophy, Institute of Education, University of London.

Alur, M. 2000. 'They Did Not Figure: Policy Exclusion of Disabled People in India'. Paper presented at the International Special Education Congress 2000, Manchester, subsequently published in 2002 in the *International Journal on Inclusive Education* 6(2): 101–12.

Alur, M. 2002. 'Status of Disabled People in India—Policy and Inclusion'. *Exceptionality Education Canada* 12(2–3): 137–68.

Alur, M. 2003. *Invisible Children: A Study of Policy Exclusion*. New Delhi: Viva Books.

Alur, M. 2007. 'Inclusive Education: The Challenge for India'. Paper presented at the Institute of Education (IOE), London.

Alur, M. 2009. 'A New Inclusive Model of Care and Rehabilitation: A Spastics Society of India Perspective'. Paper presented at the Birth Defects Conference, New Delhi.

Alur, M. 2010a, August. 'From One to a Million—Developing Sustainable Services Where There Is a Systemic Failure and Moving Towards Education for All'. Paper presented at the World Conference on Inclusive and Supportive Education Congress (ISEC) 2010, Queen's University, Belfast.

Alur, M. 2010b. 'Family Perspectives: Parents in Partnership'. In *Confronting Obstacles to Inclusion: International Responses to Developing Inclusive Education*, edited by Richard Rose, 61–73. London: A David Fulton Book.

Alur, M. 2012. 'Huge Learning Curve Ahead'. *The Indian Express*, 21 June.

Alur, M., and M. Bach. 2005a. *Inclusive Education: From Rhetoric to Reality—The North South Dialogue II*. New Delhi: Viva Books.

Alur, M., and M. Bach. 2005b. *CAPP I: Culturally Appropriate Policy and Practice: The Whole Policy Approach*. Mumbai: National Resource Centre for Inclusion, Mumbai.

Alur, M., and M. Bach. 2010. *The Journey for Inclusive Education in the Indian Sub-Continent*. New York: Routledge.

Alur, M., and M. Rioux. 2003. *Included: An Exploration of Six Early Pilot Projects for Children with Disabilities in India*. New York: UNICEF.

Alur, M., M. Rioux, and J. Evans. 2005. *CAPP II: Culturally Appropriate Policy and Practice II: The Whole Community Approach to Inclusion*. Mumbai: National Resource Centre for Inclusion.

Alur, M., and P. Natarajan. 2000. *Developing Sustainable Educational Inclusion Policy and Practice: UK, South Africa, Brazil and India: Final Report*. Mumbai: The Spastics Society of India, National Resource Centre for Inclusion.

Alur, M., and T. Booth, eds. 2005. *Inclusive Education: Proceedings of North South Dialogue I*. New Delhi: UBSPD.

Alur, M., and V. Timmons. 2005. *CAPP III: Culturally Appropriate Policy and Practice III: The Whole School Approach*. Mumbai: National Resource Centre for Inclusion.

Alur, M., and V. Timmons, eds. 2009. *Inclusive Education across Cultures: Crossing Boundaries, Sharing Ideas*. New Delhi: SAGE Publications.

Alur, S. 2012. *Report of Cognitive Research on Proposed Survey Questions for Identifying Out-of-School Children with Disabilities in India*. Mumbai: ADAPT formerly The Spastics Society of India.

Armstrong, F., and M. Moore, eds. 2004. *Action Research for Inclusive Education: Changing Places, Changing Practice, Changing Minds*. London: Routledge Falmer.

Barton, L. 1989. 'Disability and Dependency'. In *Disability, Handicap and Life Chances Series*. New York: Routledge.

Barton, L., and F. Armstrong, eds. 2007. *Policy, Experience and Change: Cross Cultural Reflections on Inclusive Education*. Dordrecht: Springer.

Barton, L., and S. Tomlinson, eds. 1984. *Special Education and Social Interests*. London: Croom Helm.

Barnes, C., I. Bynoe, and M. Oliver. 1990. *Equal Rights for Disabled People: The Case for a New Law*. London: Hurst & Co.

Baher, E. 1975. *Parents Views*. Mumbai: The Spastics Society of India.

Billimoria, R., and S. Krishnaswamy. 1986. *Prevalence of Disabilities among Children in Mumbai*. Mumbai: The Spastics Society of India.

Booth, T. 2009. 'Keeping the Future Alive—Maintaining Inclusive Values in Education and Society'. In *Inclusive Education Across Cultures: Crossing Boundaries, Sharing Ideas*, edited by Mithu Alur and Vianne Timmons, 121–34. New Delhi: SAGE Publications.

Booth, T., and M. Ainscow. 1998. *From Them to Us: An International Study of Inclusion in Education*. London and New York: Routledge.

Booth, T., and P. Potts. 1983. *Integrating Special Education*. Oxford: Blackwell.

Bordoloi, S. 2004. 'Psychological Support in Events of Mass Destruction: Challenges and Lessons'. *Economic and Political Weekly*, May 22, 2121–27.

Bose-Sethi, Junie. 1987. *Reach of Services of The Spastics Society of India: Its Affiliates & Branches* (in-house publication). Mumbai: The Spastics Society of India.

Bowley, A.H., and L. Gardner. (1980) 1989. *The Handicapped Child*. Edinburgh: Churchill Livingstone. Reprint.

Chib, M. 1978. 'Therapeutic and Educational Management of Cerebral Palsied Children'. Paper presented at the International Cerebral Palsy Society (ICPS) Conference, Saudi Arabia.

Chib, M. 2010. *One Little Finger*. New Delhi: SAGE Publications.

Cole, T. 1989. *Apart or a Part? Integration and the Growth of British Special Education*. Milton Keynes: Open University Press.

Cole, L., and C. Hones. 1989. *Teaching the First Certificate in English: A Practical Guide for Teachers of English*. London: Cassell.

Dasgupta, P.R. 1997. 'Education for the Disabled'. In *Education and Children with Special Needs: From Segregation to Inclusion*, edited by Seamus Hegarty and Mithu Alur. New Delhi: SAGE Publications.

Denzin, N., and Y.S. Lincoln. 1994. *Handbook of Qualitative Research*. Thousand Oaks, CA: SAGE Publications.

De Souza, A. 1978. *The Indian City*. New Delhi: Manohar Publications.

Desai, A.R., and S.D. Pillai. 1970. *Slum and Urbanisation*. Mumbai: Popular Prakashan.

Erb, S., and Harriss-White, B. 2002. *Outcast from Social Welfare—Adult Disability, Incapability and Development in Rural South India*. New Delhi: Jain Book Publishers.

Education World. 2005. Published by Dilip Thakore, Bangalore.

Evans, J. 2005. *CAPP—Guidelines for the Manuals*. Mumbai: NRCI.

Foucault, M. 1976. *Mental Illness and Psychology*, 1st ed. Translated by Alan Sheridan. New York: Harper & Row.

Fulcher, G. 1989. *Disabling Policies? A Comparative Approach to Education Policy and Disability*. London: Falmer Press.

Fulcher, G. 1990. 'Students with Special Needs: Lessons from Comparisons'. *Journal of Education Policy* 5: 347–58.

Fulcher, G. 1993. 'Schools and Contests: A Reframing of the Effective Schools Debate?' In *Is there a Desk With My Name On It?* edited by R. Slee, 125–38. London: Falmer Press.

Government of India. 1961. *2nd Five Year Plan*. New Delhi.

Gupta, S.K. 1984. 'A Study of Special Needs Provisions for the Education of Children with Visual Handicaps in England and Wales and in India'. Associateship study, Institute of Education, University of London.

Hegarty, S., K. Pocklington, and D. Lucas. 1982. *Integration in Action: Case Studies in the Integration of Pupils with Special Needs*. Windsor: NFER-Nelson.

Hegarty, S., L. Clumies-Ross, and A. Hodgeson. 1984. *Learning Together: Teaching Pupils with Special Educational Needs in the Ordinary School*. Windsor: NFER-Nelson and Schools Council Publication.

Hegarty, S., and M. Alur. 2002. *Education & Children with Special Needs—From Segregation to Inclusion*. New Delhi: SAGE Publications.

ICPS (International Cerebral Palsy Society). 1964. *Are There Ethnic Differences in the Attitudes to Handicap and If So, Does It Matter?* Oxford: ICPS.

Jangira, N.K. 1995, June. 'Rethinking Teacher Education.' *Prospects* 25(2): 261–72.

Khare, L. 1982. 'The Able-disabled: India's Investment: Parents' Difficulties and Changing Community Attitudes'. In *It's Ability That Counts,* edited by Mithu Alur and Leslie Gardner, 164–67. Mumbai: Unique Printers.

Kirp, D. 1982. 'Professionalisation as a Policy Choice: British Special Education in Comparative Perspective'. *World Politics* 34(2): 137–75.

Kothari Commission. 1965. *Report of the Education Commission 1964–66 Education and National Development*. Ministry of Education, Government of India, New Delhi.

Kuruvilla, S. and A.I. Joseph. 1999. 'Identifying Disability: Comparing House-to-House Survey and Rapid Rural Appraisal'. *Health Policy and Planning* 14(2): 182–90.

Laporta, R. 1978. *Mainstreaming Pre-schoolers: Children with Hearing Impairment: A guide for Teachers, Parents, and Others Who Work with Hearing Impaired Preschoolers*. Washington, D.C.: US Government Printing Office for US Office of Human Development Services, Administration for Children, Youth and Families, Head Start Bureau.

Lipsky, D.K., and A. Gardner. 1997. *Inclusion and School Reform: Transforming America's Classrooms*. Baltimore: Paul Brookes Publishing Co.

Lukes, S. 1974. *Power: A Radical View*. London: Macmillan.

McRae, H. 2010. *What Works*. Great Britain: Harper Press.

Manual. 1989. *What Everyone Should Know about Cerebral Palsy*. Mumbai: The Spastics Society of India.

Manual. 1991. *Early Language Stimulation*. Mumbai: The Spastics Society of India.

Miles, M. 1994. 'Disability, Care and Education in 19th Century India: Some Dates, Places and Documentation'. *Action Aid Disability News* 5(2 Supplement): 1–22.

Miles, M.B., and A.M. Huberman. 1994. *Qualitative Data Analysis: A Expanded Sourcebook*. New Delhi: SAGE Publications.

Ministry of Human Resources Development. 1989. *Report of the Working Group on Early Childhood Education and Elementary Education Set Up for Formulation of 8th Five Year Plan*, Government of India, New Delhi.

Ministry of Human Resources Development. 1994. *Integrated Child Development Services (ICDS)*, Department of Women and Child Development, Ministry of Human Resources Development, Government of India, New Delhi.

National Networking Seminar on Vocational Rehabilitation and Employment. 1992. Mumbai: The Spastics Society of India.

Newell, P., and P. Potts. 1984. *Under 5s with Special Needs: Pre-school Children: The New Law and Integration.* London: The Advisory Centre for Education.

OECD. 1994. *The Integration of Disabled Children into Mainstream Education: Ambitions, Theories and Practices.* Paris: OECD.

Oliver, M. 1988. 'The Social and Political Context of Education Policy'. In *The Policy of Special Educational Needs,* edited by L. Barton, 13–31. London: Falmer Press.

Pai, M. 1998a. *A Comparative Study of Infant Stimulation and Intervention Programs Followed in Mumbai.* Mumbai: The Spastics Society of India.

Pai, M. 1998b. *A Longitudinal Study for the Mobility, Manipulation and Independence among Children with Cerebral Palsy.* Mumbai: The Spastics Society of India.

Pai, M., and M. Chib. 1991. *Early Intervention: A Distinctive Advantage.* Mumbai: The Spastics Society of India.

Pai, M., and S. Balaram. 1993. *Epilepsy and Its Management. Mumbai:* The Spastics Society of India.

Perlstein, M.A. 1949. 'Medical Aspects of Cerebral Palsy'. In *The Nervous Child,* Vol. 8, edited by Ernest Harms, 128. MT: Literary Licensing, LLC.

Planning Commission. 1961. http://planningcommission.nic.in/plans/planrel/fiveyr/index3.html (Accessed on 2 August 2016).

Prabhu, A. 2004. *Inclusive Education and the Use of Aids by Students with Physical Challenges.* Mumbai: The Spastics Society of India.

Rangwalla, S. 2004 *Physical Therapy: Role and Impact on Students with Disabilities after Inclusion.* A research study done under the NRCI Project. Mumbai: The Spastics Society of India.

Ray, S. 2003. *Disabled Persons in India.* New Delhi: National Sample Survey Organisation, Ministry of Statistics and Programme Implementation, Government of India.

Registrar General of India. 2001. 'Census of India 2001'. Available at http://www.censusindia.net (Accessed on 2 August 2016).

Registrar General of India. 2013. The Office of the Registrar General and Census Commissioner, Ministry of Home Affairs is responsible for conducting the decennial Census. https://india.gov.in/official-website-registrar-general-and-census-commissioner (Accessed on 2 August 2016).

Roy, P., and S. Dasgupta. 1995. *Urbanisation and Slums.* New Delhi: Har-Anand Publications for Indian Council for Social Development.

CABE. 1944. 'Chapter IX'. In *Sargent Report of the CABE Report, Post-war.*

Schwartz, R.P. 1951, July. 'New Technic in Cerebral Palsy Treatment'. *American Journal of Nursing* 51(7): 12–13.

Sen, A. 1981. *Poverty and Famine.* Oxford: Clarendon Press.

Singh, S.D., and K.P. Pothen. 1982. *Slum Children of India.* New Delhi: Deep and Deep Publications.

Singhal, Nidhi. 2010. 'Education of Children with Disabilities in India'. Background paper prepared for the Education for All Global Monitoring Report.

Siraj-Blatchford, I. 1994. 'An Evaluation of Early Years Education and Training in the ICDS in India'. *International Journal of Early Years Education* 2(1, Spring): 52–66.

Slee, R. 1993. 'The Politics of Integration—New Sites for Old Practices?' *Disability, Handicap and Society* 8 (4): 351–60.

Sood, N. 1987. 'An Evaluation of Non formal Preschool Education Component in Mangolpuri ICDS Block'. *NIPCCD Technical Bulletin,* April 1.

Stretch, P. 1989. *Vojtaan Holistic: Approach to Cerebral Palsy.* Mumbai: The Spastics Society of India.

Stretch, P. 1992. *Intrinsic Development: New Thoughts on Therapy for Cerebral Palsy.* Mumbai: The Spastics Society of India.

Stretch, P. 1993. *Basic Medical Aspects of Cerebral Palsy.* Mumbai: The Spastics Society of India.

Stretch, P., and M. Jariwalla. 1993. *The Need of Therapy in the Life of a Child with Cerebral Palsy.* Mumbai: The Spastics Society of India.

Swaminathan, M. 1996. 'Innovating Child Care Programmes in India'. *International Journal of Early Years Education* 4(2, Summer): 41–56.

Taylor, W.W., and I.W. Taylor. 1970. *Services for the Handicapped in India*. New York: International Society for Rehabilitation of the Disabled.

Tomlinson, S. 1982. *A Sociology of Special Education*. London: Routledge and Kegan Paul.

UN. 1993. *The Standard Rule on the Equalisation of Opportunities for Persons with Disabilities*. New York: United Nations.

UNESCO. 1995. *Review of the Present Situation in Special Education*. Paris.

UPKARAN. 1982. *A Manual of Aids for the Multiply Handicapped*. Mumbai: The Spastics Society of India.

Verma, A. 1994. 'Early Childhood Care and Education in India'. *International Journal of Early Years Education* 2(2, Autumn): xxx.

Vincent, C., J. Evans, I. Lunt, and P. Young. 1996. 'Professionals under Pressure: The Administration of Special Education in a Changing Context'. *British Educational Research Journal* 22(4): 475–91.

Vulliamy, G., K. Lewis, and D. Stephen. 1990. *Doing Educational Research in Developing Countries: Qualitative Strategies*. London: Falmer Press.

Wade, B., and M. Moore. 1992. *Patterns of Educational Integration: International Perspectives on Mainstreaming Children with Special Educational Needs*. Wallingford: Triangle Books.

Wedell, K. 1982. 'Special Education and Research: A Recent Survey'. *Special Education: Forward Trends* 9(3): 19–25.

Wedell, K. 1985. 'Research Supplement 2: Future Directions for Research on Children's Special Educational Needs'. *British Journal of Special Education* 12 (1): 22–26.

Welton, J., and J. Evans. 1986. The Development and Implementation of Special Education Policy: Where did the 1981 Act Fit In? *Public Administration* 64(2): 200–27.

World Bank. 2007. *People with Disabilities in India: From Commitments to Outcomes*. South Asia: Human Development Unit.

World Bank. 2009. *People with Disabilities in India: From Commitments to Outcomes, National Action Plan for Inclusion in Education of Children and Youth with Disabilities*, page 60.

World Health Organization and the World Bank. 2007. *World Disability Report: A Summary*, World Bank Report, Washington.

www.inclusion.com/artbiggerpicture.html (Accessed on 2 August 2016).

Index

About the Author

Mithu Alur has been closely involved with education, healthcare and employment, for women and children, leading to social change, legislation and social policy for more than 50 years. Her doctoral research dissertation from the University of London was entitled 'Invisible Children—A Study of Policy Exclusion' which analyzed the Indian government's educational policy for children with disability.

Her daughter Malini Chib, who is disabled, has been the reason for her involvement with disabled children. Malini too has two Masters—in gender studies and in information technology—from the University of London.

Dr Alur set up the first model of The Spastics Society of India (SSI) in Mumbai in 1972. This was the first special school in India for children with multiple disabilities, providing them education, treatment, and looking after their socio-emotional development under one roof. Her approach emphasized *professionalism combined with care and compassion*. Children were to be treated as children first and not as handicapped children. This was a new concept in India at the time.

This path-breaking work led to the development of a very successful model of education for children with disability which spread out all over the country. This model has been replicated in 16 of the 31 states of the country. Children from the organization have moved out and become accountants, lawyers, businessmen, librarians, or have completed their PhDs. The government too has now made cerebral palsy (CP) one of the official classifications amongst the 11 categories that already exist.

Dr Alur has also served on several government committees. She is a member, Central Advisory Board for Education (CABE), New Delhi; Round Table on School Education, Ministry of Human Resources Development (MHRD), New Delhi; Round Table of Elementary Education of Disadvantaged Groups, New Delhi; Working Committee for Implementation of Right to Education (RTE), New Delhi; National Advisory Council working group on child protection, New Delhi; National Monitoring Committee for Education of Scheduled Castes, Scheduled Tribes and Persons with Disabilities. At the state level, Dr Alur has been involved in community-based projects which deal with state and municipal authorities and non-governmental agencies. She is particularly known for her work at the ground level, empowering parents, families and disabled adults.

On the international front, Dr Alur put forward the concept of a dialogue between North and South countries and organized four conferences called the North-South Dialogues (NSD) with representation from South Africa, Brazil, Bangladesh, Hong Kong (China), Canada, Norway, UK, Chile, Pakistan and Russia. The proceedings of these conferences have also been published.

In the area of pedagogy, Dr Alur has initiated several courses for teachers, therapists, administrators and parents. Presently, she is involved in a course in collaboration with the Women's Council, UK, which reaches out to master trainers in the Asia-Pacific Region. Known as Community Initiatives in Inclusion (CII) course, it has been taught for over 15 years and has trained over 230 students from as diverse countries as Mongolia, Bangladesh, Nepal, Tonga, Malaysia, Pakistan, Indonesia, Tajikistan, Tonga, Sri Lanka, China, Cambodia, Vietnam as well as India.

Researcher, author, lecturer, a national and international contributor, she has ranged over the dimension of social policy, producing cost-effective methodologies to address educational needs of children and has published extensively on issues of disability rights and the 'hows' of educating disabled and disadvantaged children within a challenging framework of exclusion.

SAGE was founded in 1965 by Sara Miller McCune to support the dissemination of usable knowledge by publishing innovative and high-quality research and teaching content. Today, we publish over 900 journals, including those of more than 400 learned societies, more than 800 new books per year, and a growing range of library products including archives, data, case studies, reports, and video. SAGE remains majority-owned by our founder, and after Sara's lifetime will become owned by a charitable trust that secures our continued independence.

Los Angeles | London | New Delhi | Singapore | Washington DC | Melbourne